Virtual Reality in Medicine

Robert Riener • Matthias Harders

Virtual Reality in Medicine

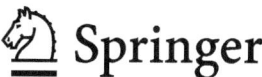 Springer

Robert Riener
Sensory-Motor Systems Lab
ETH Zurich
University Hospital Balgrist
Zürich
Switzerland

Matthias Harders
Computer Vision Lab
ETH Zurich
Zürich
Switzerland

ISBN 978-1-4471-4010-8   ISBN 978-1-4471-4011-5 (eBook)
DOI 10.1007/978-1-4471-4011-5
Springer London Heidelberg New York Dordrecht

Library of Congress Control Number: 2012936558

Printed on acid-free paper

Springer is part of Springer Science+Business Media (www.springer.com)

Preface

Virtual Reality has the potential to provide descriptive and practical information for medical training and therapy while relieving the patient or the physician. Multimodal interactions between the user and the virtual environment facilitate the generation of high-fidelity sensory impressions, by using not only visual and auditory, but also kinesthetic, tactile, and even olfactory feedback modalities. On the basis of the existing physiological constraints, this book derives the technical requirements and design principles of multimodal input devices, displays, and rendering techniques. Several examples are presented that are currently being developed or already applied for surgical training, intra-operative augmentation, and rehabilitation.

This book resulted from the lecture notes of the course Virtual Reality in Medicine, which has been taught and further developed at ETH Zurich, Switzerland, since 2003. It is well suited as introductory material for engineering and computer science students as well as researchers who want to learn more about basic technologies in the area of virtual reality applied to medicine. It also provides a broad overview to non-engineering students as well as clinical users, who desire to learn more about the current state of the art and future applications of this technology.

Many people contributed to the preparation of this book. Our thanks go to Gerald Bianchi, Basil Fierz, Philipp Fürnstahl, Marco Guidali, Johannes Hug, Seokhee Jeon, Benjamin Knörlein, Alexander König, Peter Leskovsky, Bryn Lloyd, Nikolas Neels, Bundit Panchaphongsaphak, Georg Rauter, Raimundo Sierra, Mario Sikic, Jonas Spillmann, Christoph Spuhler, Stefan Tuchschmid, and Heike Vallery. A special thanks goes to Roland Sigrist for his work in organising and performing the final editing of the book.

Zurich, Switzerland

Matthias Harders
Robert Riener

Contents

Chapter 1
Introduction to Virtual Reality in Medicine

1.1 What Is Virtual Reality?

1.1.1 Definition of Virtual Reality

The term *Virtual Reality (VR)* was popularized in the late 1980s by Jaron Lanier, one of the pioneers of the field. At the same time, also the term *Artificial Reality* [11] came up. 1982 the term *cyberspace* was coined in a novel by W. Gibson ("Burning Chrome"). The Encyclopaedia Britannica describes Virtual Reality as "the use of computer modeling and simulation that enables a person to interact with an artificial three-dimensional (3-D) visual or other sensory environment" [6]. Furthermore, it states that "VR applications immerse the user in a computer-generated environment that simulates reality through the use of interactive devices, which send and receive information and are worn as goggles, headsets, gloves, or body suits" [6]. For example, a user wearing a head-mounted display with a stereoscopic projection system can view animated images of a virtual environment. An important term is *presence* or *telepresence*, which can be described as an illusion of "being there" [6]. This illusion is enhanced by the use of motion sensors that pick up the user's movements and adjust the view on the visual display accordingly, usually in real-time; the user can even pick up and manipulate virtual objects that he[1] sees through the visual display wearing data gloves that are equipped with force-feedback modules that provide the sensation of touch [6]. Virtual reality usually refers to a technology designed to provide interaction between a user and artificially generated environments. This interaction is supposed to be more natural, direct, or real than pure simulation technologies or other previous technologies, for example those, which are based on passive mechanical phantoms. However, the simple definition of Virtual Reality derived only from its technical components and devices is not complete and, thus, not very useful, because it fails to provide an explanation for varying degrees of the Virtual Reality interaction experience. Considering this limited width of

---

[1] With the personal pronoun "he", we always address a female or male person.

R. Riener, M. Harders, *Virtual Reality in Medicine*,
DOI 10.1007/978-1-4471-4011-5_1, © Springer-Verlag London 2012

the term Virtual Reality, some engineers and scientists did not distinguish between the terms immersion and presence, i.e. between the objective contribution of the technology (*system immersion*) and the human response to the technology (presence) [21]. Therefore, the terms presence and immersion will be described in the next section, since the terminology in this area is often ambiguous.

1.1.2 Presence and Immersion

In general use, presence is defined as "the fact or condition of being present; the state of being with or in the same place as a person or thing; attendance, company, society, or association" [17], although presence has also different significations. In the early 1990s, the term presence was increasingly used to describe the subjective experience of participants in a virtual environment. A definition most often used for virtually generated environments is that of "being in one place or environment, even when one is physically situated in another" [23] or, more shortly, "being there" [7]. These kinds of definitions follow a transportation metaphor, as the user perceives to be in a different place. In addition to considering presence as transportation, the concept can be defined as social richness when used for human-human interaction in organizations, as degree of realism of the displayed environment, or as degree of immersion. Trying to find a common denominator for all these definitions, a general definition of presence was suggested to be "perceptual illusion of non-mediation" [13].

In contrast to presence, immersion is usually defined as a quantifiable system characteristic, which describes the capability of a system to display an artificially generated environment in a way that it comes close to the real experience. Features of highly immersive systems are real-time interaction, stereo vision, high frame rate and resolution, and multiple displays (visual, auditory, and haptic).

1.2 VR in Medicine

1.2.1 Need for Training in Medicine

Recent years have brought about a drastic change in patient awareness and sense of adverse effects in medical care. The combination of this process with an increasing focus on patient safety has put traditional educational paradigms in the medical area to the test. Especially in the surgical domain, the time-honored concept of theoretical education followed by supervised clinical practice—often referred to as "see one, do one, teach one"—is becoming less and less acceptable [20], wherefore innovative and complimentary methods of teaching medical knowledge are being sought. Further concerns are rooted in the high cost of teaching in a clinical environment [5]. The level of costs, complexity, risks, and

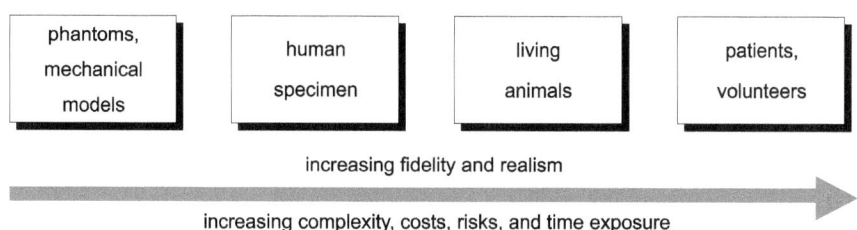

Fig. 1.1   Practical limitations in medical education

time exposure of the training process increases with the fidelity of the objects (Fig. 1.1).

Increased awareness of patient safety has for instance been stimulated by studies on surgical or medical errors, and associated health care costs. According to the seminal study carried out by the Institute of Medicine (IOM) of the US National Academies in 1999 [10], medical errors cause the deaths of an estimated 44,000 patients in US hospitals per year. The report states that mortality due to medical mistakes is higher than due to highway accidents, AIDS, or breast cancer in the USA. Moreover, an additional $8.8 billion of direct health care costs is caused, not taking into account secondary effects. While the report has been criticized due to poor study methodology and vague differentiation between preventable and non-preventable adverse effects, it still reflects a need for reducing complications in the medical area. Similar findings have been reached in a study conducted in Canada in 2000 [1]. An estimated 70,000 preventable adverse events are reported, which occurred in Canadian hospitals and resulted in 1.1 million additional hospital days. Furthermore, it is estimated that about 9,000 to 24,000 of these events resulted in death. In a related study in Australia it is indicated that an additional 3.3 million days of hospitalization became necessary due to medical error [22]. Similar trends have also been stated for a number of European countries [14, 16, 19].

According to [12], about half of medical errors occur during surgical interventions, of which 75% are preventable. Unfortunately, exact numbers of surgical error are not easy to obtain, which makes the recording of these events an important initial step. Open and anonymous discussion of errors is a valuable means for quality insurance, which is for instance practiced in the pilot community. As an example, to address these shortcomings a Critical Incident Reporting System has been established in Switzerland in 1998, providing an online tool for recording adverse events [4].

One key factor, which has been identified as a cause of such considerable numbers of surgical error, is the rapid growth of medical knowledge and the very fast turnover of new technologies, which makes it hard for practitioners to keep up. Possibly the most significant change in recent times has been the advent of minimally-invasive surgery (MIS) in the late 1980s. This technique minimizes the damage of healthy tissue during interventions on internal organs. An example of this procedure for laparoscopic interventions is depicted in Fig. 1.2. The relatively large cuts

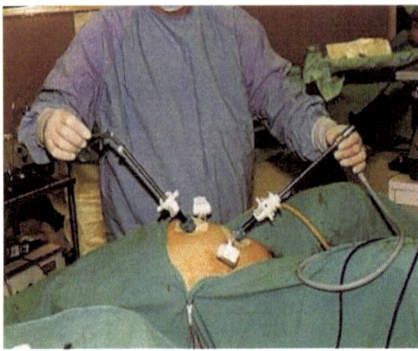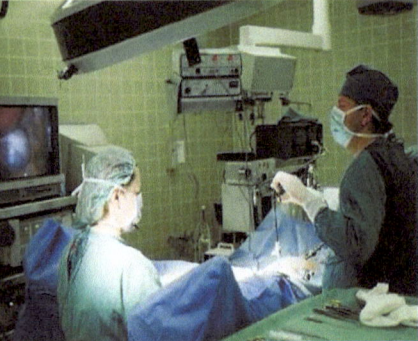

Fig. 1.2 Laparoscopic interventions in gynecology; courtesy of Clinic of Gyn., University Hospital Zurich, Prof. D. Fink

in open surgery are replaced by small incisions, through which optical and surgical instruments are inserted. Reduced tissue damage and careful selection of the entry points results in a major gain in patient recovery after operation as well as reduced scarring. The price for these advantages is paid by the surgeon who loses direct contact with the operation site. Visual information is acquired via endoscopic cameras and displayed on a monitor, thus impairing normal hand-eye coordination. In addition, much of the manipulative freedom usually available in open surgery is lost. Therefore, performing operations under these conditions demands very specific capabilities of the surgeon, which can only be gained with extensive training. Nevertheless, MIS procedures have been replacing traditional approaches in several areas. For instance, laparoscopic gallbladder surgery has largely replaced conventional interventions. Since the end of the 1980s the majority of all cholecystectomies in the US have been performed using this MIS technique. Taking all these points into consideration, the need for improved medical training and continuing education becomes apparent.

1.2.2 VR for Medical Education and Training

Casuistics, anatomy atlases, and surgical training environments can be enhanced by VR. Nowadays, novel VR technologies exist that display the anatomical information via auditory and haptic modalities additionally to the visualized data. The user can hear the sound or feel the touch from the digital body in a similar way as one would perceive it from the real interaction. This can enhance the performance, allowing the VR system to be used for advanced applications such as surgical training. For example, the hysteroscopy simulator, developed at the Computer Vision Lab, ETH Zurich, illustrates an application of a digital body that is used for simulating surgical procedures (Fig. 1.3).

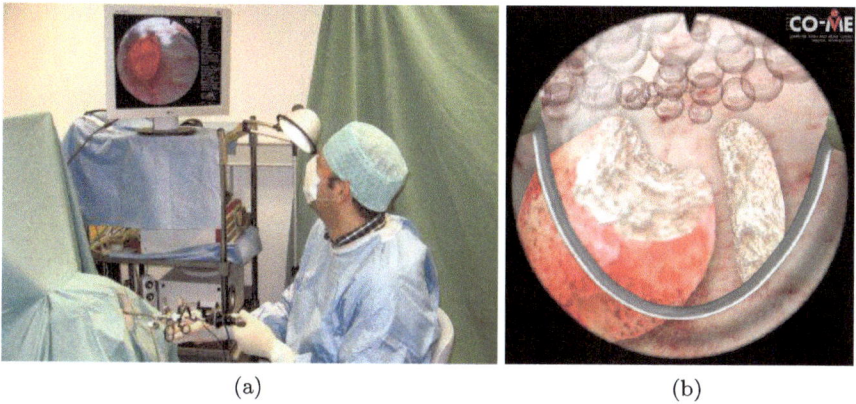

(a)   (b)

Fig. 1.3 Hysteroscopy simulator: (**a**) System setup, (**b**) Visualization; developed at the Computer Vision Lab, ETH Zurich

1.2.3 VR in Rehabilitation, Psychotherapy, and Surgery

VR in combination with rehabilitation robotics can not only relieve exhausting therapy sessions of physical therapists. It can also motivate patients to train longer in an exciting artificial environment while being supported by the robot. An example is the gait rehabilitation robot Lokomat, developed at the Balgrist University Hospital, Zurich, Switzerland, that can be combined with different VR scenarios (Fig. 1.4(a)). Moreover, VR applications can be used in psychotherapy, for example for phobia treatment such as fear of spiders [8], closed rooms [2], open spaces or fear of flying [3]. The VR system simulates the real conditions in which the user is confronted with the phobic stimulus (Fig. 1.4(b)). One of the advantages of VR is the ability to vary the degree of the different situations and the immediate termination of the procedure. VR applications are quite successful in phobia treatment, however, they should only be used in addition to traditional approaches. Intra-therapeutic augmentation, e.g. intra-operative navigation, can assist physicians during therapy or surgery. Also diagnostic and pre-therapeutic planning can be enhanced by 3D-reconstructions and graphical animations of the individual patient.

1.2.4 Benefits and Chances

There are several benefits of applying VR technology to medicine. VR is more comprehensive than books and cadavers. It is also time and case independent, as the users can train and repeat medical skills at any time they want. Surgeons can practice treatments in extreme situations without taking a risk for the patient, as no patients are directly involved. Procedures are observable and reproducible, and performance can be recorded and used for assessment or evaluation of the treatment. Moreover,

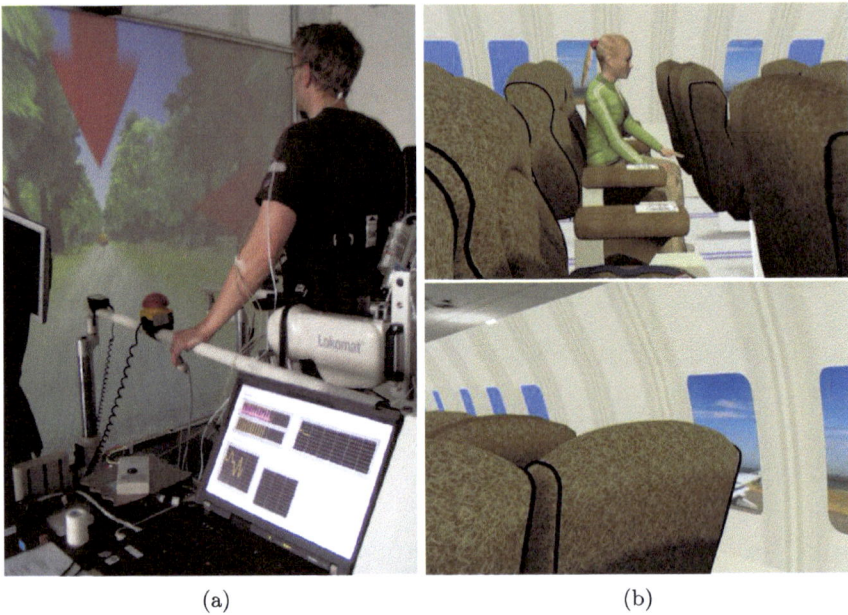

(a)   (b)

Fig. 1.4 Virtual reality used in rehabilitation and psychotherapy: (**a**) The gait rehabilitation robot Lokomat provides VR, (**b**) Graphical scenario used to treat fear of flying; by courtesy of BIOPAC Systems, Inc. www.biopac.com

augmented information can be displayed to assist the treatment or decision making. Medical applications can benefit from VR in several areas. VR in medicine aims to optimize cost, improve quality of the education and therapy, allow long and efficient training sessions, and increase safety.

1.3 Principles of Virtual Reality

1.3.1 Main Components

VR comprises two main components: the user environment and the virtual environment (Fig. 1.5). While the user interacts with the VR system, the two environments communicate and exchange information through a barrier called *interface*. The interface can be considered as a translator between the user and the VR system. When the user applies input actions (e.g. motion, force generation, speech, etc.), the interface translates these actions into digital signals, which can be processed and interpreted by the system. On the other hand, the system's computed reactions are also translated by the interface into physical quantities, which the user can perceive through the use of different display and actuator technologies (e.g. images, sounds, smells, etc.). Finally, the user interprets this information and reacts to the system accordingly.

Fig. 1.5 Bidirectional exchange of information in VR systems

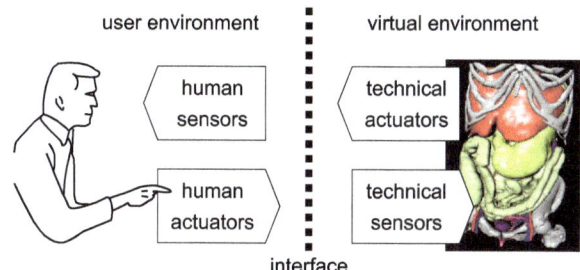

1.3.2 Importance of Multimodality

In VR applications, the exchange of different physical quantities between the user and the virtual environment occurs via different channels or *modalities*. Such modalities can be sound, vision or touch. Communicating with multiple modalities is called *multimodal interaction*. Multimodal interaction allows several types of modalities to be simultaneously exchanged between the user and the virtual environment. The goal of applying multimodal interaction is to provide a complete and realistic image of the situation, to give redundant information, for example, for safety reasons, and to increase the quality of presence.

Multi-modality plays an important role also in our daily life. In most daily situations, we interact with the real environment through multiple modalities, for example, when watching a movie (hearing and vision), painting and molding (vision and touch), making music (hearing and touch), walking (vision and balance), or ingesting (taste, smell, vision, touch, hearing). Furthermore, multi-modality can influence human behaviors and decisions. For example, the decision to buy a product may depend on the optical appearance or tactile property of the product. Or the optical appearance of a meal can influence our subjective impression of its taste. A horn of a car can warn a pedestrian when crossing a street and, thus, support other senses like vision.

Multi-modality is important for medical applications. Medical activities often involve multiple senses (e.g. touch, vision, hearing, and smell) especially in diagnosis and surgical treatments. In medical simulations, multi-modality can increase the fidelity of the encountered situations (e.g. by adding the sound of the medical device), making the situation more realistic, which increases the quality of presence and the performance of the VR system. In addition, multi-modality can provide additional instructions or warnings while the user is practicing a surgical or any other task.

1.3.3 Early Steps in Multimodal Displays

One of the first multimodal systems, whose purpose was to provide the user with a sense of presence, was created by Morton Heilig. In 1956, he built the Sensorama (Fig. 1.6(a)). It was designed as an arcade machine that provided the sensation of

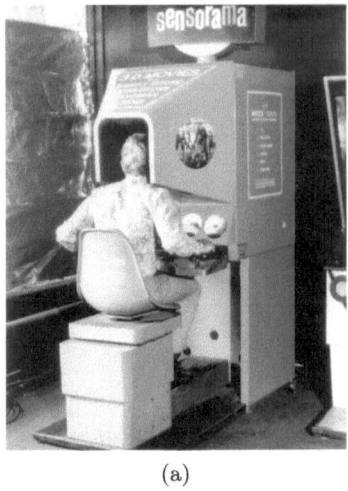
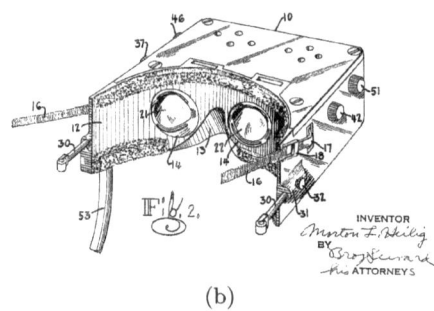

(a)   (b)

Fig. 1.6 Two display systems introduced by Morton Heilig: (**a**) Sensorama simulator, (**b**) First design of a head-mounted display (HMD); by courtesy of Marianne Heilig

riding a motorcycle through Brooklyn. The user could see a 3D movie of a motorcycle ride completed by engine vibrations, wind, and olfactory effects. Unfortunately, the user could not interact with the environment. He could only drive along a predefined path. In addition to this, in 1960, Heilig also designed a simulation mask introducing the first head-mounted display (HMD) (Fig. 1.6(b)). It should display prerecorded stereoscopic slides with wide field of view and also included stereo sound and smell.

In 1965, Ivan Sutherland suggested the concept of the Ultimate Display, a window into a virtual world. At Harvard University, he also developed a cathode ray tube (CRT) head-mounted display. A tracking system could record the position and orientation of the user's head, and a simple wire frame scene was displayed in a CRT-HMD [18] (see Sect. 3.3.3).

In the beginning of the 1980s, Jaron Lanier was one of the first who designed interface gloves (datagloves (Fig. 1.7)) to measure position and orientation of the fingers and hand, which allows a natural way of communicating with the computer using gestures.

1.3.4 Multimodal Training Simulation

A very successful application of multimodal techniques, which in fact existed long before the term VR was initially coined, is flight simulation for pilot education. Initial attempts at using simulated environments for pilot education have already been undertaken a century ago at the inception of manned flight. From the early mechanical trainers, flight simulators have grown into highly complex, fully immersive

Fig. 1.7 Example of a data glove together with a head-mounted display; by courtesy of NASA

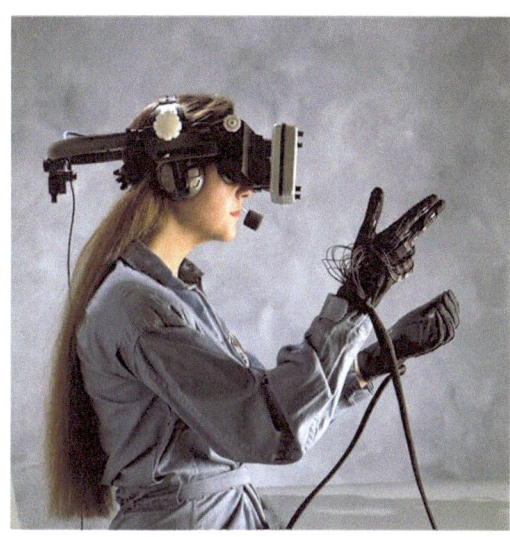

computer-based tools for teaching in aviation (Fig. 1.8). Nowadays, simulator training is an indispensable element embedded into pilot education. Aviation authorities have issued regulations how simulator training hours can be logged. Furthermore, official certification procedures for new simulators have been established. Commercial pilots are even certified for new types of aircraft based on simulator experience alone.

Similar to other VR-based training environments, flight simulators allow practicing complex or emergency situations. The reduction of airplane accidents over the last decades is partly attributed to simulator training. Already the system developed by Edward Link in the 1930s (Fig. 1.8(b)) resulted in a significant reduction of accidents in instrument meteorological conditions, i.e. flight in clouds only with reference to the flight instruments.

Flight simulation, or vehicle simulation in general, coexisted a long time unnoticed by VR. These applications actually have been around before VR even started. Immersive experience improved simulators by including motion platforms, real word mock-ups, artificial sound, or visual display.

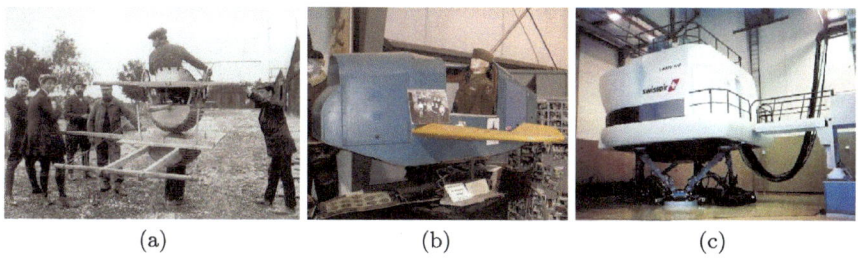

(a)   (b)   (c)

Fig. 1.8 History of flight simulation devices: (**a**) Early synthetic flight training device from 1910, (**b**) Link Trainer from the 1930s, (**c**) Contemporary high fidelity flight simulator

Fig. 1.9 VR scenarios can improve the ergonomic design of a new car; by courtesy of G. Monacelli, Product Development Methodologies, ELASIS, Italy

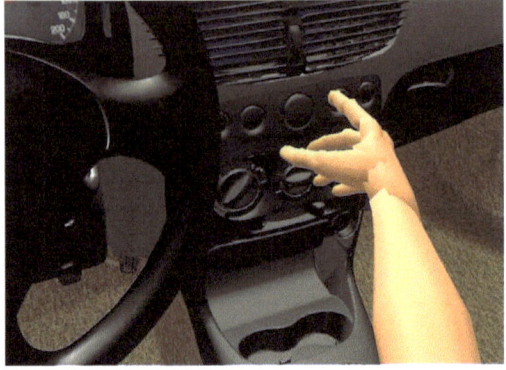

Also in the field of car design and manufacturing, VR systems are found to be an attractive tool. Development costs can be reduced dramatically, as the designs can be virtually displayed and evaluated which can save manufacturing costs of real objects (Fig. 1.9).

1.3.5 Problems

Increasing use of VR also turned up some problems due to the technology. Sometimes users experience the so-called cybersickness [9, 15] with symptoms of nausea, dizziness, eye-strain, headache, disorientation, or vomiting. Of course, the level of sickness depends on the susceptibility of the user. Symptoms can appear during the exposure to the VR and last for hours after the exposure. Technical issues may be one of the reasons for cybersickness. For example, a 15 ms lag in a head-mounted display can already induce cybersickness of the user.

1.4 Contents of the Book

In this book the basic components of virtual reality systems as well as concrete applications will be introduced. The chapters are divided into two main parts with 11 chapters in total.

In the first part, we describe the bidirectional interface between the user and a VR environment (Fig. 1.10). First, in Chap. 2 the input periphery is introduced. In the subsequent four chapters, different modalities of the output periphery are presented. This comprises the key sensory modalities—vision (Chap. 3), touch (Chap. 4), hearing (Chap. 5), as well as taste and smell (Chap. 6). In all these chapters, perceptual mechanisms, varieties of hardware solutions as well as rendering techniques are discussed. The relevance to virtual reality applications in medicine is also outlined.

In the second part, the application of VR technology in rehabilitation (Chap. 7), medical training (Chap. 8) is presented in more detail as well as for planning and

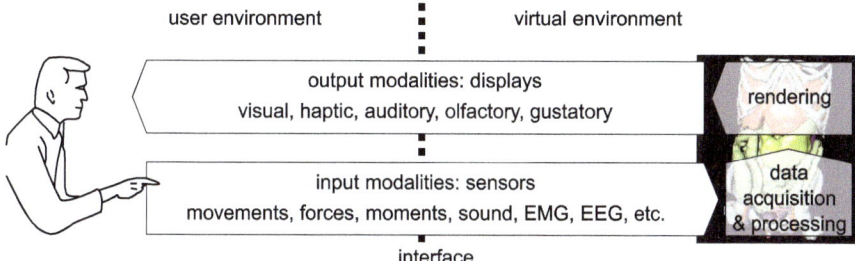

user environment   virtual environment

output modalities: displays
visual, haptic, auditory, olfactory, gustatory

rendering

input modalities: sensors
movements, forces, moments, sound, EMG, EEG, etc.

data
acquisition
& processing

interface

Fig. 1.10 Multimodal, bidirectional interaction between the user and the Virtual Environment

intra-operative support (Chap. 9). Several examples as well as key algorithms for medical model generation (Chap. 10) and soft tissue deformation (Chap. 11) are described that are currently being used in research or in commercial solutions for use in the medical community.

References

1. Baker, G.R., Norton, P.G., Flintoft, V., Blais, R., Brown, A., Cox, J., Etchells, E., Ghali, W.A., Hebert, P., Majumdar, S.R., O'Beirne, M., Palacois-Derflingher, L., Reid, R.J., Sheps, S., Tamblyn, R.: The Canadian adverse events study: the incidence of adverse events among hospital patients in Canada. Can. Med. Assoc. J. **170**(11), 1678–1686 (2004)
2. Botella, C., Banos, R., Perpina, C., Villa, H., Alcaniz, M., Rey, A.: Virtual reality treatment of claustrophobia: a case report. Behav. Res. Ther. **36**(2), 239–246 (1998)
3. Botella, C., Osma, J., Garcia-Palacios, A., Quero, S., Banos, R.M.: Treatment of flying phobia using virtual reality: data from a 1-year follow-up using a multiple baseline design. Clin. Psychol. Psychother. **11**(5), 311–323 (2004)
4. CIRS: Critical incidence reporting system. Webpage: www.cirsmedical.ch (1998). Visited Aug 2011
5. CPSI: Canadian patient safety institute—current state report on patient simulation in Canada, April (2005)
6. Encyclopædia Britannica: Virtual Reality (VR). Encyclopædia Britannica Online (2011)
7. Heeter, C.: Being there: the subjective experience of presence. Presence **1**(2), 262–271 (1992)
8. Hoffman, H., Garcia-Palacios, A., Carlin, A., Furness, A. III, Botella-Arbona, C.: Interfaces that heal: coupling real and virtual objects to treat spider phobia. Int. J. Hum.-Comput. Interact. **16**(2), 283–300 (2003)
9. Kim, Y.Y., Kim, E.N., Park, M.J., Park, K.S., Ko, H.D., Kim, H.T.: The application of biosignal feedback for reducing cybersickness from exposure to a virtual environment. Presence **17**(1), 1–16 (2008)
10. Kohn, L.T., Corrigan, J.M., Donaldson, M.S.: To Err Is Human: Building a Safer Health System. National Academy Press, Washington (1999)
11. Krueger, M.: Artificial Reality 2. Addison-Wesley Professional, Reading (1991). ISBN 0-201-52260-8
12. Leape, L.L.: The Preventability of Medical Injury, pp. 13–25. Erlbaum Publications, Hillsdale (1994)
13. Lombard, M., Ditton, T.: At the heart of it all: the concept of presence. J. Comput.-Mediat. Commun. **3**(2) (1997)

14. Makeham, M.A.B., Dovey, S.M., County, M., Kidd, M.R.: An international taxonomy for errors in general practice: a pilot study. Med. J. Aust. **177**(2), 68–72 (2002)
15. McCauley, M., Sharkey, T.: Cybersickness-perception of self-motion in virtual environments. Presence **1**(3), 311–318 (1992)
16. Ollenschlaeger, G.: Medizinische Risiken, Fehler und Patientensicherheit – Zur Situation in Deutschland. In: Schweizerische Aerztezeitung, pp. 1404–1410 (2001)
17. Soanes, C., Stevenson, A.: Oxford Dictionary of English (Dictionary), 2nd edn. Oxford University Press, Oxford (2005)
18. Sutherland, I.E.: A head-mounted three dimensional display. In: Proceedings of the December 9–11, 1968, Fall Joint Computer Conference, Part I. AFIPS '68, pp. 757–764. ACM, New York (1968)
19. Vincent, C., Stanhope, N., Crowley-Murphy, M.: Reasons for not reporting adverse incidents: an empirical study. J. Eval. Clin. Pract. **5**(1), 13–21 (1999)
20. Vozenilek, J., Huff, J.S., Reznek, M., Gordon, J.A.: See one, do one, teach one: advanced technology in medical education. Acad. Emerg. Med. **11**(11), 1149–1154 (2004)
21. Wellner, M.: Evaluation of virtual environments for gait rehabilitation and rowing. PhD thesis, ETH Zurich (2009)
22. Wilson, R.M., Runciman, W.B., Gibberd, R.W., Harrison, B.T., Newby, L., Hamilton, J.D.: The quality in Australian health care study. Med. J. Aust. **163**(9), 458–471 (1995)
23. Witmer, B.G., Singer, M.J.: Measuring presence in virtual environments: a presence questionnaire. Presence **7**(3), 225–240 (1998)

Chapter 2
Input Periphery

2.1 Human Actuators, Input Modalities

A human operator presents actions to the VR system in various forms, for instance, as positions and movements, forces and torques, speech and sounds as well as physiological quantities (see Fig. 1.10, Table 2.1). The choice of method or device to measure such information depends on the physical properties of the information to be transferred and the range of the signal to be measured (Table 2.2). In the next subchapters we will present different basic principles and technologies how to record positions and movements, forces and torques, and physiological data.

2.2 Position and Movement Recording

2.2.1 Physical Measurement Principles

For many VR applications it is required to measure positions and movements of body segments or objects used by the human operator. Measurement of positions and movements can be based on the physical sensory principles, which are described in the following sections.

2.2.1.1 Resistive Sensors

The change of electrical resistance of the sensor reflects the change of position of the object. Typical resistive sensors are potentiometers, which are variable resistors whose resistances are adjustable via a sliding contact called wiper. In general, the wiper is connected to the object being sensed. When the object changes its position, it will also change the resistance of the potentiometer. The correlating change of the circuit's voltage shows how far the object has moved (Fig. 2.1(a)). Potentiometers are available in both linear and rotary types.

R. Riener, M. Harders, *Virtual Reality in Medicine*,
DOI 10.1007/978-1-4471-4011-5_2, © Springer-Verlag London 2012

Table 2.1 Examples of different input modalities

Physiological function	Information transferred	Physical quantities	Measurement device examples
Voice, speech	sound, acoustics, words, commands	sound pressure, frequency	microphone
Muscle activities, segmental kinematics and kinetics	posture and body motion; mechanical load	position, velocity, angle, acceleration; force, moment	joystick, gonio-accelerometer
Physiological functions	cardiovascular state, thoughts, well-being	heart rate, temperature, electrophysiological quantities	thermometer, electromyogram (EMG), electroen-cephalogram (EEG), pulse oxymeter

Table 2.2 Input signal ranges

Input modality	Signal type	Typical ranges	Source
Voice, speech	sound pressure level	> 100 dB SPL	[15]
	frequency when speaking	80 Hz–9 kHz	[9]
	frequency when singing	50 Hz–4 kHz (fundamental tones)	[9]
Posture and body motion	joint angles	150°–180°	[14]
	joint angular velocities	250°/s	
	movement frequencies	12 Hz	[18]
Mechanical load	finger force	50 N	[16]
	fist force	400 N	[1]
	holding load arm	> 300 N	[10]
	joint torque (knee)	220 Nm	[17]
Physiological signal	electromyogram	2 Hz–10 kHz, 50 μV–10 mV	[8]
	electroencephalogram	0.5–100 Hz 2–100 μV	[6]

2.2.1.2 Capacitive Sensors

In capacitive sensors, the position of the object is determined by the voltage changing with the capacitance of the sensor. In general, a sensor contains two plates which are separated by a dielectric medium such as ceramic or plastic. The capacitance of the sensor changes when the distance d between the two plates, the overlapping surface area A of the plates, or the properties/homogeneity ϵ of the dielectric medium change (Fig. 2.1(b)).

Fig. 2.1 Sensing principles to record positions and movements: (**a**) Resistive, (**b**) Capacitive; $C = \epsilon * A/d$

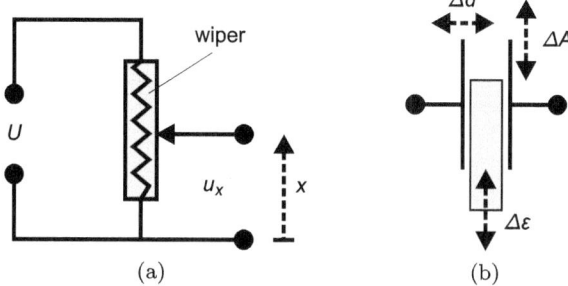

(a)   (b)

2.2.1.3 Inductive Sensors

Inductive sensors utilize an electromagnetic field to detect the position of the object. The change of the ferromagnetic core's position with respect to position of the inductive coils induces the voltage change, which yields a mutual inductance of the primary and secondary coils. One example of an inductive sensor is a linear variable differential transformer.

2.2.1.4 Ultrasound and Optical Methods

Running time differences of the sound echo or the Doppler effect can be detected to determine distance or speed, respectively. Alternatively, also light sources or images can be used to detect the position or motion of an object. Examples are cameras or photo-electrical components such as photo diodes, photo transistors, photo resistors or energy producing photo-electrical elements.

2.2.2 Position and Movement Measuring Systems

The position and movement measuring systems can be classified into three categories depending on structure and design. These are desktop systems, body-mounted systems, and contact-free systems.

2.2.2.1 Desktop Systems

Desktop measuring devices are usually placed on tables, boxes or shelves. For example, computer mice and joysticks belong to this kind of category. More complex joystick-type devices exist that allow rendering of several degrees of freedom, for example in spatial (3D) range.

Fig. 2.2 Potentiometer-based
goniometer; joint angle ϕ_k
can be determined as a
geometric functions of the
angles ϕ_1 and ϕ_2 measured
by the two potentiometers

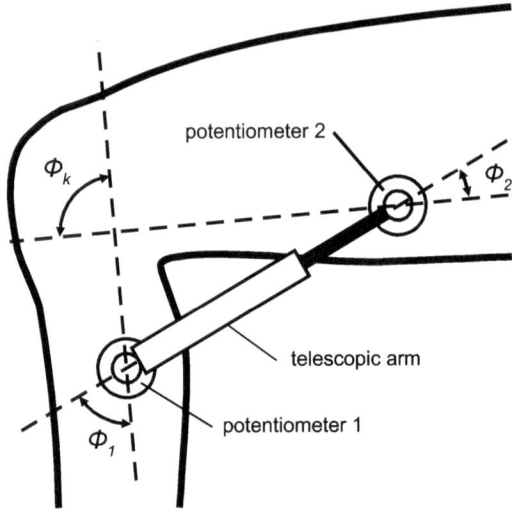

2.2.2.2 Body-Mounted Systems

Body-mounted sensing systems are usually used to measure the posture or movement of the human. The equipment needs to be attached to the body of the subject.
Examples are goniometers, gyroscopes, accelerometers and inclinometers in order
to measure angles, velocity or acceleration. Inertial sensors, such as accelerometers
and gyroscopes, are used to measure motion and orientation. Inertial sensors are
widely applied in head-mounted displays to track the angular motion of the user's
head.

Goniometers are used to measure joint angles. Many versions are based on resistive measurement principles using potentiometers. For example, goniometers with
two potentiometers can be employed to measure the knee joint angles during knee
flexion and extension (Fig. 2.2). The two angular potentiometers are attached to the
thigh and the lower leg of the subject and connected by a telescopic arm. Also flexible versions of goniometers are available such as the twin axis goniometers from
Biometrics Ltd. (Fig. 2.3). A similar flexible goniometer technology, known as *resistive bend sensor*, is integrated in the CyberGlove III (CyberGlove Systems LLC,
San Jose, CA, USA) to measure the angles of the finger joints (Fig. 2.4).

ShapeTape^{TM} (Fig. 2.5(a)) and ShapeWrap^{TM} (Fig. 2.5(b)), Measurand Inc.,
Fredericton, Canada, were developed to measure multiple joint angles with multiple
degrees of freedom. Both systems are flexible and work on the basis of a special
fiber optics. When the ShapeTape^{TM} is bent or twisted, the frequency and the intensity of the light changes. This allows detection of curvature in short elements, which
enables to reconstruct the shape of the tape. From this information one can estimate
the body posture and movement of the user.

Gyroscopes are used to measure angular speeds and are often applied in
aerospace. Recently, gyroscopes are also integrated in game controllers that allow

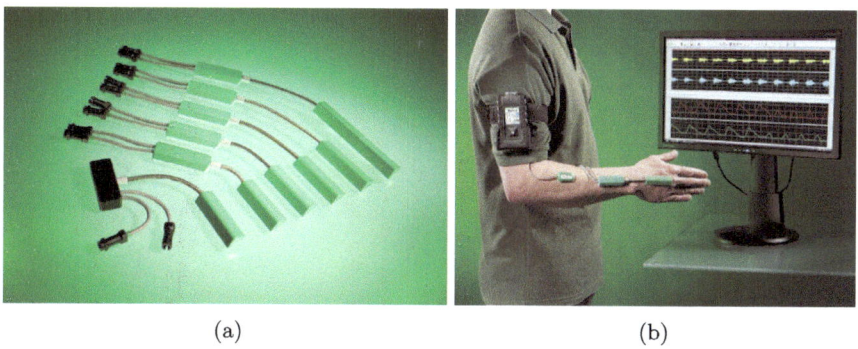

(a)   (b)

Fig. 2.3 Twin Axis Goniometers; by courtesy of Biometrics Ltd. (www.biometricsltd.com)

Fig. 2.4 CyberGlove III
including 18 to 20 sensors; by
courtesy of CyberGlove
Systems LLC

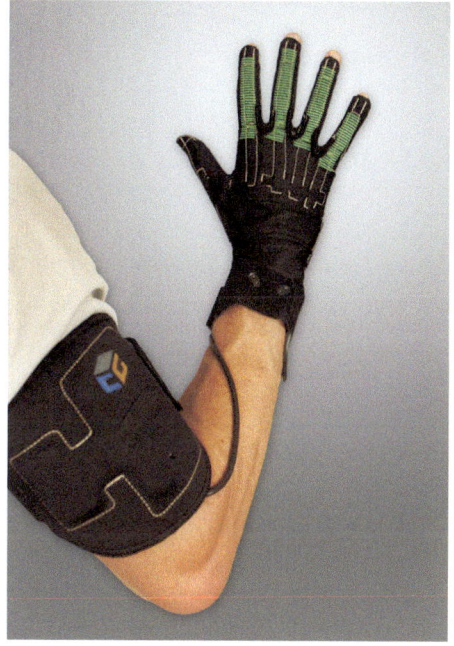

users playing games by just moving the wireless controller. Conventional gyro-scopes are made by a rotating mass. Smaller versions contain a vibrating bar, which is equipped with piezoelectric actuators generating vibrations and piezoelectric sensors measuring gyro effects induced by angular movements.

Accelerometers contain a small mass and measure the inertial force produced on the mass during movements. So called multi-axis accelerometers are designed to detect magnitude of acceleration in different directions. Inclinometers are special kinds of accelerometers that allow the measurement of angles of an object with respect to gravity.

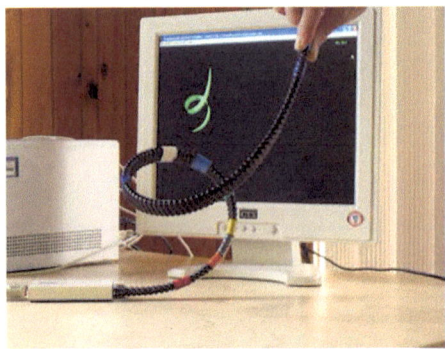

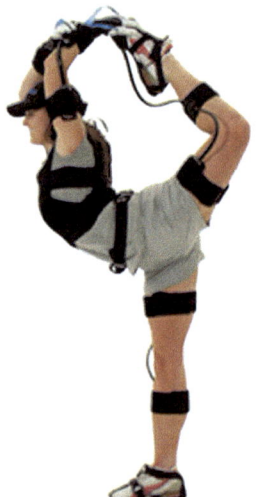

(a) ShapeTape™   (b) ShapeWrap™   III
                                                            Plus

Fig. 2.5   Multiple joint angle measurement: (**a**) ShapeTape™, (**b**) ShapeWrap™ III Plus; by courtesy of Measurand Inc., Fredericton, New Brunswick, Canada

2.2.2.3   Contact-Free Systems (Remote Systems)

Contact-free systems (remote systems) can capture the position and motion of the
body in space without mechanical contacts between the subject and the sensing unit.
This type of sensing system is often preferable since it gives a large scope and the
users are normally not encumbered by wires and bulky components. Most systems
are based on optical, acoustic or magnetic measuring principles.

- **Optical systems** The first optical contact-free system was introduced by Ead-
  weard Muybridge already in the 19th century. The system consisted of two cameras placed orthogonally to each other to capture the motion of subjects from
  different directions. A grid wall located behind the subject enabled movement
  quantification. In modern systems, at least two cameras are used to detect 3D positions of optical markers, which are attached to the body of the subject (Fig. 2.6).
  The markers can be either active (LEDs) or passive indicators (self reflective,
  color dots). A redundant number of cameras can help to avoid losing the tracking
  of single markers when the vision is blocked by obstacles or when the markers
  are getting out of a camera's field of vision. Optical systems are quite sensitive,
  reaching position accuracy below 1 mm.
- **Acoustic systems** Acoustic or ultrasound systems use a set of microphones to
  detect the signal from acoustic emitters, which are attached to the body of the
  subject. The position in space of each emitter is calculated from the time difference that the signal needs for traveling from the emitter to the microphones,
  whose positions are known. A minimum set of three microphones is required

Fig. 2.6 A contact free opto-electronical motion capture system; by courtesy of Qualisys AB, Gothenburg, Sweden

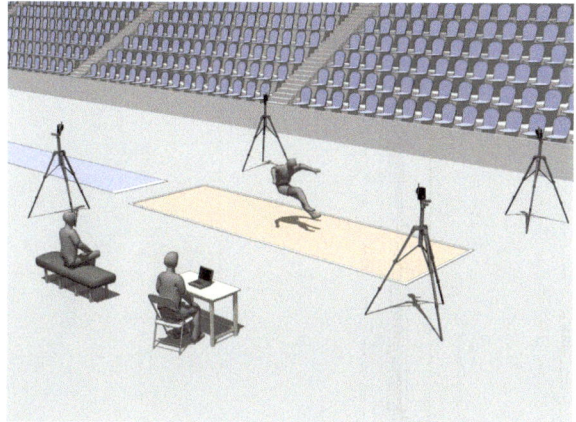

to acquire spatial information of the microphone markers through triangulation. Sound reflections as well as variations in room temperature and humidity usually worsen the tracking accuracy compared to optical systems.

- **Magnetic systems** Magnetic systems consist of markers based on small electrical coils. The markers are attached to the body of the subject and a transmitter placed in the vicinity, which generates a strong magnetic field through the entire workspace. When the markers are moved inside the magnetic field, inductive effects produced in the marker coils allow determining the marker orientation and location. Thus, the system can measure up to six DOF for each marker. The system works even if there are visual obstacles between markers and transmitter. However, ferromagnetic material inside the workspace distorts the magnetic field resulting in measurement errors. Therefore, the accuracy of magnetic systems is in general lower than that of optical or acoustic systems.

2.2.3 Eye-Tracking Systems

Eye-tracking systems are used to detect and record the positions and movements of one or both eyes of the viewer while looking at any real or virtual object, e.g. on a screen. Most popular eye tracking technologies are based on image processing approaches. Other solutions use magnetic coils placed into special contact lenses, or they are based on electrooculographical recordings.

2.2.3.1 Optical Systems

The positions and movements of the eye are tracked by a camera or special optical sensor. Most eye-trackers in this category use the center of the pupil and a corneal reflection to detect eye movement. These optical systems are rather popular because

Fig. 2.7 Head-mounted eye
trackers: EyeLink II; by
courtesy of SR Research Ltd.,
Ottawa, Ontario, Canada

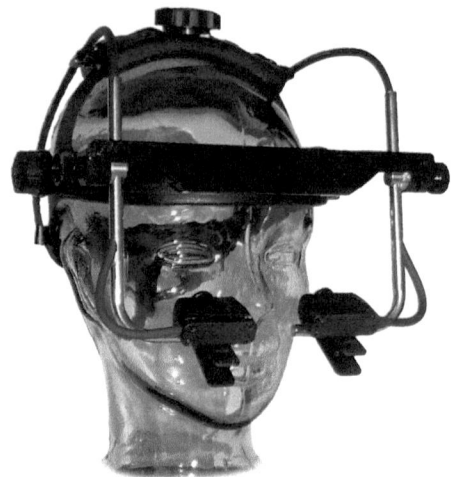

they work non-invasively and they are relatively inexpensive. One example of optical eye tracking systems are remote cameras which are, for example, connected to
a computer screen. The eye movements are captured and interpreted by image processing techniques. Other examples are eye trackers that are integrated in computer
monitors or head-mounted eye tracker systems (Fig. 2.7).

2.2.3.2 Magnetic Systems

A magnetic coil sensor is embedded into a contact lens. The subject is surrounded
by a magnetic field. Thus, movements of the eye induce currents in the coil, which
allows determining the eye movements and viewing angle.

2.2.3.3 Bioelectrical Systems

The eye positions can also be detected by electrodes attached around the eye measuring the electrical potential produced by the electrical dipole of the eye ball (Fig. 2.8).
When the eye moves, a potential is detected between a horizontal and/or a vertical
pair of electrodes, producing the signal that is called electrooculogram (EOG). The
eye position can be derived from the potential [4].

2.3 Force and Torque Recording

Whenever a user is touching and manipulating objects, forces and torques are interacting between the user and the object. Sensing user interaction forces and torques is
important especially for force feedback controllers implemented in haptic devices.

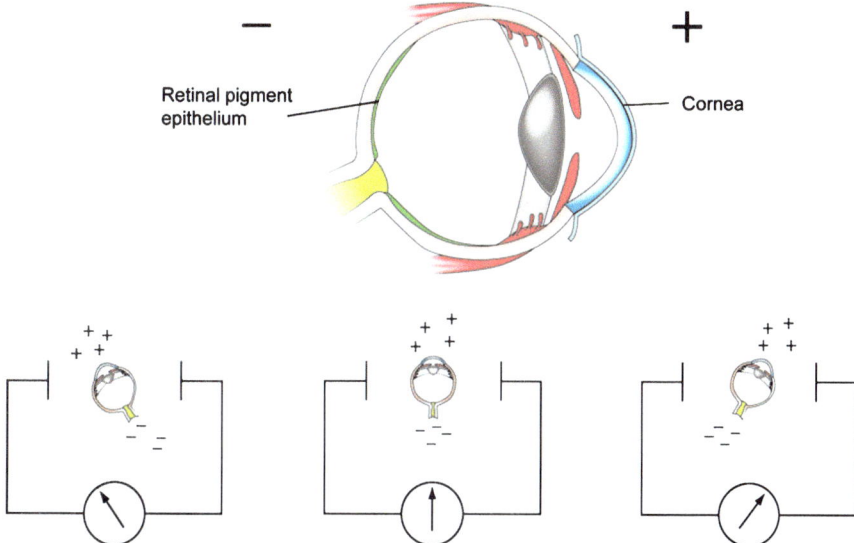

Fig. 2.8 Dipole that can be detected with electrooculogram (EOG) measurement systems; © ADInstruments Pty Ltd. Reproduced with permission

Several physical recording principles to measure these quantities are described in the following sections.

2.3.1 Resistive Methods

Most resistive methods to record forces and torques are based on strain gauges. A strain gauge is an electronic component used for measuring deformation of the object to which the gauge is attached. The resistance of the strain gauge varies in proportion to the deformation of the object caused by mechanical strain. The resistance change can usually be measured using a Wheatstone bridge circuit. A strain gauge contains a long thin fiber arranged in a meander pattern (Fig. 2.9). The strain gauge is usually attached to the surface of the object being sensed. When the object is deformed or subjected to strain in fiber direction, it will cause a change of resistance. Combinations of strain gauges, specially arranged on a mechanical structure, allow measuring force and moment up to six degrees of freedom.

2.3.2 Piezoelectric Methods

Piezoelectric sensors are made of piezoelectric crystals, which deliver an electrical charge when mechanically loaded. The crystal is placed between two conductive

Fig. 2.9 Illustration of a
strain gauge

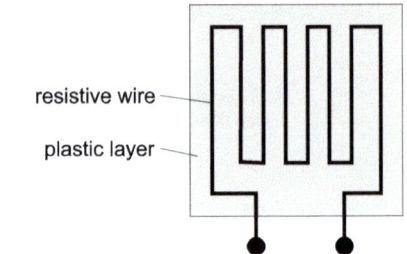

resistive wire

plastic layer

Fig. 2.10 Force plates can
measure ground reaction
forces and torques (by
courtesy of Kistler
Holding/Instrumente AG,
Switzerland)

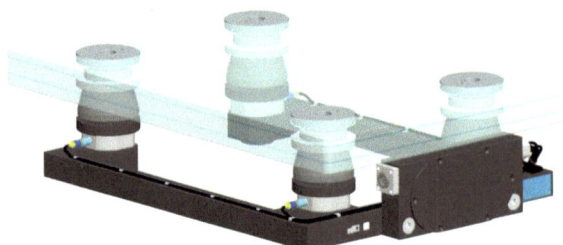

plates in order to lead the charge to a high-resistive voltage recorder. The amount
of charge is related to the magnitude of force. Layers of three crystal rings of plates
allow measuring three orthogonal components of a force. Piezoelectric 3-component
force sensors are used in force plates to record ground reaction forces, e.g. in gait
analysis (Fig. 2.10).

2.3.3 Optical Systems

Optical systems contain light sources, mirrors, and receivers. When a force is applied, it causes the flexible part of the sensor to move slightly. One can estimate
the amount of the forces from the change of light intensity recorded by the internal
receivers (Fig. 2.11).

2.3.4 Capacitive Methods

Capacitive pressure sensors use flexible thin conductive diaphragms as plates of a
capacitor. Silicone oil or any non-conductive flexible material (e.g. plastic foam)
is used as dielectric medium. The diaphragm is exposed to the active pressure on
one side and to a reference pressure on the other side. Changes in pressure cause
it to deflect, which changes the capacitance, and, thus, the voltage at the capacitor.
Instrumented insoles can measure pressure distributions of the foot during stance
phase of gait by the means of capacitive methods (Fig. 2.12) [13].

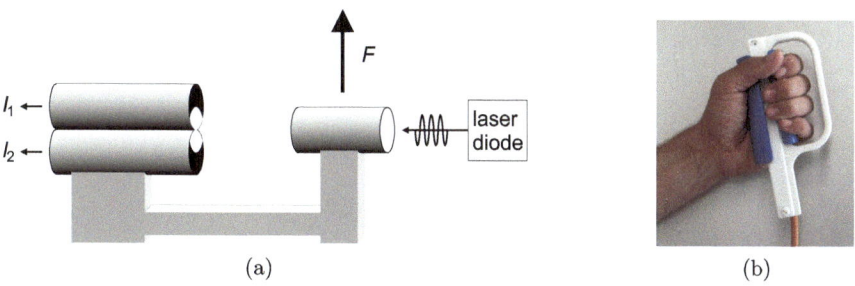

(a) (b)

Fig. 2.11 Optical force sensor can be integrated in handgrips of MRI-compatible dynamometers: (**a**) Principle (I = intensity; F = force), (**b**) MRI-compatible dynamometer; ETH Zurich

Fig. 2.12 Schematic diagram
of an instrumented insole

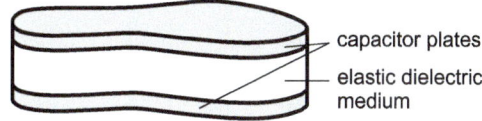

2.4 Sound and Speech Recording

There is a large variety of sound and speech recording systems available. They differ from each other in terms of their setup (mounted on a desk, a wall, or the user's head), their connection (with wires or wireless), the number of recording channels (mono, stereo or array of microphones) [3, 7], and the processing technology (e.g., sound detections or speech analysis) [5].

2.5 Physiological Data Recording

Also physiological signals from the human body can be used as input modality for VR systems, for example, to detect if the user of any VR scenarios gets emotionally involved or even stressed. Measurable quantities are, for example, muscle activity, nerve signals, cardiovascular signals, metabolic signals, respiratory variables, body temperature, and skin conductance [2, 12].

2.5.1 Electromyography (EMG)

Electromyography (EMG) is the electrical recording of muscle activity. Muscles are stimulated by signals from nerve cells called motor neurons, which causes muscle contraction. This electrical activity can be detected by electrodes inserted into the muscle or attached to the skin and connected to a recording device. The EMG signals can be used to detect muscle function and activity, for diagnostic purpose or as input signal to drive a device or VR environment, respectively. There are two basic types of electrodes, i.e. self-adhesive surface electrodes and needle electrodes (Fig. 2.13).

Fig. 2.13 Electromyography, EMG; © ADInstruments Pty Ltd. Reproduced with permission

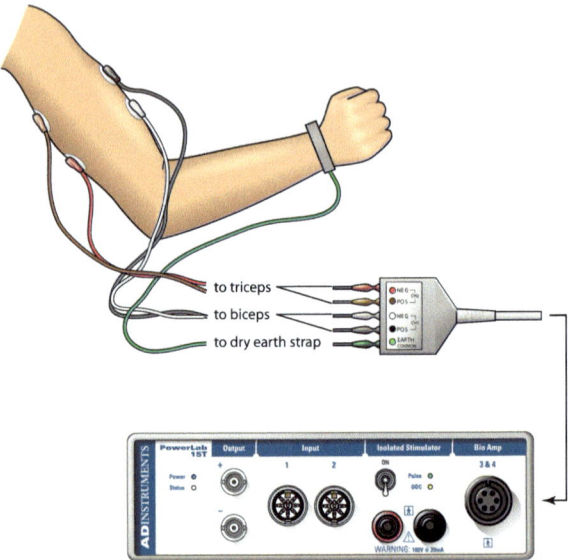

2.5.2 *Electroencephalography (EEG)*

Electroencephalography (EEG) records the electrical activity of the brain by electrodes placed on the scalp (Fig. 2.14(a)). EEG can also be used for brain-computer-interfaces (Fig. 2.14(b)) in order to drive any device or system "just by thoughts".

2.5.3 *Electrocardiography (ECG)*

Electrocardiography (ECG) is a method that measures electrical potentials associated with heart muscle activity (Fig. 2.15). It is usually applied to detect and diagnose heart abnormalities. An example of an ECG readout is shown on Fig. 2.15(b). The ECG allows to determine heart rate, heart rate variability and other parameters to detect the physical and mental involvement of the user.

2.5.4 *Blood Pressure Measurement*

Blood pressure can be measured invasively or non-invasively. Invasive arterial pressure measurement with intravascular cannula involves direct measurement of arterial pressure by placing a cannula needle in an artery. The cannula is then connected to a sterile, fluid-filled system, with an electronic pressure transducer. The advantage of this system is that pressure is constantly monitored on a beat-to-beat basis,

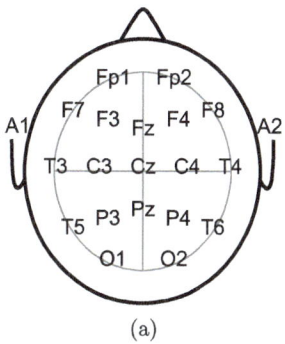

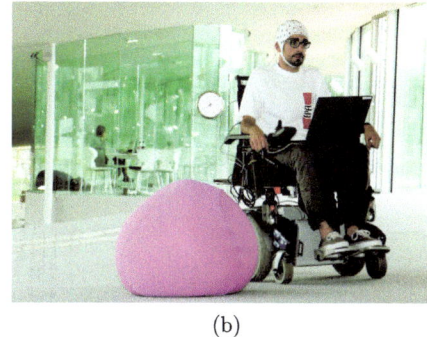

(a)   (b)

Fig. 2.14 Electroencephalographic (EEG) methods: (**a**) International 10-20 system of electrode placement [11], (**b**) EEG-based brain-computer interface; by courtesy of Dr. José del R. Millán

Fig. 2.15 ECG recording and readout: (**a**) The voltage source is assumed to be in the center of the triangle, (**b**) Typical readout of a bipolar Einthoven II ECG-derivation. The intervals between R-waves (RR-interval) is used to determine heart rate and heart rate variability; © ADInstruments Pty Ltd. Reproduced with permission

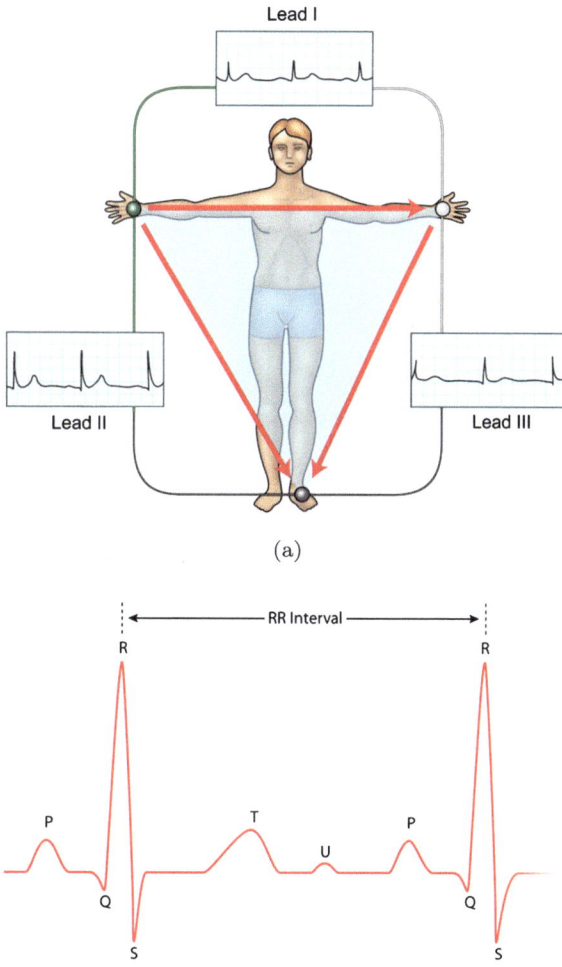

Fig. 2.16 Non-invasive
blood pressure measurement
principle by Riva-Rocci:
(**a**) Setup to measure blood
pressure, (**b**) Blood pressure
measurement;
© ADInstruments Pty Ltd.
Reproduced with permission

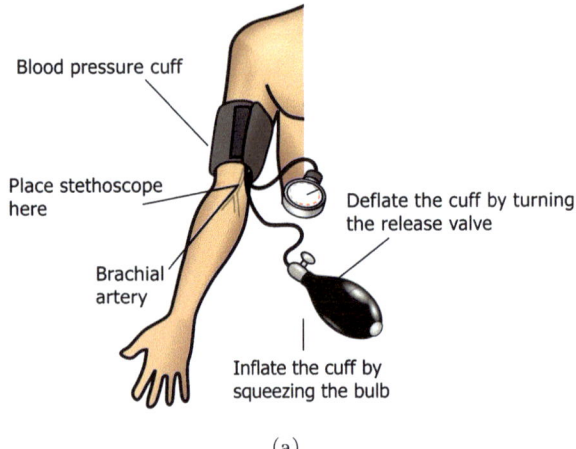

(a)

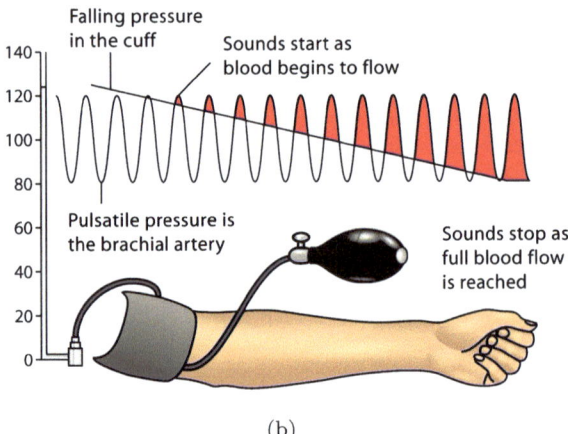

(b)

so that the quasi-continuous time course of the pressure can be displayed. The non-invasive Riva-Rocci method uses a stethoscope and an inflatable cuff placed around the upper arm at roughly the same vertical height as the heart (Fig. 2.16). The cuffs are attached to a pressure measuring manometer. This approach does not allow continuous measurements.

2.5.5 Pulse Oximetry

A pulse oximeter is a medical device that determines the amount of oxygen in the blood. It displays the percentage of arterial hemoglobin in the oxyhemoglobin configuration. Typically, it is based on a pair of small light-emitting diodes facing a photodiode through a translucent part of the patient's body, usually a fingertip or an ear-

Fig. 2.17 Sensory belt to
measure respiration;
© ADInstruments Pty Ltd.
Reproduced with permission

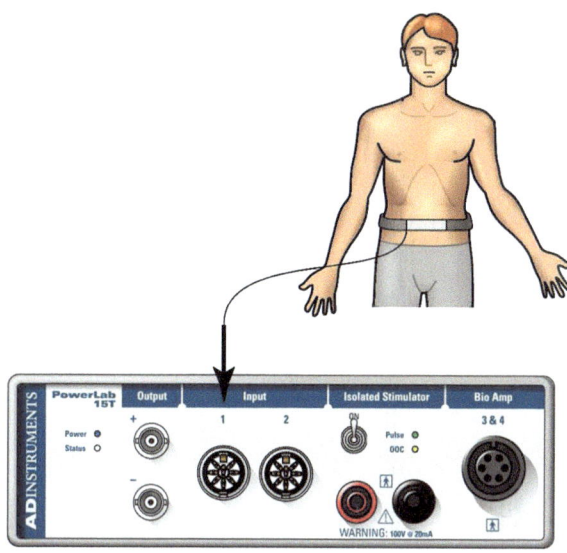

lobe. One LED sends red and the other one infrared light. Absorption at these wave-lengths differs significantly between oxyhemoglobin and its deoxygenated form, so that the oxy/deoxyhemoglobin ratio can be calculated from the ratio of the absorption of the red and infrared light.

2.5.6 Respiratory Measurements

Respiratory gas and other variables of the respiratory system (respiration frequency and breath volume) serve as indicator for metabolic strain during exercise (Fig. 2.17). The average pair of human lungs can hold about six liters of air, but only a small amount of this capacity is used during normal breathing (vital capacity). Breathing mechanism is called *tidal breathing*. Tidal volume and vital capacity can be measured directly with a spirometer (Fig. 2.18).

2.5.7 Skin Conductance

The skin conductance is one of the fastest responding measures of stress response. It is a robust and non-invasive physiological measure of autonomic nervous system activity. The activation of sweat glands leads to changes in the electrical conductance due to sweat production. Skin conductance is measured by passing current through the skin and recording the electrical resistance (Fig. 2.19). Skin conductance is one of the signals used by lie detectors.

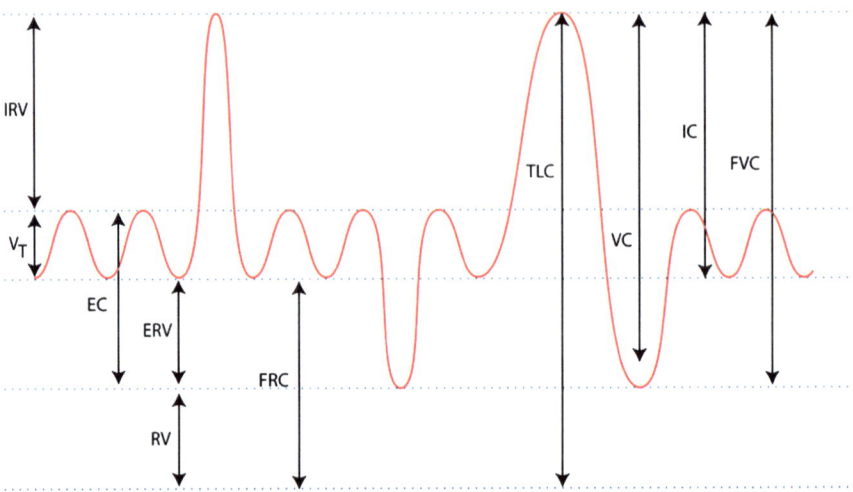

Fig. 2.18 Respiration measurement with a special measurement belt and output graph of measurement with a spirometer (*IRV*: Inspiratory Reserve Volume; V_T: Tidal Volume; *EC*: Expiratory Capacity; *ERV*: Expiratory Reserve Volume; *RV*: Residual Volume; *FRC*: Functional Residual Capacity; *TLC*: Total Lung Capacity; *VC*: Vital Capacity; *IC*: Inspiratory Capacity ; *FVC*: Forced Vital Capacity); © ADInstruments Pty Ltd. Reproduced with permission

Fig. 2.19 Galvanic skin response (GSR) is usually measured on the fingers; © ADInstruments Pty Ltd. Reproduced with permission

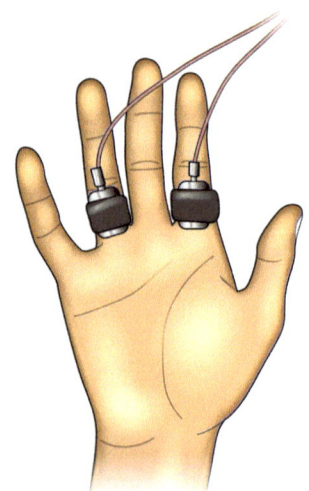

References

1. An, K.N., Askew, L.J., Chao, E.Y.: Biomechanics and functional assessment of upper extremities. In: Trends in Ergonomics/Human Factors III, pp. 573–580 (1986)
2. Andreassi, J.L.: Psychophysiology: Human Behavior and Physiological Response, 5th edn. Lawrence Erlbaum Associates, Inc., Mahwah (2007). http://books.google.ch/books?id=

mPE20OeU0poC&lpg=PP1&ots=TYhkFUcKi2&dq=andreassi%20psychophysiology&pg=
PR4#v=onepage&q&f=false

3. Ballou, G.: Handbook for Sound Engineers. Focal Press, Waltham (2005)
4. Barea, R., Boquete, L., Mazo, M., López, E.: System for assisted mobility using eye movements based on electrooculography. IEEE Trans. Neural Syst. Rehabil. Eng. **10**(4), 209–218 (2002)
5. Benzeghiba, M., De Mori, R., Deroo, O., Dupont, S., Erbes, T., Jouvet, D., Fissore, L., Laface, P., Mertins, A., Ris, C., Rose, R., Tyagi, V., Wellekens, C.: Automatic speech recognition and speech variability: a review. Speech Commun. **49**(10–11), 763–786 (2007). doi:10.1016/j.specom.2007.02.006. Intrinsic Speech Variations
6. Bronzino, J.D.: The Biomedical Engineering Handbook. CRC Press LLC and Springer-Verlag GmbH&Co and IEEE Press, Boca Raton (1995)
7. Eargle, J.: The Microphone Book. Focal Press, Waltham (2005)
8. Eichmeier, J.: Medizinische Elektronik. Springer, Berlin (1991)
9. Eska, G.: Schall und Klang: Wie und Was Wir Hören. Birkhäuser, Basel (1997)
10. Hwang, S.L., Barfield, W., Chang, T.C., Salvendy, G.: Integration of humans and computers in the operation and control of flexible manufacturing systems. Int. J. Prod. Res. **22**(5), 841–856 (1984)
11. Jasper, H.H.: The ten twenty electrode system of the international federation. Electroencephalogr. Clin. Neurophysiol. **10**(2), 371–375 (1958)
12. Koenig, A., Omlin, X., Zimmerli, L., Sapa, M., Krewer, C., Bolliger, M., Mueller, F., Riener, R.: Psychological state estimation from physiological recordings during robot assisted gait rehabilitation. J. Rehabil. Res. Dev. **48**(4), 367–386 (2011)
13. Kumar, N., Singh, D.P., Kumar, A., Sohi, B.S.: Spatiotemporal parameters measurement of human gait using developed fsr for prosthetic knee joint. Int. J. Med. Eng. Inform. **2**(4), 389–394 (2010)
14. Leonhardt, H., Tillmann, B., Töndury, G., Zilles, K.: Anatomie des Menschen, Lehrbuch und Atlas. Thieme Verlag, Stuttgart (1987)
15. Schmidt, R.F., Thews, G.: Die Physiologie des Menschen. Springer, Berlin (1990)
16. Sutter, P.H., Iatridis, J.C., Thakor, N.V.: Response to reflected-force feedback to fingers in teleoperations. In: Proceedings of the NASA Conference on Space Telerobotics (1989)
17. van Eijden, T.M., Weijs, W.A., Kouwenhoven, E., Verburg, J.: Forces acting on the patella during maximal voluntary contraction of the quadriceps femoris muscle at different knee flexion/extension angles. Acta Anat. **129**(4), 310–314 (1987)
18. Winter, D.A.: Biomechanics and Motor Control of Human Movement, 3rd edn. Wiley, New York (1990)

Chapter 3
Visual Aspects

3.1 What Is Computer Graphics?

Computer graphics deals with artificially creating and manipulating image content. Commonly the term refers to three-dimensional scene representations in real-time, however, also the offline generation of single, high-quality images belongs to this area. Both directions involve scene rendering, i.e. the generation of artificial images based on a computational model. In this context it is useful to distinguish between interactive real-time and offline rendering. The former is used in virtual reality, and more commonly in computer games, while the latter is typically applied, for instance, in the movie industry or in digital architecture. Depending on the application area, different approaches for generating artificial images are followed, which will be discussed in more detail below.

The underlying methods and paradigms in computer graphics comprise diverse related research fields. Following is a brief list of, not necessarily distinct, domains which provide some of the building blocks for computer graphics.

- **Photography** The process of generating artificial images is closely related to acquiring photographs with a real camera. This denotes for instance aspects of reflection of light, projective geometry, and depth of field.
- **Mathematics** In order to generate computer-based images, mathematical descriptions of the image formation process are required. This for example includes geometrical transformation through matrix vector multiplications, as well as idealized functions of light-matter interaction, e.g. the bidirectional reflectance distribution function [19].
- **Geometry** An important component of computer graphics is the representation of scene geometry. A common technique is the approximation of object surfaces with piecewise linear triangular elements. Alternatives are parametric polynomial surfaces, e.g. based on B-splines [9], or implicit descriptions, such as quadrics.
- **Mechanics** The physical behavior of objects in dynamics simulation is often a key element in computer graphics. The movement and/or deformation of bodies

R. Riener, M. Harders, *Virtual Reality in Medicine*,
DOI 10.1007/978-1-4471-4011-5_3, © Springer-Verlag London 2012

due to external forces has to be computed via methods from classical mechanics. A typical example is the draping of cloth [32].

- **Psychology** The capabilities and limitations of human users have a direct influence on computer graphics, e.g. on the required computational complexity. A typical example is the perceptual illusion of motion induced by fast succession of still images. Also in computer graphics a series of individual frames is generated to evoke the illusion of motion. This is done at fast update rates to make flicker imperceptible. A refresh rate of 30 Hz is often considered to be sufficient.
- **Design** Aspects of design also play a role in interactive visualization systems. This mainly denotes the development of user interfaces for steering an application [14]. The type of input/output interface used for user interaction can also be considered in this context [7].

A number of typical application areas exist for computer graphics, which are outlined in the following.

- **Entertainment** The entertainment sector is currently the largest application area of computer graphics, comprising for instance animated movies, special effects, as well as computer games. Especially the latter have a strong influence. For instance, the development of commercial graphics processing units (GPUs) is often tailored to meet the requirements of this large consumer field.
- **Data visualization** Another important application domain of computer graphics is the visualization of data. This ranges from the display of acquired medical images, via results of physical simulations, to weather forecasts. Visualization is sometimes considered to be distinct from computer graphics. Nevertheless, both directions have considerable similarities.
- **Graphic design** Computer graphics is also a powerful means to support computer-based design. A key direction in this context is digital prototyping, which allows the creation of new products in-silico (thus considerably reducing development time).
- **Marketing** Related to the field of entertainment, computer graphics techniques are also often employed for marketing or advertising. The applied technologies usually stem from the movie industry.
- **Virtual environments** Computer graphics are an important component of virtual reality applications. A key focus is on the immersiveness of the visual rendering, while maintaining high update rates. Also, different types of display hardware are used. Typical interactive simulations, e.g. for surgical or flight training, can also be considered in this category.

This chapter will first briefly overview the human visual sense, followed by a discussion of typical visual display technology. Thereafter, a general introduction into rendering in computer graphics is provided and related key concepts are presented. An in-depth discussion of all technologies and trends in computer graphics is, however, out of the scope of this chapter.

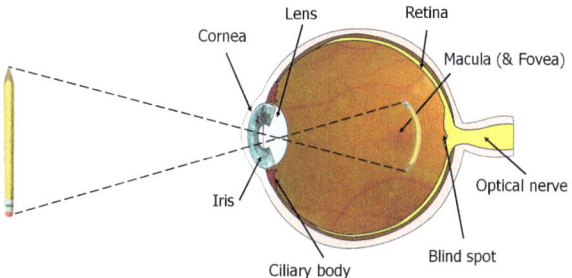

Fig. 3.1 Schematic depiction of the structure of the human eye

3.2 Visual Sense and Perception

The visual sense plays a key role in the perception of and interaction with our environment. Consequently, in the development of virtual reality setups a large focus has been on providing, analyzing, as well as enhancing visual feedback. At the current state, the realistic and real-time display of virtual scenes is a standard feature in Virtual Reality (VR). In order to better understand some of the concepts related to the visual aspects of a VR setup, the human visual sense should first be examined. Therefore, the structure of the human eye, color vision, and depth perception will be introduced in the following sections.

3.2.1 Structure of the Human Eye

The eye is the key sensing element in human vision. Its receptors are sensitive to a part of the electromagnetic spectrum, turning incoming light into electrochemical impulses in the neural system. Signals are sent through the optical nerve and neural visual pathways to the primary visual cortex (as well as other sections) in the brain. In the following we will only focus on the early, low-level process of human vision taking place in the eye. The overall structure of the human eye is illustrated in Fig. 3.1.

The function of the eye can be likened to a camera. Cornea and lens provide the refractive power to focus incoming light onto the retina. Note that the geometry of the cornea is fixed, while the shape of the lens is adjustable through activation of the ring-shaped ciliary muscles. Thus, the refractive power of the cornea is constant, while that of the lens can be changed to allow focusing at different depths. It is interesting to note that the majority of the refractive power of the eye (about 70%–80%) originates from the cornea. In addition to this, cornea and lens also absorb ultraviolet and infrared components of the electromagnetic spectrum. The amount of light entering the eye is controlled via the iris. The latter consists mainly of smooth muscles, and changes its shape to adjust the size of its central opening, the pupil. Its function can be compared to the aperture of a camera. At the back of the eye the retina is located, housing the light-sensitive photoreceptors, as well as additional neural cell layers and vessels. There are two types of receptors—the rods and the cones (more details on the structure of the retina will be provided below). The cones are key for color and high resolution vision. The majority of them are located in the central region of the eye, the macula which has a diameter of about 5 mm. The area of highest visual acuity is in the center of the macula, in the fovea (centralis). It exhibits the highest density of cones, and is free of vessels or additional cell layers. The diameter of the fovea is about 0.5 mm. It is interesting to note that the fovea only covers a small fraction of the retinal surface, but is represented in a disproportionately large area in the primary visual cortex. The fovea is responsible for high acuity vision, used for instance in reading, driving, etc. When an object is focused by the eye, then its image is projected onto this central region. Another special area in the retina is the blind spot, i.e. the region where the optical nerve and the vessels exit and/or enter the eye [35]. No photoreceptors are located in this area, therefore, the corresponding region in the visual field is not directly perceived in that eye. Various mechanisms are, however, used to fill in this blind spot. Additional visual information is obtained via the second eye as well as through saccadic eye movements. In addition, empty spots are also filled-in during high-level processing in the visual cortex.

3.2.2 Photoreceptors in the Retina

As already mentioned, there are two types of photoreceptors in the retina—rods and cones (both named according to their typical cell shapes). The rods are central for vision in dim light conditions, especially for night vision. They are also important for motion detection in peripheral vision. There are about 100 million rods in the retina, mainly located in the non-central regions. The second category, the cones, is sensitive to bright light. In addition, the cones are central to color vision. There are about 7 million cones in the retina, mostly located in the macula (with the highest density in the fovea). It is conjectured that there are three types of cones, which are sensitive to different parts of the light spectrum (in the ranges of long, medium, and short wavelengths). Figure 3.2(a) depicts a simplified illustration of the retinal structure. As can be seen, the photoreceptors are connected to further layers of neurons. These

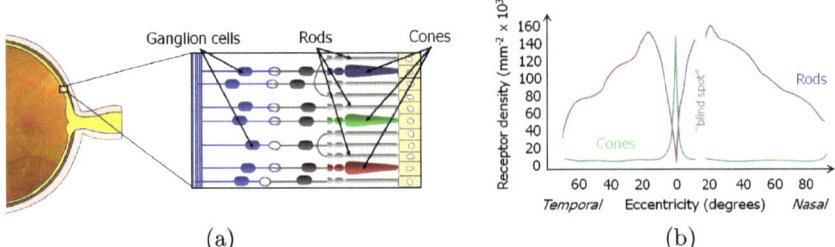

Fig. 3.2 Receptors in the retina. (**a**) Cross-section of retina with different receptors; (**b**) Changing receptor density in relation to eccentricity (adapted from [20])

Fig. 3.3 Electromagnetic radiation and the visible spectrum

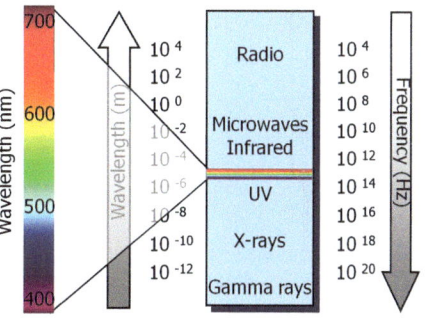

receive as input stimuli from groups of varying numbers of photoreceptors. These are then sent through Ganglion cells (note that various interneurons have been omitted for simplicity) as neural impulses via the optical nerve to the brain. The receptor density of cones and rods in the retina [20] is shown in Fig. 3.2(b). The density is plotted in relation to the eccentricity, i.e. with regard to the geodesic distance from the fovea in the transverse plane (measured in degrees). Note that there is a high density of cones in the fovea with almost no rods present. The blind spot is located at about 15 degrees horizontal eccentricity in nasal direction.

3.2.3 Electromagnetic Waves

As mentioned above, the photoreceptors are stimulated by electromagnetic (EM) radiation at certain wavelengths. Following quantum mechanical principles, EM radiation exhibits both wave and particle properties (wave-particle duality). In the following mainly the wave properties will be considered. Electromagnetic radiation manifests as self-propagating, oscillating waves travelling along a specific direction. EM radiation can be classified according to its wavelength λ and frequency f, which are inversely proportional. The waves propagate in vacuum (without any external forces) at the speed of light $c = \lambda \cdot f$. The visible part of the EM spectrum is in the range of $\lambda = 380$–750 nm. Longer wavelengths (in ascending order) comprise infrared, microwaves, and radio waves; the shorter ones contain ultraviolet, followed by ionizing radiation such as X-rays or gamma rays. Figure 3.3 depicts the complete EM spectrum.

An oscillating EM wave exhibits an electric field vector **E** and a magnetic field vector **M**. **E** and **M** are perpendicular to each other, as well as to the direction of propagation. The amplitudes of the changing field vectors are denoted by $\|\mathbf{E}\|_{max}$ and $\|\mathbf{M}\|_{max}$, respectively. A further property of an EM wave is its polarization, i.e. the orientation of the field oscillations (usually considering the electric field vector). If the field vectors oscillate in a plane, then the wave is called linearly polarized. This situation is illustrated in Fig. 3.4(a). If, instead, the field vectors rotate around the propagation vector, then the wave is called circularly polarized. Note that this could occur with clockwise or counterclockwise orientation. The third

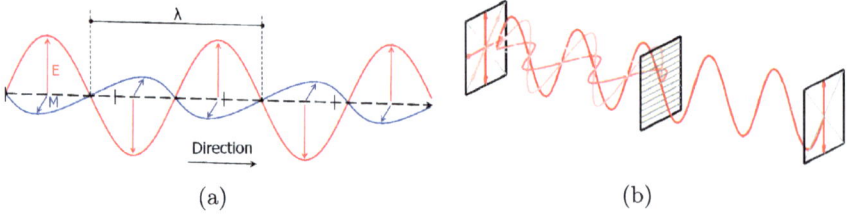

Fig. 3.4 Electromagnetic waves and their linear polarization with wire-grid polarization filters.
(**a**) Electromagnetic wave (linearly polarized); (**b**) Linear polarization of EM wave

type of polarization is in between the other two special cases. In this form the tip
of the field vector follows an elliptical path when projected perpendicular to the
propagation direction. Note that most light sources create unpolarized light (i.e. light
of a normal light bulb is made up of varying uncorrelated polarization types and
angles).

Considering human vision, it is useful to examine, which of the discussed properties can actually be observed. The wavelength of visible light determines its color
due to the varying stimulation of the three types of cones. Moreover, the square of
the wave amplitude is proportional to the light intensity. In this context, note that
there are different definitions of intensity in radiometry and photometry. The former examines observer-independent quantities, whereas the latter targets perceived
brightness. Finally, the propagation direction trivially determines visibility, since
only light entering the eye is visible. In contrast to this, the human eye has not
evolved for discriminating polarization. Therefore, this property can be used for various purposes in display technology. In the later sections various examples of this
will be provided. Nevertheless, it should be mentioned that certain insects or animals are capable of discerning celestial polarization, which for instance aids them
in navigation.

In order to exploit polarization of light in hardware solutions, ordinary light first
has to be polarized. A typical approach is to use a polarization filter for this. The
simplest solution is an absorptive, wire-grid polarizer. These filters consist of parallel metallic wires embedded into transparent material. An EM wave with a component of its electric field vector parallel to the wires will partly be absorbed and
reflected. Only the perpendicular component, i.e. perpendicular to the wires, will
pass through the wire-grid, thus, resulting in linearly polarized light. Figure 3.4(b)
illustrates this process. Note that the polarization orientation is perpendicular to the
wires. Also, light intensity is usually reduced. If a second polarizer (also called an-
alyzer) is placed in sequence with the first, then the amount of light transmitted
through the assembly depends on the relative orientation between the polarizers. If
the respective planes of polarization are perpendicular to each other, then the light
is fully blocked. If the planes are parallel, then all light passing through the first is
also transmitted by the second filter. Thus, changing the relative orientation allows
to control the amount of light passing through.

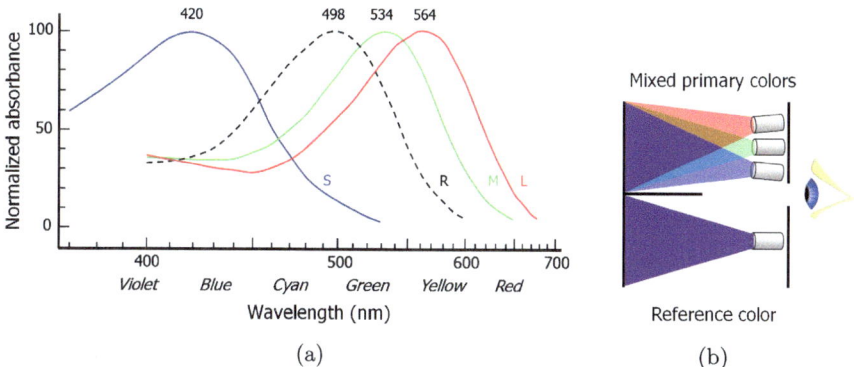

Fig. 3.5 Absorbance of photoreceptors and CIE color matching experiment. (**a**) Normalized absorbance of three types of cones as well as rods (adapted from [6]); (**b**) CIE experiment matching three primary colors with reference color

3.2.4 Color Vision

The three types of cones in the retina are sensitive to different parts of the visible spectrum of electromagnetic radiation. The combined response of the cones to light at different wavelengths leads to the perception of color. Figure 3.5(a) shows the normalized degree of absorbance of the cones [6] with regard to different wavelengths (note that the absorbance of the rods (R) is also shown for completeness). The cones have their respective peaks in the short (S), medium (M), and long (L) wavelengths. The cones are sometimes also labeled as B (blue), G (green), and R (red) type, however, the peaks are located in somewhat different color regions. For instance, the peak of the L cones is in the yellowish-greenish area. Also note that the curves of the receptors overlap. The overall highest sensitivity of human photoreceptors is at a wavelength of about 550 nm.

The perception of a specific color arises from the stimulation of the cones by incoming light that is composed of a mixture of various wavelengths, i.e. with a specific spectral power distribution. It is important to note that different light spectra can lead to the perception of the same color. This effect is called metamerism, and the respective colors are named metamers. It was early on conjectured that color could in principle be described by three parameters (trichromatic color theory), which was later on confirmed by the discovery of three different types of color receptors. Following this notion, in the late 1920s a user experiment has been carried out focusing on matching of colors in order to determine a first, theoretical color space [28]. Three monochromatic, i.e. single-wavelength base colors (primaries) were projected onto one half of a screen. On the other half, a single monochromatic reference color was projected. The observers were then asked to adjust the intensity of the primary colors to match any presented reference colors. Figure 3.5(b) illustrates the experimental setup. The study revealed that most of the reference colors could be reproduced by a combination of three primary colors (note that in some cases one of the

Fig. 3.6 Additive color
space. (**a**) Additive mixing of
colored light; (**b**) RGB color
space represented as a cube

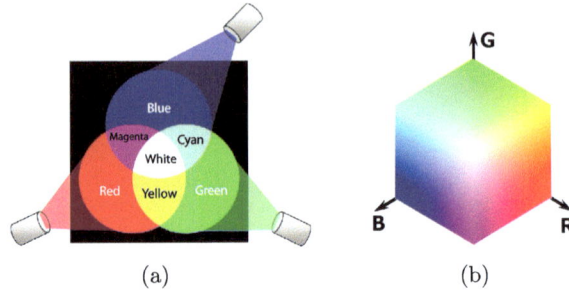

(a)   (b)

primary colors had to be added to the reference color, wherefore it was considered
as a negative value). Based on this experiment the first color space—the CIE 1931
XYZ space—was defined by the Commission Internationale de l'Eclairage (CIE),
i.e. the International Commission on Illumination.

3.2.5 RGB Color Space

Mixing together three primaries to create a wide spectrum of visible colors is the
underlying principle used in most display hardware (e.g. computer monitors or projectors) as well as in computer graphics. Such a color space follows the notion of
additive mixing of colors. Figure 3.6(a) presents this idea. In computer graphics colors are defined by a three-dimensional vector composed of the three primary channels, representing the red, green, and blue (RGB) components. Thus, the rendering
computations that will be introduced below in Sect. 3.4.3 have to be carried out for
each of the three channels separately. A typical way to specify a color is by giving
each component a value in a normalized range between 0.0 and 1.0. However, in
computer graphics libraries a color is usually represented by an integer value. Using 8 bits per channel allows to encode about 16.7 million (256^3) different colors.
This digital 24-bit RGB representation is known as the TrueColor format. In order
to visualize the RGB color space, the obtained additive colors are often depicted in
a cube (see Fig. 3.6(b)). Shades of grey are found on the diagonal between black
(0.0, 0.0, 0.0) and white (1.0, 1.0, 1.0).

As already mentioned, the idea of additive mixing of base colors is also the basic
principle used in color displays. Each display pixel on a screen is actually represented by a number of smaller subpixels (typically three (R, G, B) subpixels). Note
that depending on the underlying technology different geometrical layouts of these
subpixels are used. For instance, a geometry commonly encountered in LCD screens
is parallel stripes.

Fig. 3.7 Principle of twisted nematic liquid crystal cell in ON (*left*) and OFF state (*right*)

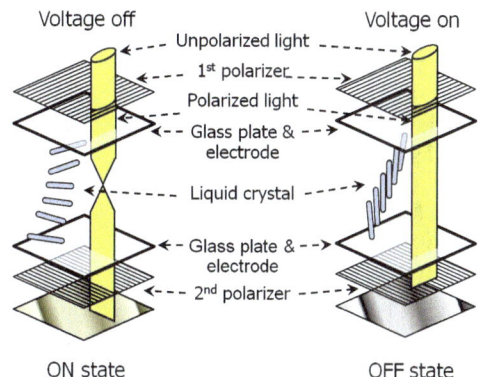

3.2.6 Liquid Crystal Display

In order to exemplify the process of image creation in a contemporary computer screen a closer look at liquid crystal displays (LCDs) will be taken. The key component in the latter is liquid crystals. These molecules exhibit properties of crystals as well as of liquids. Their structure changes depending on the presence or absence of an electric field. Figure 3.7 shows the key functional element of a LC display, the (twisted nematic) liquid crystal cell. The latter function much akin to valves. In these elements, the process of light polarization plays a key role. As depicted, light is first linearly polarized before it passes through the liquid crystal. One of the key properties of twisted nematic LCs is their effect on this polarization. In the inactive state, the liquid crystals are arranged in a twisted fashion. The molecules act much like an optical wave guide, changing the plane of polarization of the linearly polarized light by 90 degrees. Due to this change the light can pass through a second, rotated polarization filter located behind the LC cell. This is the fully ON state. However, when an electric field is applied, the molecules align with the field and change their structure. Due to this, the polarization changing effect is lost. Since the second static polarizer is rotated, all light is now blocked. This is the fully OFF state. Note that by altering the voltage the amount of polarization change can be controlled, and thus the amount of light passing through the complete element. These liquid crystal cells are used in a color LC display to control the brightness of the three (i.e. RGB) sub-pixels of a screen pixel. The initially unpolarized light is provided by a backlighting system. The subpixels are colored by simple color filters. An important characteristic of an LCD is the pixel response time, i.e. the time it takes to change a LC cell from one brightness level to another. This is especially important for fast changing scenes.

3.2.7 Further Colorspaces

So far we have introduced the additive RGB color space. There exist, however, a number of additional color spaces, a few of which will be examined in the follow-

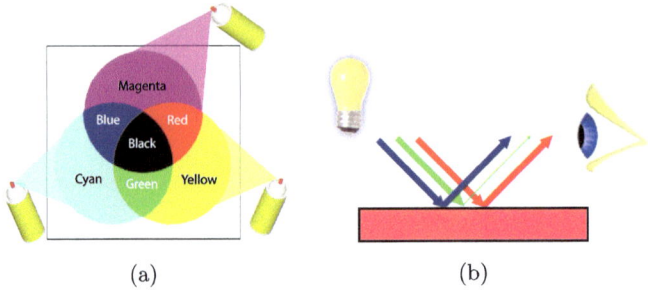

(a)   (b)

Fig. 3.8 Subtractive color model. (**a**) Subtractive color by mixing colored inks; (**b**) Absorption of color

ing. The dual of the principle of additive mixing is the subtractive color model, which is mainly applied in color printing. The underlying notion of this model is the absorption of parts of the spectrum of visible light by color pigments. Different colors are created by mixing together different inks, thus, changing the reflected light spectrum (and in turn the perceived color). Figure 3.8 illustrates the principle. The basic colors used are cyan (C), magenta (M), and yellow (Y). Therefore, the model is denoted as the CMY color space. Magenta ink, for instance, filters out wavelengths perceived as greenish tones, while yellow ink filters out bluish tones. Thus, the combination of the two would appear as red, since only those wavelengths remain. The combination of all three inks would create black color. However, to obtain a rich black tone (and also to reduce the amount of ink used) the CMY model is usually extended to include a fourth dimension for a black component (K), thus, resulting in the CMYK model. In order to convert an RGB image to a CMY image, a simple conversion formula can be applied:

$$\begin{bmatrix} 1 \\ 1 \\ 1 \end{bmatrix} - \begin{bmatrix} R \\ G \\ B \end{bmatrix} = \begin{bmatrix} C \\ M \\ Y \end{bmatrix}. \tag{3.1}$$

At this point it should be noted that the appearance of a color image is device dependent. Depending on the actual wavelengths of the used primaries a displayed (or printed) image might appear different. An exact physical description of color would actually require specifying (and then reproducing) its exact spectral power distribution.

While the previously introduced RGB color space is appropriate to define colors, it is not very intuitive to use. For instance, it is not straightforward to determine the required amounts of red, green, and blue to obtain a desired mixed color. Furthermore, it is also not clear how a less saturated version of a specific color has to be defined in RGB-coordinates. Therefore, alternative color models have been developed which attempt to follow more closely the way a human might attempt to specify a color. One example of this is the HSV color model, which defines a color by its hue (H), saturation (S), and value (V). The hue defines the type of color (e.g. red, yellow, green, etc.). Saturation determines the richness of the color (in a

Fig. 3.9 HSV color space

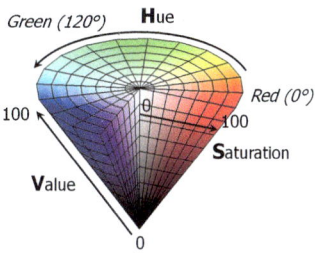

simplified sense the amount of white added). Value represents the intensity of the color (in a simplified sense the amount of black added). Hue is often specified in a 0–360 degree range, while saturation and value take a range of 0–100%. Figure 3.9 shows the HSV color cone. Note that the space is actually cylindrical, however, at low values the saturation levels become visually less distinct. Therefore, the color space is often represented by a cone. Colors with a saturation of 0 are desaturated, and, thus, greyscale tints. Pure colors have maximal saturation and value.

A final point to consider is the transformation between RGB and HSV color spaces. In order to convert normalized RGB values to HSV one can apply the following formalism:

$$M = \max(R, G, B), \qquad N = \min(R, G, B) \tag{3.2}$$

$$H = \begin{cases} 0 & M = N \\ 60 \cdot \frac{G-B}{M-N}, & M = R \\ 60 \cdot \frac{B-R}{M-N} + 120, & M = G \\ 60 \cdot \frac{R-G}{M-N} + 240, & M = B \end{cases} \tag{3.3}$$

$$H = H + 360 \quad \text{if } H < 0 \tag{3.4}$$

$$S = \begin{cases} 0 & \text{if } M = 0 \\ 100 \cdot (1 - \frac{N}{M}) & \text{else} \end{cases}$$

$$V = 100 \cdot M.$$

Note that for greyscale values hue is undefined, and, thus, set to zero. In addition, for black also saturation is set to zero. Moreover, consider that the resulting values sometimes do not correspond to exact integers (and, thus, might have to be rounded). The inverse step from HSV to RGB can be carried out using another algorithm:

$$H_i = \left\lfloor \frac{H}{60} \right\rfloor \bmod 6, \qquad f = \frac{H}{60} - H_i, \qquad S' = S/100, \qquad V' = V/100 \tag{3.5}$$

$$p = V' \cdot (1 - S'), \qquad q = V' \cdot (1 - (S' \cdot f)), \qquad t = V' \cdot (1 - (S' \cdot (1 - f))).$$

$$R = V', \qquad G = t, \qquad B = p, \qquad \text{if } H_i = 0$$
$$R = q, \qquad G = V', \qquad B = p, \qquad \text{if } H_i = 1$$
$$R = p, \qquad G = V', \qquad B = t, \qquad \text{if } H_i = 2$$
$$R = p, \qquad G = q, \qquad B = V', \qquad \text{if } H_i = 3$$
$$R = t, \qquad G = p, \qquad B = V', \qquad \text{if } H_i = 4$$
$$R = V', \qquad G = p, \qquad B = q \qquad \text{if } H_i = 5.$$

A final point to consider is color interpolation. Note that interpolating between two different colors (e.g. red and blue) will yield different intermediate values when done in RGB or HSV color space, since the transformation between the two is non-affine.

3.2.8 Depth Perception

The concept of immersion into a virtual environment has been introduced in Chap. 1. Immersion can be a critical factor for the effectiveness of a VR setup. A key element to create immersion is to provide appropriate visual cues. With regard to immersion and interaction, the perception of depth is critical. Since most display technologies show a scene as a 2D projection, appropriate cues need to be artificially added to provide users with a sense of depth.

Depth perception is the ability to appreciate spatial relationships and to perceive distances. Various cues provide humans with information about object distance. The former can be divided into three categories—monocular, oculomotor, and binocular cues.

3.2.8.1 Monocular Cues

Monocular depth cues are obtained using input from only one eye. These can be further categorized as static or dynamic. Static (pictorial) cues denote visual information present in a still image that provide hints about depths of objects (see Fig. 3.10 for an overview).

- **Retinal image size** Similar objects are often assumed to be of similar size (this effect is known as size constancy). Thus, if an instance of an object in an image appears to be smaller than another one, then it is assumed to be at a larger distance from the viewer (e.g. the bottles and plates in the example image). Moreover, if previous knowledge about the size of an object is available, then a single object is already sufficient for a rough distance estimation.
- **Linear perspective** Due to perspective projection, parallel lines appear to converge at infinity in a single point on the horizon—the vanishing point—thus also providing distance cues. This effect is also related to the already mentioned retinal image size. It is often used by artists in paintings to convey depth.

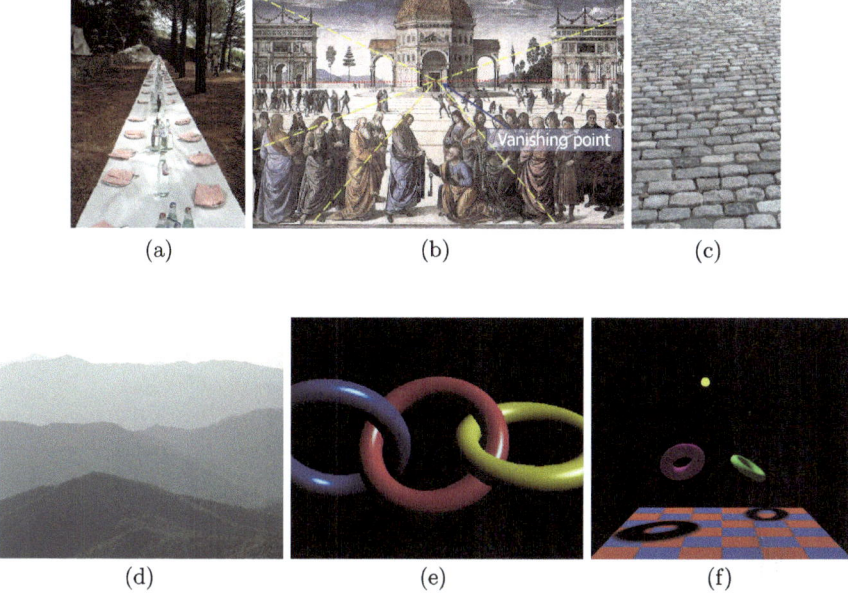

Fig. 3.10 Static monocular depth cues. (**a**) Retinal image size; (**b**) Linear perspective; (**c**) Texture gradients; (**d**) Aerial perspective; (**e**) Occlusion; (**f**) Shadows

- **Texture gradients** The change in appearance of surface texture can also provide depth information. Texture details are more visible if an object is closer. Note that additional depth cues might also be provided within a texture (e.g. linear perspective, retinal image size).
- **Aerial perspective** Light is scattered by the atmosphere, causing distant objects to appear with reduced contrast. Moreover, color shifts to shorter wavelengths of the spectrum also provide depth information. Such effects are usually noticeable in an outdoor environment and at large distances (e.g. views of distant mountains). Such strategies are occasionally implemented in computer graphics (e.g. distance fog) to add depth information in a scene.
- **Occlusion** Object interposition provides an important clue about relative object depth, i.e. the order of objects, since objects in front of others occlude the latter. Thus, the blocking object is assumed to be closer than the overlapped one.
- **Shadows** The depth of an object can be judged by examining the shadows cast on other objects or surfaces. As an example, adding the shadows of a 3D cursor in a virtual environment already facilitates navigation considerably.

Dynamic monocular depth cues originate from motion of objects or the observer. A typical example is motion parallax. Focusing on an object at a certain depth, while changing the viewing position, results in an apparent relative movement of other objects located at different depths (see Fig. 3.11(a)). For instance, fixating an object and moving the head to the side causes an apparent movement of more distant objects in the same direction, while closer objects exhibit a relative displacement to

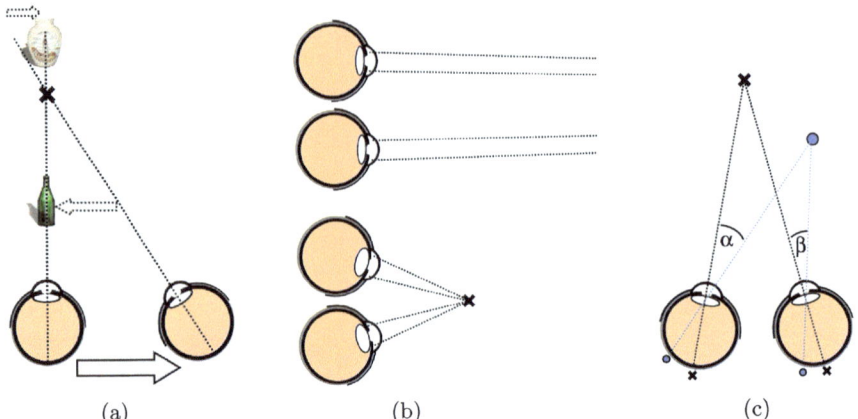

Fig. 3.11 Dynamic, oculomotor, and binocular depth cues. (**a**) Apparent movement of objects at different depths due to motion parallax; (**b**) Change in accommodation and convergence for distant (*top*) and near (*bottom*) focus; (**c**) Stereopsis due to different projections on retina

the opposite side. A similar effect is observed when driving in a vehicle, i.e. closer objects pass by faster than more distant ones. Motion parallax is a key mechanism for some animals (e.g. pigeons) to judge depth, usually by frequent change of head position. A further dynamic cue is the kinetic depth effect. 3D structures can be inferred by the motion of 2D patterns. For instance, a human shape can be discerned just by observing the motion of individual body markers (visualized as dots) in a motion tracking system. Furthermore, continuous illumination and shadow changes also result in similar effects. Note that the described dynamic cues all require movement in some form.

3.2.8.2 Oculomotor Cues

Oculomotor depth cues are related to the function of the eye. Muscular activity and eye movement provide subliminal distance information. The related key processes are accommodation and convergence. The former denotes the change of the lens shape to focus at a certain depth. This is achieved by activation of the ciliary muscle in the eye. The lens of a healthy young human eye can change from far to near vision in about 400 ms; however, this ability degrades with age. Note that in the relaxed state the lens exhibits a flat shape, thus, focusing at distant objects. The state of muscle activation is interpreted by the brain to infer depth. This is most effective in near vision. In this context it should also be considered that the change in optical power of the lens leads to blurring effects. The other related oculomotor cue is convergence. This term refers to the inward movement of both eyes when focusing on close-by objects. Again the related muscle activation provides cues to infer depth. This cue is also most effective in near vision. Figure 3.11(b) compares accommodation and convergence when focusing on far and near objects.

3.2.8.3 Binocular Cues

Binocular depth cues require information from both eyes. The most prominent one in this category is stereopsis, which arises from binocular disparity. Since our eyes are located at slightly different positions on a horizontal plane in our head, different images of the environment are projected onto the respective retinas (see Fig. 3.11(c)). A fixated point is found on corresponding locations of the retina (i.e. the fovea), while objects at different depths will be projected onto noncorresponding retinal locations. This difference is termed disparity. Based on the latter, the brain extracts depth information (thus, actually solving a correspondence problem). In addition, note that the brain fuses the double images into a single visual percept. Stereopsis is an important cue for our depth perception. The effect is strongest in near vision, since the disparity diminishes over distance. Furthermore, it should be mentioned that up to 10% of the population are (fully or partially) stereo-blind, i.e. difficulties are experienced in perceiving stereo images. This can somewhat be compensated by relying on other depth cues. Note that the previously mentioned process of convergence can also be considered as a binocular cue since both eyes are involved.

3.3 Visual Display Technology

Various hardwares exist for the visual display of computer-generated images. Key technological solutions will be presented in the following, with a focus on visual rendering in virtual reality. First, various approaches to provide stereoscopic cues will be examined, followed by a discussion of typical VR display hardware.

3.3.1 Stereoscopic Rendering

Visual cues contributing to human depth perception were overviewed in Sect. 3.2.8. In the following, solutions targeted at these cues will be presented. The former are required since most displays only provide 2D images.

Static monocular depth cues have to be generated during the rendering stage. Most of the required effects are automatically part of the standard rendering pipeline, such as linear perspective, texturing, occlusions, etc. Additional effects, such as shadows or distance fog can also easily be added. Dynamic monocular depth cues such as motion parallax are, however, not included in the standard rendering. A computer-generated image of a 3D scene displayed on a screen does not adjust when a viewer alters his position. A possible solution in this case, is the tracking of a user's head. This allows updating the rendered images according to the head motion (see Fig. 3.12). In addition, it should be noted that the rendering of a scene also provides dynamic depth cues when motion is simulated, for instance when riding a

Fig. 3.12 Dynamic depth
cues from motion parallax

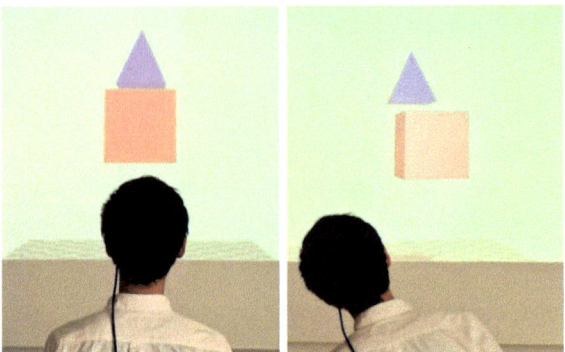

vehicle. In contrast to the mentioned effects, oculomotor cues are difficult to include
and commonly not taken into account.

One of our strongest depth cues in near vision is stereopsis. Unfortunately, it
is more complicated to provide a technical solution in a VR system for this effect
than for monocular cues. The general approach is to compute and display two images, one for each eye. In addition, it has to be ensured that a specific image is only
visible to the corresponding eye. The basic concept of the dual rendering is illustrated in Fig. 3.13(a). Points on a 3D object are displayed at different locations on
the screen, depending on whether the image is rendered for the left or the right eye
(note that a mechanism to exclusively render an image to a specific eye is not shown
in the picture). A critical point to consider is the incongruence between convergence
and accommodation. The eyes converge to an apparent depth of the focused object,
while accommodation occurs for the depth of the screen. This difference is assumed
to be one potential source of cybersickness.

Depending on the stereo pairs shown, an object will appear at a certain depth with
respect to the screen (see Fig. 3.13(b)). Points whose projections coincide in the two
images are said to have zero parallax and appear to be in the screen plane. An object
located behind the screen is said to have positive parallax. In this case, the projection
of a point in the image is shifted to the right for the right eye, and to the left for the
left eye, respectively. The shift between the projections should optimally be smaller
than the inter-pupillary distance. Stereo renderings with negative parallax require

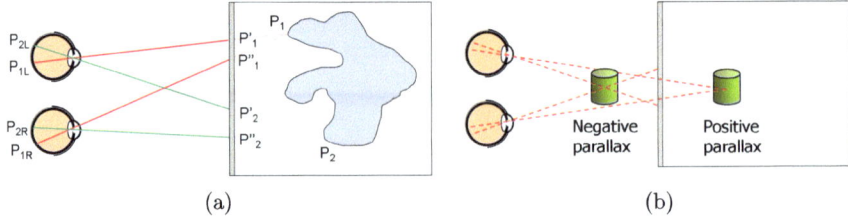

(a)   (b)

Fig. 3.13 Stereoscopic display concepts. (**a**) Rendering of stereo-pairs on the screen for stereoscopic display; (**b**) Location of objects rendered in stereo appears to be in front of or behind the
screen

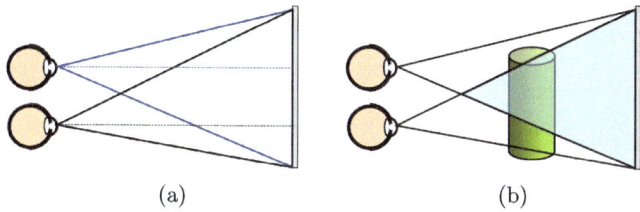

(a)   (b)

Fig. 3.14 Rendering stereo-pair images for stereoscopic display. (**a**) Oblique perspective projection for creating stereo pairs; (**b**) Border effects when using negative parallax

the eyes to be rotated further inwards. In this case, points appear to be floating in front of the screen. The projections shown on the screen are shifted to the left for the right eye, and vice versa. When objects rendered in stereo are brought too close to the viewer, at some point the images will separate and appear as two. This is due to the visual system not being able to fuse the stereo pairs anymore, thus, also breaking down the stereo impression.

The stereo image pairs are created via standard computer graphics rendering. However, there are a few pitfalls that should be avoided. In order to create the two images, the scene has to be rendered from two different viewpoints representing the eyes. For both views the same projection plane, i.e. the screen plane, needs to be used. Therefore, an off-axis, oblique perspective projection has to be applied (see Fig. 3.14(a)). A further point to consider is the varying inter-pupillary distance of different viewers. Depending on the former the perceived depth of an object can differ. However, this effect is minor and can usually be neglected. A more critical problem is the screen border effect possibly occurring for objects with strong negative parallax (Fig. 3.14(b)). This is encountered when an object is too large to be displayed on the screen. The screen borders seemingly clip the object, resulting in conflicting visual cues (in the example the lower part of the cylinder is clipped in both views). According to stereopsis the object appears to be in front of the screen, while according to the occlusion (i.e. the clipping) the screen and its borders appear to be in front. This situation should be avoided. Related to this, with negative parallax a part of an object might be visible in one of the stereo renderings, but not visible in the other (in the example the top part of the cylinder). Considering these points, positive parallax is usually preferable.

3.3.2 Stereoscopic Display Hardware

The final point to consider for stereo rendering is mechanisms to present the correct stereo image to the respective eye. Light polarization (see Sect. 3.2.3) often plays a key role in currently available solutions.

One common approach is using a so-called passive stereo setup. The key idea is to encode the images for the respective eyes via light polarization. Filters are em-

Fig. 3.15 Hardware
solutions for stereoscopic
display. (**a**) Passive stereo
glasses. Stereo image for a
specific eye encoded by
polarization; (**b**) Active stereo
glasses. Opposite eye blocked
out synchronized with display
via emitter

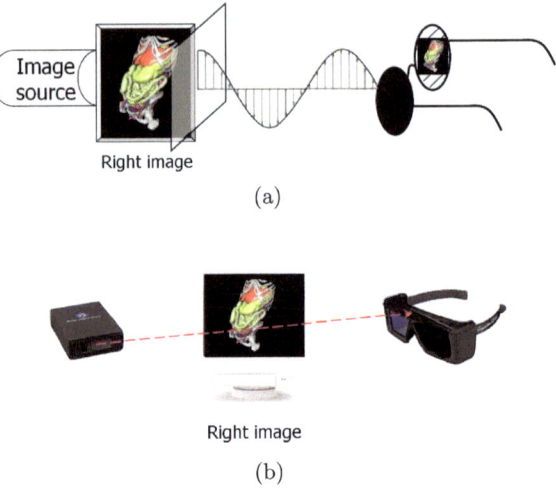

Right image

(a)

Right image

(b)

ployed to distinctly polarize the left- and right-eye stereo image. Users don glasses
with corresponding polarization filters, thus letting only the appropriately polarized
rendering pass each filter. Figure 3.15(a) depicts this approach. This display strategy can for instance be implemented by using two projectors equipped with rotated
linear polarizers. The rendered images are projected simultaneously onto the same
surface. Passive stereo glasses are worn, which contain matching rotated linear polarizers. Note that this approach usually requires a special projection surface which
does not depolarize the reflected light, e.g. a silver or aluminized screen. A further
concern is the required tight synchronization between the two projections. An alternative technical solution is to use an active polarization shutter placed in front of
a screen or a projector. The shutter is based on liquid crystal technology, allowing
to change the polarization of the passing light. According to the displayed image
the shutter polarization is switched. This requires additional hardware to synchronize the polarization change with the display. Moreover, the switches have to be
carried out in fast succession to avoid perception of flicker. Note that standard LCD
screens might not be optimal for this, since the displayed images are already polarized. Moreover, some screens might not be capable of providing the required fast
refresh rates.

A second class of stereoscopic systems are the so-called active stereo setups.
These also employ liquid crystal-based active polarization shutters that are synchronized with the displayed images. However, in this case a user wears special glasses
containing the active LC shutter. The LC layer in front of each eye is switched
to opaque according to the image displayed on the screen. A transmitter (e.g. infrared or bluetooth) connected to the graphics card is used to synchronize the shutter glasses with the rendering. Figure 3.15(b) illustrates the approach. Note that the
update again has to be carried out at high frequencies to avoid flicker, thus requiring
appropriate display hardware. Usually batteries are employed to provide the voltage

for activating the liquid crystal layer in the glasses. The cost of active shutter glasses is considerably higher than for passive stereo systems.

A critical point to consider in stereo displays is the effect of crosstalk or ghosting. This denotes the effect of the image for one eye becoming visible in the other, and vice versa. This is for instance encountered when using linear polarization in passive stereo. When a user starts tilting the head, ghost images of the other views become increasingly visible. This problem can be avoided by using circular polarization of opposite handedness. This solution has recently found increasing application for displaying 3D motion pictures in movie theaters. The mentioned ghosting effects can also be encountered when active polarization shutters are not exactly synchronized with the display. A further drawback to consider is that light polarization reduces the overall image brightness.

In addition to the discussed setups, other technologies exist to provide stereoscopic images, such as autostereoscopic screens not requiring any glasses or holographic projections. However, these are not commonly used in VR applications. A further solution is head-mounted displays, which will be discussed in more detail below. Since a separate screen is available for each eye, appropriate stereo images can easily be displayed.

3.3.3   Virtual Reality Displays

The display hardware used in virtual reality systems can be categorized with regard to the attainable degree of immersion. Three main classes exist, which will be introduced in the following.

- **Desktop VR** The simplest solution for a VR setup is to combine a desktop-based display device, for instance a standard computer screen, with additional components, such as stereoscopic rendering and head tracking (to provide motion parallax). Often a desktop-based haptic interface is also included in such a setting (see Fig. 3.16(a)). It is occasionally questioned whether such setups should be considered as "true" VR or not, since the user is not fully immersed into the virtual world. Nevertheless, gaming applications using even less sophisticated hardware have already shown the potential to elicit a very high degree of immersion. Since the virtual world is viewed through a small window (i.e. the screen), such setups are also referred to as fish-tank VR [36].
- **Projective VR** A straightforward extension of desktop VR is the enlargement of the display area. This widens the provided field of view, thus, increasing the sense of immersion. Moreover, additional users can participate in the viewing of the presented VR content. Such setups usually employ one or more projectors for displaying on flat or curved surfaces. A typical interface in this category is the so-called Responsive Workbench [17] (see Fig. 3.16(b)). Stereoscopic rendering and head tracking is usually integrated into these setups. However, in multi-user settings it has to be considered that a correct view needs to be rendered for each

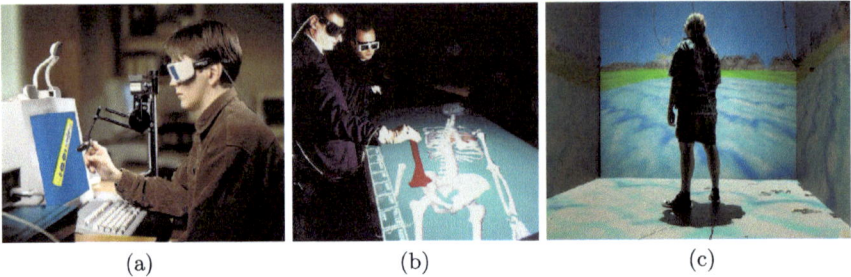

(a)   (b)   (c)

Fig. 3.16   Types of virtual reality display hardware setups. (**a**) Multimodal desktop VR (from [2]); (**b**) Projective VR on a Responsive Workbench (courtesy of Bernd Fröhlich); (**c**) Immersive VR in a CAVE (courtesy of Electronic Visualization Laboratory, University of Illinois at Chicago)

viewer [1]. If only the head of one person is tracked, then correct perspective is only generated for this viewer, while the others will experience image distortions.

- **Immersive VR** The target of immersive displays is to place a user inside of a virtual world, while blocking out cues from the real environment. This is related to the sense of presence, i.e. the feeling of actually being in the simulated environment. Two key examples in this category are CAVE-like setups and head-mounted displays. In the former a user stands inside a small room, whose walls are used as projection surfaces. The virtual world is displayed on the latter via rear-projection (see Fig. 3.16(c)). In the other immersive display type, a head-mounted setup is worn, which houses small screens in front of the eyes. By tracking head movements of a user, the views of the virtual world are updated according to the changes in viewing position and orientation. These immersive technologies are sometimes considered as being "true" virtual reality interfaces. In the following the advantages and disadvantages of both solutions will be discussed in more detail.

3.3.3.1 CAVE

The CAVE (Cave Automatic Virtual Environment) is an immersive virtual reality display setup. It usually comes in the form of a cube-shaped room, whose walls are used as projection screens for displaying the virtual world. The first CAVE setup was developed at the Electronic Visualization Laboratory of the University of Illinois at the beginning of the 1990s [8]. It should be noted that the term *CAVE* has been registered as a trademark by the University of Illinois, and is being licensed to VR hardware manufacturers. Nevertheless, similar technological solutions have been produced by other groups. These are also commonly referred to as CAVEs. Up to six walls of a CAVE can be used as display surfaces, the majority of existing systems having four. The highest degree of immersion is achieved when a user is fully surrounded by the virtual environment. The CAVE is driven by a main user, whose head position is tracked. This allows generating correct renderings, usually including stereoscopic images as well as motion parallax. Note that in this setup the

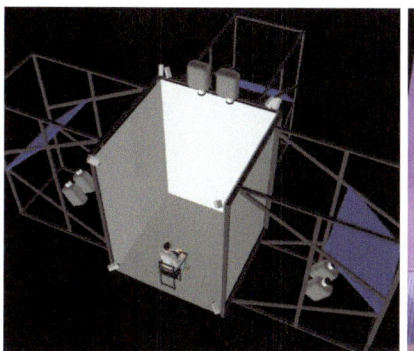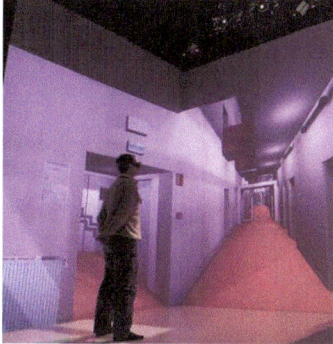

Fig. 3.17 Cave Automatic Virtual Environments (CAVE) (courtesy of Daniel Mestre, MVRC)

perspective is only correct for the main viewing position, and the views will only be updated according to the main driver's movements. Thus, additional persons inside the CAVE usually experience visual artefacts. For stereoscopic display normally active shutter glasses are employed. In order to interact with the virtual environment, special input devices are required. These can, for instance, be tracked gloves or 3D mice. Since the latter provide multiple functionality and are often shaped like a rod, they are commonly referred to as wands. An alternative is to control a VR application by speech commands. Advanced sound systems are also used to provide audio feedback in a CAVE. Figure 3.17 shows examples of CAVE setups.

Various drawbacks have to be taken into consideration when building or using a CAVE. First of all, the considerable setup cost should be mentioned. Multiple high-fidelity projectors, specialized projection screens, fast rendering hardware, tracking and input devices are required. While the cost has decreased since the first installations in the 1990s, building high-quality setups still requires a significant investment. This also includes maintenance and the space requirement for the CAVE. Concerning the latter, note that usually mirrors are employed to reduce the overall footprint. CAVEs also have a limited portability due to the considerable setup time. The latter also comprises the system calibration, which is necessary to compensate for any distortions in the tracking. A further technical issue to consider is interreflections at edges and corners between the walls due to light scattering. These effects can be compensated by adjusting the rendered images before displaying. A typical approach in this context is to solve an inverse radiosity problem. Further, it should be noted that actual locomotion within the virtual world inside a CAVE is limited. Although some technical solutions have been proposed, such as (omnidirectional) treadmills [29] or walking-in-space [27, 31], unconstrained, fully natural walking for exploration is not yet possible.

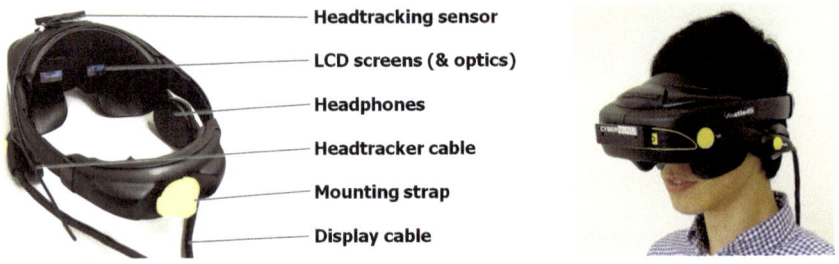

Fig. 3.18   Head-mounted displays—key components (*left*) and user wearing an HMD (*right*)

3.3.3.2   Head-Mounted Displays

The second display hardware solution typical for immersive VR is head-mounted displays (HMDs). In these systems a user wears an assembly directly on his head containing small screens in front of the eyes. A further key component is the tracking of the user's head. The view displayed on the screens is updated according to the head movements. The first HMD-based VR system was developed in 1968 by Ivan Sutherland [30]. It used CRT displays and a mechanical linkage for head tracking. The displayed virtual world only consisted of simple wireframe models. Note that in normal usage it had to be suspended from the ceiling due to its weight. Another key element of HMDs is the optical system. It provides magnification as well as collimation, thus, letting the image appear further away than just a few centimeters in front of the eye. Another common element of a HMD is stereo headphones. Figure 3.18 depicts the main components of a typical HMD.

Various concerns arise when using a HMD for immersive VR. User comfort plays a critical role in this respect. HMDs are often too heavy and uncomfortable for prolonged usage. Moreover, the head-mounted device is often connected via cables (for tracking and rendering), which limits movement. Nevertheless, some attempts are currently made to provide wireless solutions. Cables are also not visible while wearing the HMD, thus, a user might accidentally trip on them. In fact, since the real environment is fully blocked out, a user also cannot see his own body in the virtual world (unless some form of body tracking is provided) [26]. In this context, using a HMD is usually a single user experience. A further point to consider is the mismatch between the human field of view (about 200 degrees horizontally and 130 degrees vertically) and the usually much smaller one provided by a HMD [10]. A larger FOV of the HMD increases user immersion. In this context image resolution also has to be taken into account. With a limited number of pixels available, a trade-off has to be made between the field of view and visual acuity. Moreover, the head-mounted system has to be adapted for each single user. This usually includes the adjustment of the optical system according to the inter-pupillary distance of a user. Another critical point is the unavoidable lag between head movements and the corresponding update of the displayed images. This latency is another potential source of cyber sickness [23].

Fig. 3.19 Schematic
depiction of image formation

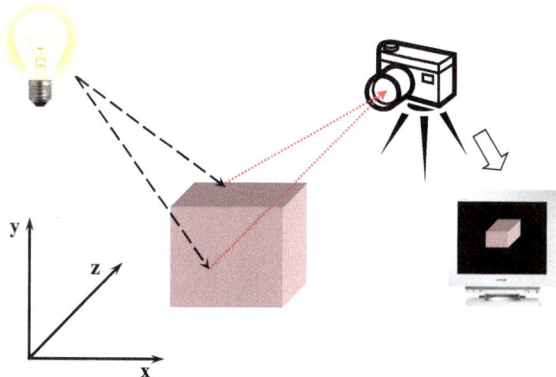

3.4 Rendering in Computer Graphics

The formation of images in computer graphics is akin to the processes taking place in photography (or human vision). Typical elements required for rendering are sources of light, objects in the environment, and the camera (or eye) viewing the scene. Moreover, physical processes, e.g. light reflection and image formation in the camera, are also essential components. These basic ingredients can be found in most standard rendering approaches. However, note that in some specialized cases, e.g. volume rendering (see [15] for an overview), different image creation paradigms are followed.

The real physics underlying the mentioned processes are complex, wherefore often simplifications are made. This is especially true, if real-time performance is required. This can be seen as a trade-off between photorealism and interactivity. In the following we will examine how rendering takes place in a basic, simplified model in computer graphics. The presented principles are typical for contemporary graphics libraries, for instance the Open Graphics Library (OpenGL)—a widespread, platform-independent, cross-language API (application programming interface) for creating 3D renderings (see for instance [25] for a general, although partly deprecated introduction and [22] for more recent extensions).

A schematic depiction of the image formation process is shown in Fig. 3.19. Note that the coordinate system is defined as left-handed. This is for instance in contrast to OpenGL, which uses a right-handed system. In the following the key components are examined in more detail.

3.4.1 Object Representations

The first step for creating images in computer graphics is the description of the objects in the scene. Various strategies can be followed here, the most common one being the approximation of object surfaces via simple, piecewise linear polygons (or faces). The latter are usually triangles. Other representations, such as quadran-

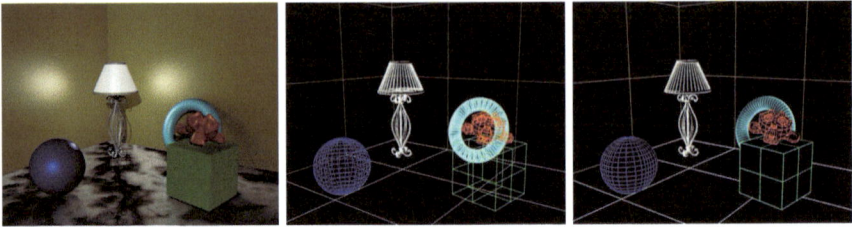

Fig. 3.20 Object representation with polygons (*left*). The underlying mesh is also shown as a wireframe rendering (*middle*) and as wireframe with hidden line removal (*right*)

Table 3.1 Polygon model of a cube

Vertex	Coordinates	Polygon	Indices
v_1	$-1, 1, -1$	P_1	$1, 2, 4, 3$
v_2	$-1, -1, -1$	P_2	$1, 3, 7, 5$
v_3	$1, 1, -1$	P_3	$5, 7, 8, 6$
v_4	$1, -1, -1$	P_4	$2, 4, 8, 6$
v_5	$-1, 1, 1$	P_5	$3, 4, 8, 7$
v_6	$-1, -1, 1$	P_6	$1, 5, 6, 2$
v_7	$1, 1, 1$		
v_8	$1, -1, 1$		

gles, also exist, but these are often converted to triangle representations internally. Moreover, some additional difficulties arise with non-triangular faces, for instance coplanarity of all polygon vertices has to be ensured. Figure 3.20 shows the underlying mesh structure of an artificial scene (left). The mesh is also shown as a wireframe model (middle). In this representation, only the polygon edges are depicted (in this case also colored appropriately). An advanced depiction of a wireframe model is also shown where a hidden line removal has been performed (right). With this technique only the actually visible edges of polygons are rendered.

A common approach to define a mesh is to specify a list of vertices (i.e. by their positions) as well as the mesh topology through indices. This results in so-called indexed face sets. The mesh of a cube—with edge length two and quadrangles as basic elements—is defined in this form by eight vertices and six polygons (see Table 3.1).

The polygons, i.e. quadrangles, are defined by the indices of their four vertices according to the vertex list. In addition to these elements, another essential component of object meshes are the surface normals. Normal vectors are used in several stages of the rendering process, for instance to determine the orientation of the face with regard to the incoming light, and, thus, the amount of light reflected by the polygon. In the general case, mesh normals are defined per face, given by a vector orthogonal to the latter. In some cases, however, normals are specified per vertex

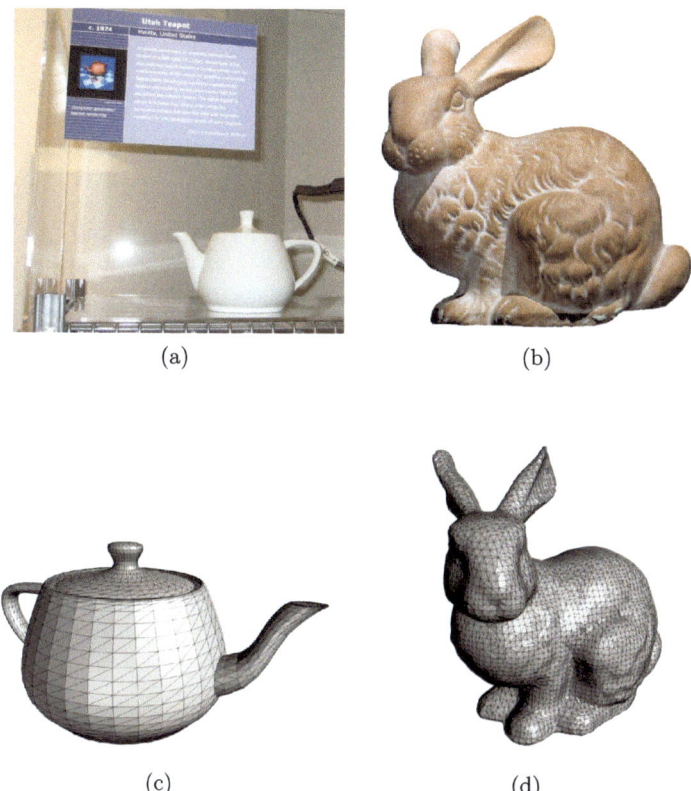

(a)   (b)

(c)   (d)

Fig. 3.21 Well-known examples of reference triangle models. (**a**) Original Utah teapot at the Computer History Museum (courtesy of Michael Plitkins); (**b**) Original Stanford bunny (courtesy of Stanford Computer Graphics Laboratory); (**c**) Teapot triangle mesh; (**d**) Bunny triangle mesh (courtesy of Stanford Computer Graphics Laboratory)

(so-called vertex normals) by averaging the normals of all adjacent polygons. In addition, the normal vectors are normalized to unit length.

It should be noted that a normal of a face does not have a unique direction. The vector can point inwards or outwards. Often, however, a consistent normal direction is required, for instance, in collision detection routines where point-in-polygon tests are performed. A typical way to determine an outward facing normal is by taking the polygon orientation into account. By convention, faces are considered as outside facing, if their vertices appear in counterclockwise order.

The generation of detailed polygon meshes of objects can be a laborious process. More details on the involved steps are given in Chap. 10. For the presentation of general concepts or testing of new algorithms in computer graphics some standard models have emerged and been used in the past. Two well-known examples are the Utah teapot and the Stanford bunny, shown in Fig. 3.21. Both triangle models were generated by scanning real objects (note that the original teapot is larger than its digital representation. This is due to a frame buffer used for early renderings having non-square pixels. The height was down-scaled by a value of 1.3, and this change was never removed subsequently).

3.4.2 Geometry Transformations

After defining object meshes, it is desirable to transform, e.g. position, them in scene space. Typical transformations that are carried out are translations, rotations, or scaling. For a simple translation in 3D space, a translation vector $\mathbf{t}$ is added to all mesh vertices.

$$\mathbf{v}' = \mathbf{v} + \mathbf{t} \quad \rightarrow \quad \begin{bmatrix} x' \\ y' \\ z' \end{bmatrix} = \begin{bmatrix} x \\ y \\ z \end{bmatrix} + \begin{bmatrix} t_x \\ t_y \\ t_z \end{bmatrix}. \tag{3.6}$$

Componentwise scaling relative to the origin with factors s_i can be achieved by multiplication with a diagonal matrix.

$$\mathbf{v}' = \mathbf{S} \cdot \mathbf{v} \quad \rightarrow \quad \begin{bmatrix} x' \\ y' \\ z' \end{bmatrix} = \begin{bmatrix} s_x & 0 & 0 \\ 0 & s_y & 0 \\ 0 & 0 & s_z \end{bmatrix} \cdot \begin{bmatrix} x \\ y \\ z \end{bmatrix}. \tag{3.7}$$

Note that a scaling matrix could also be used to reflect (and scale) an object across an axis by choosing a negative scaling value.

A simple rotation by θ degrees around one of the main coordinate axes is also carried out by a matrix multiplication.

$$\mathbf{v}' = \mathbf{R}_x(\theta) \cdot \mathbf{v} \quad \rightarrow \quad \begin{bmatrix} x' \\ y' \\ z' \end{bmatrix} = \begin{bmatrix} 1 & 0 & 0 \\ 0 & \cos\theta & -\sin\theta \\ 0 & \sin\theta & \cos\theta \end{bmatrix} \cdot \begin{bmatrix} x \\ y \\ z \end{bmatrix}. \tag{3.8}$$

Since a rotation matrix is orthogonal, an inverse rotation is given as $\mathbf{R}^{-1}(\theta) = \mathbf{R}^T(\theta)$. Also note that rotations are length preserving:

$$\|\mathbf{v}'\|^2 = (\mathbf{v}')^T \mathbf{v}' = (\mathbf{R}\mathbf{v})^T \mathbf{R}\mathbf{v} = \mathbf{v}^T \mathbf{R}^T \mathbf{R}\mathbf{v} = \mathbf{v}^T \mathbf{v} = \|\mathbf{v}\|^2. \tag{3.9}$$

Moreover, angles between arbitrary vectors are also preserved.

While rotation and scaling can be represented by a matrix multiplication, the translation requires a vector summation. In order to also work with multiplication in the latter case in computer graphics usually homogeneous coordinates are used. These were introduced by the mathematician August Ferdinand Möbius [18]. They allow affine transformations to be represented by matrix multiplications. 3D vectors are represented in homogeneous coordinates by a four-dimensional vector by adding a component w.

$$(x, y, z, w)^T \rightarrow \left(\frac{x}{w} \ \frac{y}{w} \ \frac{z}{w} \right)^T. \tag{3.10}$$

Note that for computer graphics in general $w \neq 0$ ($w = 0$ denotes a plane at infinity). Moreover, for any $a \neq 0$ all points $(x, y, z, w)^T$ and $(ax, ay, az, aw)^T$ represent the same 3D vertex. Nevertheless, for simplicity w is usually set to 1.

Using homogeneous coordinates allows to represent a translation by a matrix.

$$\mathbf{v}' = \mathbf{T} \cdot \mathbf{v} \quad \rightarrow \quad \begin{bmatrix} x' \\ y' \\ z' \\ 1 \end{bmatrix} = \begin{bmatrix} x + t_y \\ y + t_y \\ z + t_z \\ 1 \end{bmatrix} = \begin{bmatrix} 1 & 0 & 0 & t_x \\ 0 & 1 & 0 & t_y \\ 0 & 0 & 1 & t_z \\ 0 & 0 & 0 & 1 \end{bmatrix} \cdot \begin{bmatrix} x \\ y \\ z \\ 1 \end{bmatrix}. \tag{3.11}$$

Scaling and rotation matrices are modified accordingly.

$$\mathbf{S} = \begin{bmatrix} s_x & 0 & 0 & 0 \\ 0 & s_y & 0 & 0 \\ 0 & 0 & s_z & 0 \\ 0 & 0 & 0 & 1 \end{bmatrix}, \quad \mathbf{R}_x(\theta) = \begin{bmatrix} 1 & 0 & 0 & 0 \\ 0 & \cos\theta & -\sin\theta & 0 \\ 0 & \sin\theta & \cos\theta & 0 \\ 0 & 0 & 0 & 1 \end{bmatrix}. \tag{3.12}$$

For combining transformations, the different matrices can be multiplied together. Note, however, that matrix multiplication is generally not commutative, i.e. $\mathbf{T} \cdot \mathbf{R} \neq \mathbf{R} \cdot \mathbf{T}$.

A combination of translation and rotation matrices allows performing a rotation around one of the coordinate axes (in this example the x-axis) with an arbitrary rotation center $\mathbf{v}_c$.

$$\mathbf{v}' = \mathbf{M} \cdot \mathbf{v} = \mathbf{T}(\mathbf{v}_c) \cdot \mathbf{R}_x(\theta) \cdot \mathbf{T}(-\mathbf{v}_c) \cdot \mathbf{v}. \tag{3.13}$$

In this concatenation of transformations, an object is first translated to the origin, then rotated around the x-axis, and finally translated back to the original position. Note the order of the matrices in the example. The rightmost matrix is applied first. The transformation matrix in detail is given by:

$$\mathbf{M} = \begin{bmatrix} 1 & 0 & 0 & v_{c,x} \\ 0 & 1 & 0 & v_{c,y} \\ 0 & 0 & 1 & v_{c,z} \\ 0 & 0 & 0 & 1 \end{bmatrix} \cdot \begin{bmatrix} 1 & 0 & 0 & 0 \\ 0 & \cos\theta & -\sin\theta & 0 \\ 0 & \sin\theta & \cos\theta & 0 \\ 0 & 0 & 0 & 1 \end{bmatrix} \cdot \begin{bmatrix} 1 & 0 & 0 & -v_{c,x} \\ 0 & 1 & 0 & -v_{c,y} \\ 0 & 0 & 1 & -v_{c,z} \\ 0 & 0 & 0 & 1 \end{bmatrix}. \tag{3.14}$$

A rotation around an arbitrary (normalized) vector $\mathbf{u}_0$ by an angle α can be performed similarly. The underlying idea is to rotate the arbitrary rotation axis around one coordinate axis onto a coordinate surface (e.g. spanned by the x- and y-axis), and thereafter rotate it onto one of the coordinate axes. Then a basic rotation around an axis by α is carried out, and finally the initial rotations are undone. Thus, our transformation matrix is given by the concatenation:

$$\mathbf{M} = \mathbf{T}(\mathbf{v}_c) \cdot \mathbf{R}_z(-\theta_z) \cdot \mathbf{R}_y(-\theta_y) \cdot \mathbf{R}_x(\alpha) \cdot \mathbf{R}_y(\theta_y) \cdot \mathbf{R}_z(\theta_z) \cdot \mathbf{T}(-\mathbf{v}_c). \tag{3.15}$$

In order to carry out this transformation the two rotation matrices $\mathbf{R}_z(\theta_z)$ and $\mathbf{R}_y(\theta_y)$ need to be determined. As an example, the former will be derived. First,

Fig. 3.22 Derivation of
trigonometric terms in
rotation matrix for rotations
around an arbitrary vector

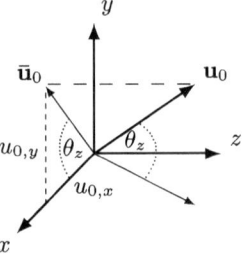

note that the unit vector can be represented through direction cosines:

$$\mathbf{u}_0 = (u_{0,x}, u_{0,y}, u_{0,z})^T = (\cos\psi_x, \cos\psi_y, \cos\psi_z)^T, \tag{3.16}$$

where the ψ_i represent the angle of the vector with the respective coordinate axis.

Next, in order to construct $\mathbf{R}_z(\theta_z)$, we will derive $\cos\theta_z$. The angle between vector $\mathbf{u}_0$ and the x–z plane is equal to the angle of the (orthogonally onto the x–z plane) projected vector $\bar{\mathbf{u}}_0$ with the x-axis (see Fig. 3.22). Thus, we find $\cos\theta_z = u_{0,x}/\|\bar{\mathbf{u}}_0\|$ and $\sin\theta_z = u_{0,y}/\|\bar{\mathbf{u}}_0\|$. Therefore, we can avoid to directly determine the angle θ_z and just use the rotation matrix

$$\mathbf{R}_z(\theta_z) = \begin{bmatrix} u_{0,x}/\|\bar{\mathbf{u}}_0\| & -u_{0,y}/\|\bar{\mathbf{u}}_0\| & 0 & 0 \\ u_{0,y}/\|\bar{\mathbf{u}}_0\| & u_{0,x}/\|\bar{\mathbf{u}}_0\| & 0 & 0 \\ 0 & 0 & 1 & 0 \\ 0 & 0 & 0 & 1 \end{bmatrix}. \tag{3.17}$$

The second rotation matrix $\mathbf{R}_y(\theta_y)$ can be derived similarly. By multiplication with the remaining transformation matrices, we finally obtain the rotation matrix $\mathbf{M}$ which yields our desired operation.

Note that next to the representation of rotations by orthogonal matrices other alternatives exist [11]. One example we have already implicitly encountered. Euler's Rotation Theorem states that any rotation can be expressed as a single rotation around an arbitrary vector. Thus, instead of giving the matrix $\mathbf{M}$, the rotation can also be defined by the rotation axis $\mathbf{u}_0$ and the rotation angle α. Thus, given a rotation matrix, the Euler axis/angle representation can be obtained by computing

$$\alpha = \arccos\left(\frac{\mathrm{tr}(M)-1}{2}\right) \wedge \mathbf{u}_0 = \frac{1}{2\sin\alpha}\begin{bmatrix} M_{3,2} - M_{2,3} \\ M_{1,3} - M_{3,1} \\ M_{2,1} - M_{1,2} \end{bmatrix}. \tag{3.18}$$

Another common and useful representation of rotations is quaternions. A quaternion can be specified as a normalized four-dimensional vector. The vector components can for instance be derived from the Euler vector and angle representation.

$$\mathbf{q} = \begin{bmatrix} q_1 \\ q_2 \\ q_3 \\ q_4 \end{bmatrix} = \begin{bmatrix} \cos(\alpha/2) \\ u_{0,x}\cdot\sin(\alpha/2) \\ u_{0,y}\cdot\sin(\alpha/2) \\ u_{0,z}\cdot\sin(\alpha/2) \end{bmatrix}. \tag{3.19}$$

Note that for this unit quaternion $\|\mathbf{q}\| = 1$. Also, the cos term is sometimes written as the last component of the vector with the remaining ones preceding in the same order.

A basis of the quaternion algebra is customarily given by the elements $1, i, j, k$ with $i^2 = j^2 = k^2 = ijk = -1$. This definition can be considered as an extension of complex numbers, where only one component $i^2 = -1$ is used. A quaternion is uniquely written as $q_1 + q_2 i + q_3 j + q_4 k$ with the q_i being real numbers.

Two quaternions, each specified by a scalar component q_1 and a vector component $(q_2 \, q_3 \, q_4) = \mathbf{q}^*$, can be multiplied in order to obtain a concatenation of the two rotations. Quaternion multiplication is carried out as:

$$\left(q_1, \mathbf{q}^*\right) \cdot \left(\tilde{q}_1, \tilde{\mathbf{q}}^*\right) = \left(q_1 \tilde{q}_1 - \mathbf{q}^* \tilde{\mathbf{q}}^*, q_1 \tilde{\mathbf{q}}^* + \tilde{q}_1 \mathbf{q}^* + \mathbf{q}^* \times \tilde{\mathbf{q}}^*\right). \tag{3.20}$$

Note that quaternion multiplication is not commutative, i.e. $\mathbf{q} \cdot \tilde{\mathbf{q}} \neq \tilde{\mathbf{q}} \cdot \mathbf{q}$.

Working with the quaternion representation of rotations yields several advantages. An important advantage is the interpolation between rotations, which is for instance needed in animations. Interpolation of unit quaternions results in smooth motions [24]. A key technique in this context is the so-called SLERP (spherical linear interpolation). Furthermore, discontinuous jumps can be avoided, which appear in three-dimensional representations. Also, there is no problem with gimbal locking. Finally, trigonometric functions are not required in the calculations and round-off errors are reduced. Unfortunately, quaternions are not easy to be visualized and usually need to be converted to a different representation.

3.4.3 Light Sources and Reflection

The next components required for generating computer-based images are sources of light. Light in a scene can either be emitted or result from a reflection of light on an object surface. In the following we will examine different basic types of light sources as well as models to characterize light reflection commonly used in computer graphics libraries.

Light sources are specified through a few basic properties. The first is the emitted light spectrum, i.e. the intensity of energy emitted at each wavelength of the visible spectrum. In order to reduce the complexity of the computations, real-time computer graphics usually only uses three primary color channels, i.e. red (R), green (G), and blue (B). This is motivated by Young-Helmholtz trichromatic color theory. Additional details have been discussed in Sect. 3.2.5. We will assume that an emitted color is defined by its RGB components. Since each of the three channels is treated the same way, we will in the following only consider one separate (abstract) channel.

A further component describing a light source is its geometrical attributes. This can include the position, the light direction, or even the shape of a light cone. A final parameter is the attenuation of light intensity over distance.

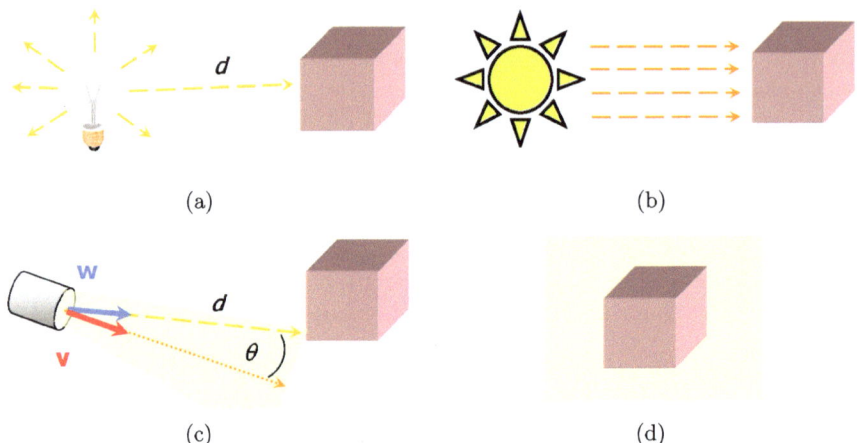

Fig. 3.23 Types of light sources in real-time rendering. (**a**) Point light; (**b**) Directional light; (**c**) Spot light; (**d**) Ambient light

The following list introduces four basic types of light sources that can usually be found in computer graphics. The light in a scene is often approximated by using a combination of these basic light sources. Relations are given to determine the intensity of light (i.e. of the separate color channel) arriving on the surface of an object.

- **Point light** A point light is defined by its position $\mathbf{p}$ in the scene, the emitted light intensity I_0, and the attenuation constants k_1, k_2, k_3 (Fig. 3.23(a)). The intensity of the light arriving at a point on the surface of a lit object I_L is related to the distance d to the light source.

$$I_L = \frac{I_0}{k_1 + k_2 d + k_3 d^2}. \tag{3.21}$$

  An example of a point light is a light bulb. Note that in addition to the light intensity, the angle of incidence of the incoming light will be required to determine the amount of reflected light.
- **Directional light** This type of light source is considered to be far from the scene (i.e. at infinity), shining evenly at all objects at a specific constant angle (Fig. 3.23(b)). The intensity is independent of the distance, i.e. the light intensity arriving at a point on an object surface is unmodified $I_L = I_0$. However, the orientation of the parallel light rays $\mathbf{v}$ lighting the scene is required to determine the reflected light on surfaces. A typical example of this category is sunlight.
- **Spot light** A spot light is akin to a point light, with the extension that light is only shining in a cone along a specific direction $\mathbf{v}$. The light intensity is highest along the central axis of the cone and drops off to the border. The light intensity arriving at a point on a surface is determined by the cosine of the angle between the cone orientation and the vector $\mathbf{w}$ between the light source position and the

lit surface point (Fig. 3.23(c)). Specifying these vectors with unit-length allows to conveniently determine the cosine by the dot product. Similar as with the point light, the intensity is also scaled by the distance to the source.

$$I_L = \frac{I_0(\mathbf{vw})}{k_1 + k_2 d + k_3 d^2}. \tag{3.22}$$

Note that often as additional parameters a cutoff angle can be specified as well as a spot exponent, which controls the light concentration. Usually, there is no light beyond a 90° cutoff angle. Again, the orientation of the incoming light is required for reflection calculations. Typical examples of this class are bedside lamps or theater spotlights.

- **Ambient light** The final source represents the ambient lighting of a scene. This one does not have a specific source, location, or direction. It can be regarded as an equal illumination of the entire scene with $I_L = I_0$. Since in real-time graphics reflected light is not considered further as a source of light, the ambient components represent diffuse light scattered in the scene. It is, for instance, used to partly illuminate surfaces not directly facing any of the previous light sources, which would otherwise be dark.

Note that for real-time computer graphics a number of simplifications have to be made. As already mentioned, only the direct lighting of object surfaces is taken into account. Indirect illumination by any reflected light is not incorporated. Moreover, in the standard model shadowing is not included. There are, however, advanced techniques to also include shadows in the rendering. Further, the exact geometry of light emitters is not taken into account. In addition, light sources are by themselves usually not visible in a scene, unless they are represented by an object geometry.

The previously discussed light sources illuminate the scene. The next step in the rendering is to determine how this light is reflected by object surfaces into the viewing camera.

Several parameters influence the reflection of light from a surface. Firstly, position and orientation of a surface patch with respect to a light emitter have to be considered. Further, the reflectance spectrum, i.e. the intensity of energy reflected at each wavelength of the visible spectrum has to be known. This defines the absorption of light, and thus the color appearance of a surface. Again, similarly to the light sources, this is specified by three RGB values. A final element determining surface appearance can be small surface structures or patterns, such as bumps or wrinkles. Since it would be computationally too expensive to model surface detail at small scale with actual polygons, they are usually approximated by local perturbations of surface normals. This technique, known as bump mapping, requires the definition of a bump map representing the smaller surface details [5].

Typically, reflections are modeled by three components—a diffuse, a specular, and an ambient part.

- **Diffuse reflection** This reflection component represents rough, so-called Lambertian, surfaces. Incoming light is scattered uniformly in all directions due to an uneven sub-surface structure (Fig. 3.24). The intensity of the reflected light is proportional to the angle of incidence, i.e. the angle between the incoming light

Fig. 3.24 Diffuse reflection model. (**a**) Lambertian reflection; (**b**) Sphere with diffuse reflection; (**c**) Angle of incidence

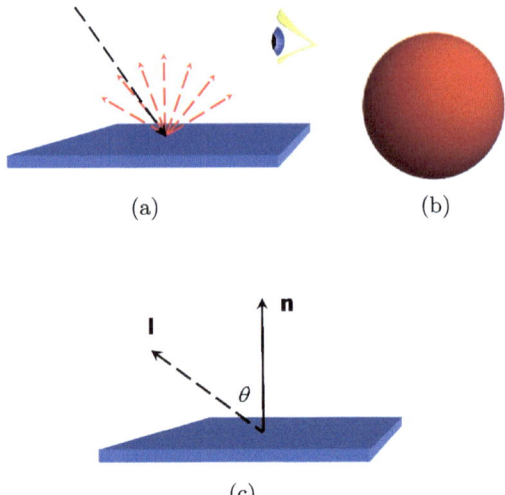

(a)   (b)

(c)

l and the surface normal **n** of the surface patch. However, the intensity is independent of the viewing position. The reflection is determined by the cosine of the angle of incidence, i.e. the reflection becomes larger the closer to perpendicular the light source is located to the surface. Again using unit vectors, the reflected light intensity can be determined.

$$I_D = k_D I_L (\mathbf{n} \cdot \mathbf{l}).\tag{3.23}$$

Note that the reflected intensity is adjusted by a scaling factor k_D. Moreover, at angles of incidence beyond $90°$, i.e. when the dot product is smaller than zero, no reflection is determined. Diffuse reflective surfaces appear somewhat dull, for instance chalk.

- **Specular reflection** Smooth surfaces show specular highlights, which are dependent on the viewpoint. In the specular component, light is not reflected equally in all directions, but instead concentrated around a perfect reflection vector (Fig. 3.25). In the model the intensity reaching a viewing position depends on the angle of incidence ϕ of the incoming light and the viewing angle. The intensity is greatest if a viewer is looking directly from a position along the reflection vector **r**, and becomes smaller when the angle between the reflection and the viewing vector increases.

$$I_S = k_S I_L (\cos \phi)^{n_s} = k_S I_L (\mathbf{v} \cdot \mathbf{r})^{n_s}.\tag{3.24}$$

Again the reflected specular component is modified by a scaling factor k_S. Further, the reflection vector has to be determined for each point on the surface.

$$\mathbf{r} = \big(2(\mathbf{n} \cdot \mathbf{l})\big)\mathbf{n} - \mathbf{l}.\tag{3.25}$$

The shape of the highlight, i.e. the shininess of the surface, is further controlled by the exponent n_s. It influences the falloff of the cosine term, and, thus, the

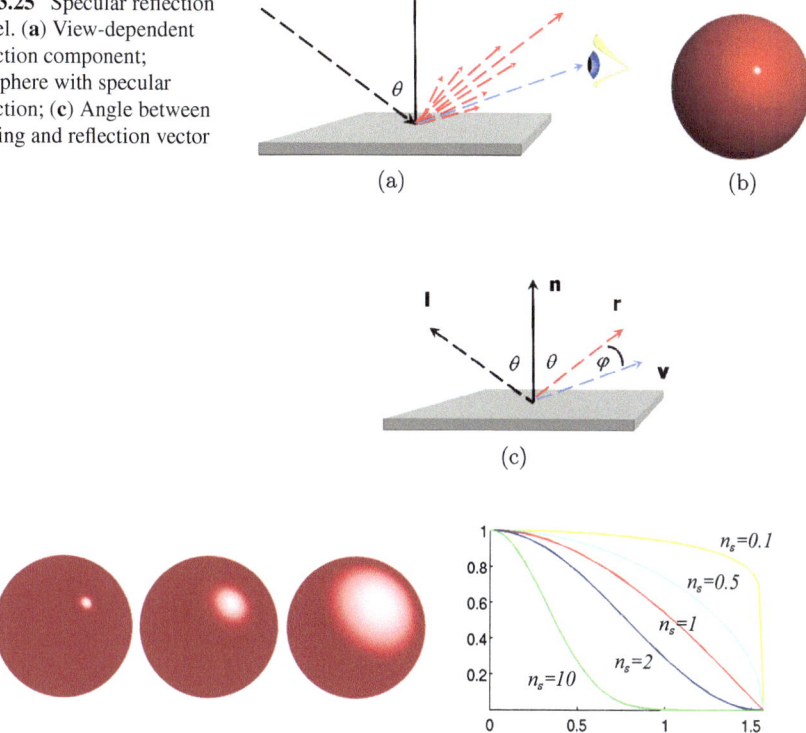

Fig. 3.25 Specular reflection model. (**a**) View-dependent reflection component; (**b**) Sphere with specular reflection; (**c**) Angle between viewing and reflection vector

(a)   (b)

(c)

Fig. 3.26 Shininess coefficient. Examples with decreasing coefficient (*left*) and shapes of the adapted cosine term (*right*)

sharpness of the highlight. Figure 3.26 depicts the influence of the shininess co-efficient. The effect of a decreased shininess coefficient on the highlight on a specular sphere is shown. Examples of objects showing specular reflections are metals or wet surfaces.

Obtaining the specular reflections using **r** is computationally expensive. A simplification has been proposed by Jim Blinn [4]. The so-called halfway vector h is determined by the light and the viewing vector.

$$\mathbf{h} = \frac{\mathbf{l} + \mathbf{v}}{|\mathbf{l} + \mathbf{v}|}. \tag{3.26}$$

The dot product $\mathbf{v} \cdot \mathbf{r}$ is replaced by $\mathbf{n} \cdot \mathbf{h}$, thus, avoiding the calculation of **r**. If light source and viewer are at a fixed position far from the scene, then the halfway vector remains constant for each light source, and only has to be computed once at the beginning. However, the angle between normal and halfway vector ψ is different from the angle ϕ between reflection and viewing vector. If **v** lies within the same plane as **r** and **n**, then $2\psi = \phi$. In order to compensate for this difference, the shininess exponent n_s is usually adjusted.

- **Ambient reflection** The final component of light reflection is an ambient term which is complementing the previously introduced ambient light source. The reflected light is independent of angle of incidence as well as viewing position. It is mainly used to represent scattered light in the scene bouncing of objects, as well as to light surfaces not directly illuminated by any source. The only parameter is a scaling factor k_A.

$$I_A = k_A I_L. \tag{3.27}$$

Combining these three reflection components results in the Phong lighting Model (named of Bui-Tuong Phong), which gives the total reflected light on a surface patch [21].

$$I_G = k_A I_L + \sum_{i=1}^{\#lights} I_L \big(k_D(\mathbf{n} \cdot \mathbf{l}_i) + k_S(\mathbf{v} \cdot \mathbf{r}_i)^{n_s}\big). \tag{3.28}$$

Note that the diffuse and specular component are evaluated per light source. In addition, as previously indicated the reflected light intensity needs to be determine for each of the three RGB channels separately. Moreover, note that in the original Phong model the reflection vector $\mathbf{r}$ is used for the computations. Applying the halfway vector instead results in the Blinn-Phong lighting model. The latter is implemented for instance in the OpenGL graphics library. Finally, it should be mentioned that a few other lighting models exist, which are computationally more expensive but give better results.

3.4.4 Viewing Projections

The methods discussed so far allow the representation of objects by meshes, the definition of light sources, the positioning of elements in the environment (including a viewing camera), and the illumination of objects by the light sources. All steps have been carried out in the 3D environment. In the next step, the 3D scene has to be projected onto the 2D image plane of the virtual camera. An important element in this step is the projection of the 3D objects into 2D space. In order to derive the underlying relations, principles of optics will first be presented.

Figure 3.27 depicts the model of a camera with a lens of negligible thickness. Incoming parallel light beams are focused by the lens at a point lying on the lens axis (the focal point). The distance of the lens center to this point is called the focal length f of the lens. The focal length is used in the thin lens equation to relate object distance z_O to image distance z_I.

$$\frac{1}{f} = \frac{1}{z_I} + \frac{1}{z_O}. \tag{3.29}$$

Assuming that the focal length of the camera and the distance of the image plane to the lens is fixed, the distance z at which objects are exactly in focus can be deter-

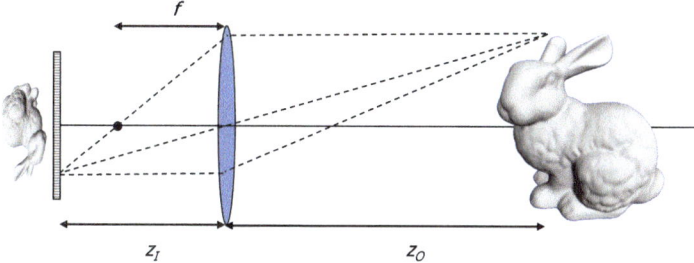

Fig. 3.27 Image projection in the thin lens camera model

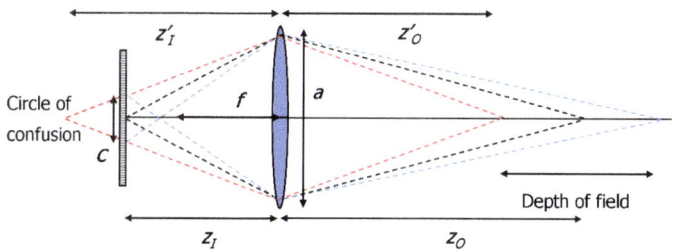

Fig. 3.28 Depth of field in thin lens camera model

mined.

$$z = \frac{z_I f}{z_I - f}. \tag{3.30}$$

Points at a distance different from z will not be exactly focused at a point on the image plane. This leads to the so-called circle of confusion. Light coming from a point source is imaged as a blurred disc on the image plane. In practice, however, a range of distances will be projected with an acceptable sharpness, which is due for instance to a finite resolution of the imaging sensor. This range of acceptable distances is known as the depth of field.

In the following a formula for the depth of field will be determined. Figure 3.28 shows the involved quantities. Only the near depth of field, i.e. the limit distance closer to the lens, will be derived. Let the closest distance with acceptable sharpness be z'_O, and the in-focus projection be z'_I. For these distances, also the thin lens equation holds.

$$\frac{1}{f} = \frac{1}{z'_I} + \frac{1}{z'_O}. \tag{3.31}$$

The diameter of the circle of confusion beyond which point projections appear out of focus on the image plane is designated as c. This value can be related to the height of the lens aperture a via the principle of congruent triangles (see also

Fig. 3.28).

$$\frac{a}{z'_I} = \frac{c}{z'_I - z_I}.$$

(3.32)

Using Eqs. (3.29), (3.31), and (3.32), the maximum distance a point can move closer to the lens $\Delta z'_O = z_O - z'_O$ without becoming blurred can be determined. First, Eq. (3.31) is rearranged.

$$z'_O = \frac{z'_I f}{z'_I - f}.$$

(3.33)

Equation (3.32) is then transformed to

$$z'_I = \frac{a z_I f}{a - c}$$

(3.34)

and inserted into Eq. (3.33). Finally, z_I is replaced using Eq. (3.29), yielding the formula for the maximal distance a point can move closer to the lens while still remaining in focus.

$$\Delta z'_O = z_O - z'_O = \frac{z_O(z_O - f)}{(z_O - f) + (a/c)f}.$$

(3.35)

One option to increase the depth of field is lowering a. However, note that in this case also less light would reach the image plane. Nevertheless, this is a common method to adjust the depth of field in cameras.

In the limit case, aperture and lens become infinitesimally small, leaving us with an ideal pinhole camera. The first constructed cameras were implementations of this model. In a pinhole camera no lenses are used for focusing and light is projected about a single point (i.e. the pinhole opening). Note that an ideal pinhole camera is only a theoretical model, while in practice deviations from this ideal case are encountered. Figure 3.29 illustrates the image projection in a 2D pinhole camera model. A point at distance z at height x_O is projected by a pinhole camera with focal length f to

$$x_I = \frac{f x_O}{z}.$$

(3.36)

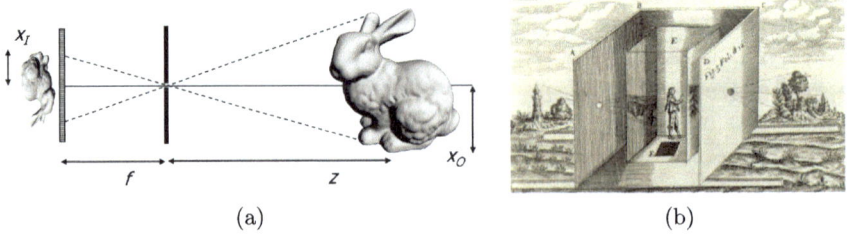

(a)   (b)

Fig. 3.29 Pinhole camera model. (**a**) Projection in pinhole camera; (**b**) Early depiction of a Camera Obscura (from [16])

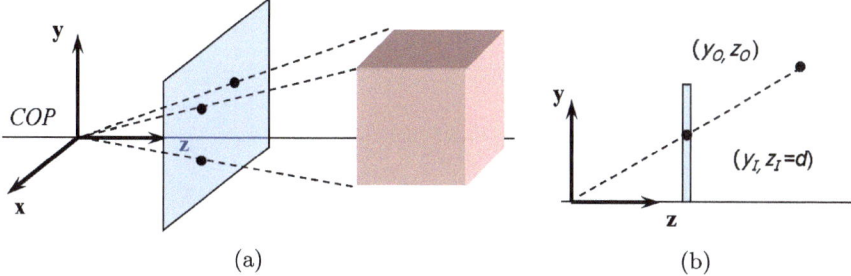

Fig. 3.30 Perspective projection. (**a**) Perspective projection onto image plane; (**b**) 3D-2D mapping in the yz-plane

This relation is simply derived based on the two similar triangles sharing a part of the projection line as hypotenuses. Due to its simplicity, a modified pinhole camera model is often used as the camera projection model in computer graphics libraries. Figure 3.30 illustrates the perspective projection process of 3D shapes onto a 2D image plane. Note that the image plane is located in front of the center of projection (at a fixed distance d along the z-axis). In order to determine the coordinates of a 3D point (x_O, y_O, z_O) projected onto the image plane, we again use triangle similarity. For instance, the y-coordinate of the projection is given by

$$y_I = \frac{y_O}{z_O/d}. \tag{3.37}$$

The x-coordinate is derived analogously. Note that these equations are non-linear. The division by z_O is related to perspective foreshortening, i.e. images of objects farther from the image plane are reduced in size. The previously introduced geometry representation via homogeneous coordinates allows to encode the perspective projection through a matrix $\mathbf{P}_{per}$.

$$\mathbf{p}_I = \begin{bmatrix} x_I \\ y_I \\ d \\ 1 \end{bmatrix} = \begin{bmatrix} x_O \\ y_O \\ z_O \\ z_O/d \end{bmatrix} = \begin{bmatrix} 1 & 0 & 0 & 0 \\ 0 & 1 & 0 & 0 \\ 0 & 0 & 1 & 0 \\ 0 & 0 & 1/d & 0 \end{bmatrix} \cdot \begin{bmatrix} x_O \\ y_O \\ z_O \\ 1 \end{bmatrix} = \mathbf{P}_{per} \cdot \mathbf{p}_O. \tag{3.38}$$

Recall that in homogeneous coordinate representation, a 3D point is obtained by dividing the first three vector components by the fourth. Also note that due to the mapping to the image plane all z-coordinates are constant. Furthermore, due to the pinhole camera approach there is no depth of field in this simplified projection, i.e. all points appear in focus on the image plane without any blurring. However, the latter can be introduced by advanced rendering techniques. Moreover, the amount of light reaching the image plane is also not considered in this basic model.

In addition to perspective projection, a further common projection model in computer graphics is orthographic projection. In the latter the projection lines are parallel to each other, which can be considered as shifting the center of projection to

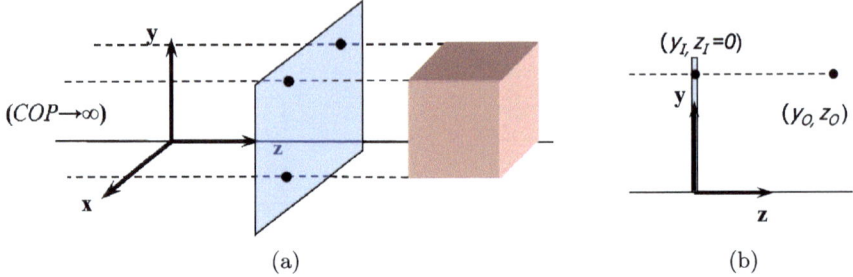

(a)   (b)

Fig. 3.31 Orthographic projection. (**a**) Orthographic projection onto image plane; (**b**) 3D-2D mapping in the yz-plane

infinity. Figure 3.31 illustrates this projection model. For simplicity of derivation we will assume that the image plane is located at the origin ($z_I = 0$). Again, this projection can be represented by a 4×4 matrix $\mathbf{P}_{ort}$.

$$
\mathbf{p}_I = \begin{bmatrix} x_I \\ y_I \\ 0 \\ 1 \end{bmatrix} = \begin{bmatrix} x_O \\ y_O \\ 0 \\ 1 \end{bmatrix} = \begin{bmatrix} 1 & 0 & 0 & 0 \\ 0 & 1 & 0 & 0 \\ 0 & 0 & 0 & 0 \\ 0 & 0 & 0 & 1 \end{bmatrix} \cdot \begin{bmatrix} x_O \\ y_O \\ z_O \\ 1 \end{bmatrix} = \mathbf{P}_{ort} \cdot \mathbf{p}_O. \tag{3.39}
$$

Note that in contrast to perspective projection an orthographic projection is an affine transformation, thus it preserves colinearity and ratios of distances. However, for obtaining realistic renderings orthographic projection is usually not applied.

3.4.5 Surface Shading

The final step in the simplified rendering pipeline is the drawing of the 2D projections onto the screen. This requires a so-called rasterization process, i.e. based on the projected geometry primitives the color of individual pixels has to be determined (see Fig. 3.32). The drawing of the screen pixels usually takes place in a line-by-line fashion. A single row of pixels on the screen is called a scan line.

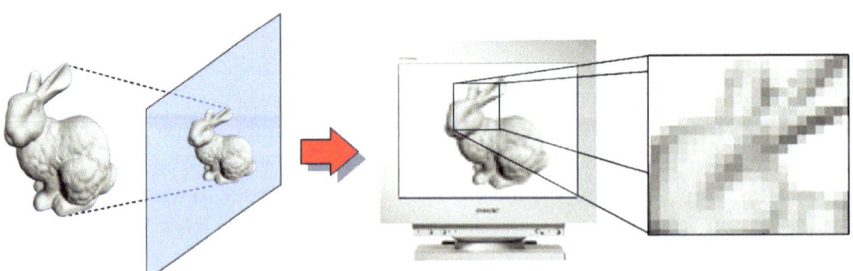

Fig. 3.32 Filling of individual screen pixels during rasterization stage

Fig. 3.33 Flat, Gouraud, and
Phong shading of the
polygonal approximation of a
sphere

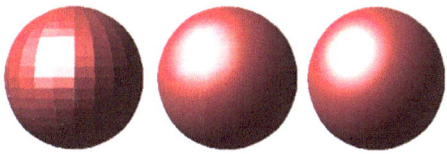

In the projection step, individual geometrical primitives, such as triangles or quadrangles, are mapped into screen coordinates via projection of their vertices. The colors of the image pixels covered by a projected primitive are determined via the previously described Phong lighting model. In order to evaluate the illumination equations information about the surface normals is required. This color information is then used to fill the projected triangles on the screen. This step is summarized via the term shading. There are different approaches to carry out the shading of polygons, mainly differing by the number of evaluations of the lighting equation. These approaches will be examined in detail below (see Fig. 3.33 for examples).

3.4.5.1 Flat Shading

In the simplest case, only one color is used for all pixels of a polygon, i.e. the lighting equation is only evaluated once to determine the polygon pixel color. In this case a constant normal per polygon is assumed. The normal can for instance be determined for a co-planar polygon (e.g. a triangle) through the vector cross product of two non-parallel edges. Note that the normal could be pointing inwards or outwards. Usually, the outward facing normal will be obtained, since the directional information is also used for determining outside and inside surfaces. Figure 3.34 depicts the concept of flat shading.

While flat shading is the fastest shading approach, it results in several artifacts. Since a constant color per polygon is used, individual elements usually become clearly visible in the rendering. This is a key concern since curved surfaces are only roughly approximated by a limited number of flat polygons. The visibility of the edges is also further amplified by the optical Mach band illusion, which is perceived as an increased contrast at an intensity discontinuity. This effect is due to lateral inhibition of retinal receptors, i.e. spatial filtering taking place in early human vision.

The described difficulty could potentially be alleviated by greatly increasing the number of polygons. However, the computational cost would also increase accordingly. Using one of the other shading approaches would be a more appropriate step

Fig. 3.34 Constant color per
polygon in flat shading

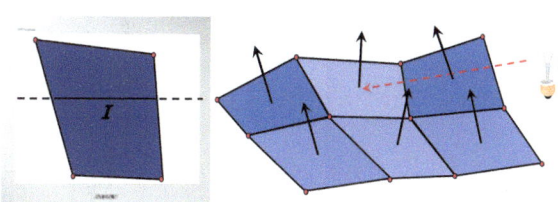

Fig. 3.35 Color interpolation between vertices in Gouraud shading

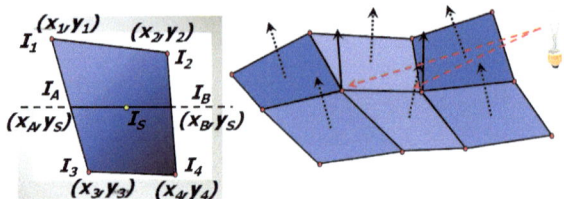

in this case. Finally, it should be noted that in some cases it might actually be desired to see the individual polygons as seen on the left in Fig. 3.33, for instance when rendering a polyhedron shape (or even a "disco ball").

3.4.5.2 Gouraud Shading

Improved shading of polygons can be achieved by using interpolation strategies for the pixel colors [13]. In Gouraud shading (named after Herni Gouraud) the lighting equation is evaluated at the vertices of a polygon. For the other pixels of the polygon the color values are found by interpolation. For this approach the normals in a mesh have to be defined per vertex. In general, the vertex normals are obtained from the normals of the adjacent faces.

$$\mathbf{n}_{ver} = \frac{\sum_{i=0}^{\#adj} \mathbf{n}_i}{\left\| \sum_{i=0}^{\#adj} \mathbf{n}_i \right\|}. \tag{3.40}$$

Note that alternative strategies exist to determine vertex normals. For instance, the geometric contribution of an adjacent face can be included in the formula by weighting a face normal by the magnitude of the incident angle. A further extension is to also include information about lengths of incident edges. Such strategies can be used when elements in a mesh differ considerably in size.

After evaluating the light equation, pixel colors are determined by interpolation. While colors are encoded in an RGB vector, we will in the following description again only examine a single intensity value. The approach, however, can analogously be applied to three-dimensional color vectors. As an example we will consider the interpolation process for pixels in screen coordinates in the case of a quadrangular element as shown in Fig. 3.35. First the intensities $I_{1,...,4}$ at the polygon vertices are determined via the lighting equation. On an arbitrary scan line passing through the polygon, we then determine the intensities of the edge intersection pixels I_A and I_B via interpolation.

$$I_A = \frac{1}{y_1 - y_3} \left[I_1(y_S - y_3) + I_3(y_1 - y_S) \right] \tag{3.41}$$

$$I_B = \frac{1}{y_2 - y_4} \left[I_2(y_S - y_4) + I_4(y_2 - y_S) \right]. \tag{3.42}$$

Fig. 3.36 Normal interpolation in Phong shading

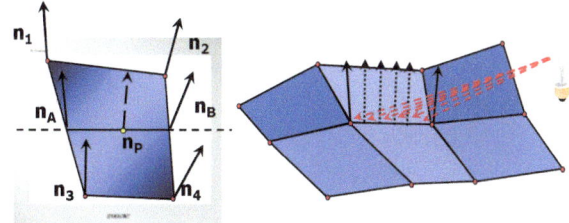

Interpolation is also used in order to fill the pixels on the scan line between the determined values. Since this process is taking place incrementally, computation time can be reduced by determining the required linear change per pixel beforehand.

$$\Delta I_s = \frac{\Delta x}{x_B - x_A}(I_B - I_A). \tag{3.43}$$

This delta value is then used to progressively fill the pixels in the scan line.

$$I_{S,n} = I_{S,n-1} + \Delta I_s. \tag{3.44}$$

Using Gouraud shading a smaller number of polygons is required to obtain smoothly shaded meshes. Nevertheless, a number of difficulties still exist. Since the lighting equation is only evaluated at the vertices, followed by linear interpolations, specular highlights will not be visible when located within a larger polygon. Also, the underlying mesh structure still becomes apparent for large highlights. This again could be alleviated by increasing the number of polygons, which would again increase computation time. Gouraud shading (and flat shading) are both supported in the standard OpenGL implementation.

3.4.5.3 Phong Shading

The interpolation of the light intensities from the vertices of a polygon results in a large improvement over the flat shading method. However, it is still an approximation causing some artifacts. A further improved strategy is followed in Phong shading [21], also named after Bui-Tuong Phong. Note that this should not be confused with the Phong reflection model. The approach works similar to Gouraud shading, but instead of interpolating the light intensity of the vertices of a polygon, the surface normal is interpolated directly. The lighting equation is then evaluated per pixel, using for each a unique interpolated normal. Note that this approach is computationally much more expensive. The standard implementation of OpenGL does not include this method, however, some modern graphics cards are now capable of supporting real-time Phong shading. The result is a much smoother shading with better rendering of specular highlights and no visible borders between polygons.

Both Gouraud and Phong shading yield reasonable results. Nevertheless, a number of artifacts can still be encountered. While both methods give the appearance

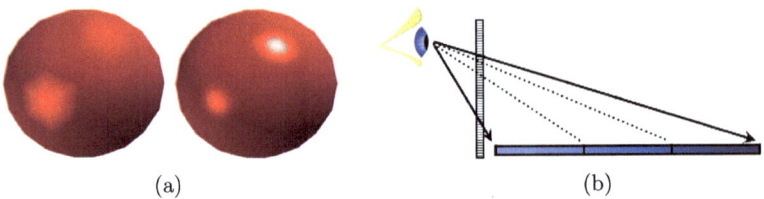

(a)   (b)

Fig. 3.37 Shading artifacts. (**a**) Mesh resolution apparent near silhouette; (**b**) Interpolation error in screen coordinates

of smoothly curved surfaces—even for meshes with low numbers of polygons—it cannot be avoided that a low mesh resolution becomes evident near object silhouettes. This is exemplified in Fig. 3.37(a), where the piece-wise approximation of the sphere surface is noticeable, independent of the shading technique. A further artifact can appear due to shading taking place in screen coordinates. As shown in Fig. 3.37(b), linear interpolation in screen space does not correspond to linear interpolation in 3D space due to perspective foreshortening (i.e. uniform steps in screen space do not correspond to uniform steps in 3D space). This causes a non-linear change in the color gradient. However, when a smooth color transition takes place, the human visual sense often does not notice the error. A final artifact is the rotation-dependency of linear scan line interpolation in quadrangular elements. However, this difficulty does not appear in triangles, which are the common basic element in mesh representations.

The methods discussed above—object representations, transformations, light sources and reflection, viewing projections, and surface shading—represent the most basic components required for rendering a simple scene in real-time computer graphics. As already discussed, numerous simplifications have to be made in order to achieve real-time feedback. Note that several additional elements exist in a standard rendering pipeline, which have not been presented further. For instance, clipping of polygons that are not visible in the current view, scan conversion of overlapping polygons using the depth buffer, anti-aliasing, etc.

As mentioned, due to the real-time requirements, numerous effects are not part of the basic pipeline, for instance shadowing, depth of field, light refraction, etc. Nevertheless, several of these phenomena can be included into the standard rendering paradigm via advanced techniques. One simple extension to provide the appearance of highly detailed surface structures is the use of texturing, i.e. the mapping of texture images to object meshes. This approach will be covered further in Sect. 10.11. It should also be noted that with the recent development of high-fidelity, consumer-level graphics cards, more and more of the advanced effects are added also in real-time applications. However, there are other techniques to obtain more realistic renderings, which do not target real-time performance. Two examples will be introduced below.

Fig. 3.38 Comparison of
rendering paradigms.
(**a**) Conventional rendering;
(**b**) Ray tracing technique

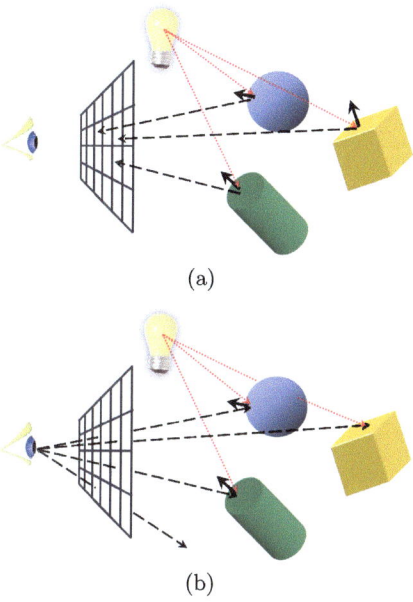

(a)

(b)

3.4.6 Advanced Rendering Techniques

Real-time rendering techniques use a simplified model of computing light interaction in a scene. Several effects are not captured in these simplifications. Interreflections, light scattering, shadowing, or refraction are usually not considered. In order to obtain more realistic images, advanced rendering techniques can be applied. The two most common examples in this category are ray tracing [3, 37] and radiosity [12]. The computations in these methods are usually very time-intensive and often not possible to be carried out in real-time. Nevertheless, recent improvements in rendering hardware have made these methods more interactive (see [33] for an overview). The underlying paradigms of the approaches will briefly be introduced in the following. However, they are only seldom applied in virtual reality applications.

3.4.6.1 Ray Tracing

In the basic rendering approach, light of various sources is reflected from polygons, which are projected into screen coordinates to determine the pixel colors in the final image (see Fig. 3.38(a)). This technique does not take into account effects such as shadowing or interreflections between objects. A possible approach to include the latter effects could be the tracing of light rays that are scattered from surfaces further into the scene. However, the computational burden of such a forward ray tracing approach would grow immensely. Moreover, most of the scattered light would possibly not reach the screen, thus computational resources would be wasted.

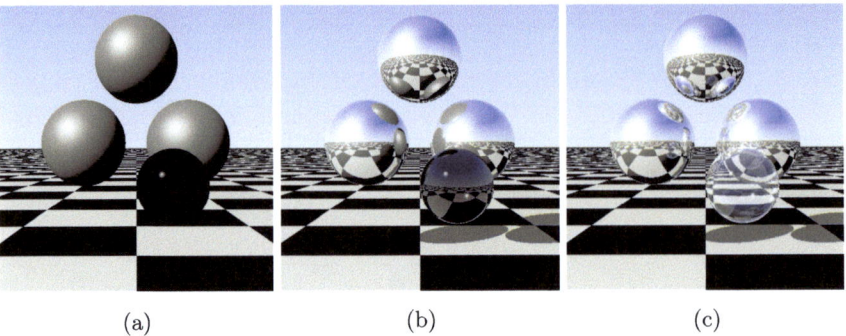

Fig. 3.39 Different rendering results at various recursion depths in ray tracing. (**a**) Recursion depth 1 (with shadows disabled); (**b**) Recursion depth 2; (**c**) Recursion depth 5

Instead, it is of advantage to reverse the light propagation in the scene. That is, instead of tracing light from light sources through the scene, rays are cast from the viewing position into the scene (see Fig. 3.38(b)). This process is termed backward ray tracing or just ray tracing. In the most basic version, one ray per screen pixel is cast into the 3D scene. These rays then either hit an object, a light source, or go to infinity. In the latter case a background color value is assigned. When a ray hits an object, it must be determined whether the surface at this location is lit or in shadow. This is done by sending so-called feeler (or shadow rays) from the intersection point to each light source. If the latter intersect other objects, then the considered point is in shadow. In this way, shadowing effects are easily integrated into the scene. The color of an illuminated surface is finally computed again using the Phong equation.

The key notion of the method is, however, to recursively propagate reflections further. To this end, the ray is split up into a reflection and a transmission part. These are further traced in the scene, potentially hitting other surfaces. Intersecting rays are further processed recursively, up to a pre-specified depth. The complexity of the first recursion step is *#pixels* × *#objects*. Depending on the recursion depth different amounts of surface reflections are included in the scene. Figure 3.39 illustrates a ray traced scene at different recursion depths. Note that at depth 1 no interreflections between the spheres are computed. With shadows disabled, this rendering is similar to a traditional scan line rendering. Depth 2 provides the first level of reflection. However, note that refracted rays have not yet passed through transparent objects, wherefore the lower right, transparent sphere in the example is not rendered correctly, yet. At recursion depth 5 multiple reflections as well as the transparent sphere are rendered appropriately.

A key ingredient of ray tracing implementations is ray-scene intersection tests. The efficient implementation of these is central to speeding up the computation of the process. Moreover, due to the inherent parallelism, ray tracing can easily be distributed on parallel computing architectures. Ray tracing yields more realistically rendered scenes than scan-line rendering. The technique is best-suited for highly reflective and transparent objects. A drawback is the computational burden of the rendering; however, recent GPUs can reach real-time performance for this method.

An example of an open source software for generating ray traced images is the POV-Ray package (Persistence of Vision Raytracer—http://www.povray.org).

A limitation of standard ray tracing is the fact that diffuse scattering of light is not taken into account. Surfaces appear strongly reflective and shadows have hard borders. Some advanced techniques exist to alleviate these artifacts, however, again add computational burden. These mentioned shortcomings are handled by a second advanced rendering approach briefly introduced in the following.

3.4.6.2 Radiosity

The key element of this advanced rendering technique is the computation of the diffuse exchange of radiation between surface patches in a scene. This allows to capture effects of light scattering and indirect illumination, as well as soft shadowing. Figure 3.40 shows a comparison for the same virtual scene—rendered once using conventional real-time techniques (with added shadowing effects) and once using radiosity.

The main strategy of radiosity is the subdivision of the scene elements into differently sized surface patches of constant color (see Fig. 3.41(a)). The light energy leaving a patch during a fixed time interval can be determined for each one via the patch equation.

$$B_i = E_i + \rho_i \sum_j B_j F_{ij}, \qquad (3.45)$$

where B_i is the energy leaving (i.e. the radiosity of) patch i, E_i is the emitted energy, ρ_i is the reflectivity over the patch (assumed to be constant), and F_{ij} is the so-called form factor. This is a constant value that specifies how visible patch i is from patch j. It is usually dependent on distance, orientation, and occlusion. These form factors have to be precomputed for all patch pairs, which can be quite time-intensive. However, various approaches have been suggested to accelerate these computations

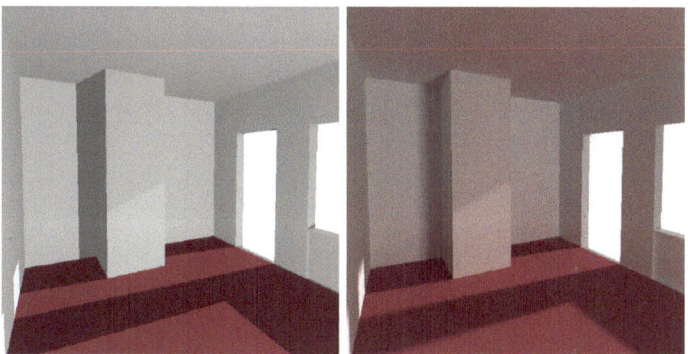

Fig. 3.40 Comparison of standard rendering using direct illumination and hard shadows (*left*) to radiosity rendering with soft shadows (*right*)

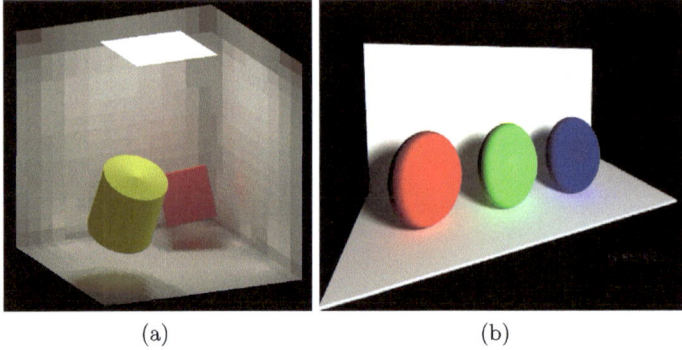

(a)   (b)

Fig. 3.41 Properties of the radiosity rendering technique. (**a**) Subdivision of surfaces into patches; (**b**) Effects of indirect diffuse reflection (color bleeding on the floor)

or to obtain approximations. Thereafter, all equations for n patches can be compiled to obtain a linear system of equations.

$$
\begin{bmatrix}
1 - \rho_1 F_{11} & -\rho_1 F_{12} & \cdots & -\rho_1 F_{1n} \\
-\rho_2 F_{21} & 1 - \rho_2 F_{22} & \cdots & -\rho_2 F_{2n} \\
\vdots & \vdots & \ddots & \vdots \\
-\rho_n F_{n1} & -\rho_n F_{n2} & \cdots & 1 - \rho_n F_{nn}
\end{bmatrix}
\cdot
\begin{bmatrix}
B_1 \\ B_2 \\ \vdots \\ B_n
\end{bmatrix}
=
\begin{bmatrix}
E_1 \\ E_2 \\ \vdots \\ E_n
\end{bmatrix}. \tag{3.46}
$$

This system is solved for the unknown light energies B_i. Note that the current computation is only mono-chromatic. In order to create color images, one system has to be solved per color channel.

The radiosity computation is independent of viewing position. Thus, once the equation system has been solved, images of new views can be generated within the scene. This method is well suited for creating walkthroughs of a virtual model, for instance in architectural presentations.

An advantage of the radiosity technique is the accurate reproduction of diffuse indirect lighting effects. An example rendering is shown in Fig. 3.41(b). Note the colored reflections of the spheres on the floor. Nevertheless, the method is not appropriate for rendering glossy or transparent material. Also, hard-edged shadows cannot be easily generated. Finally, since the strengths of radiosity and ray tracing are complementary, attempts have also been made to combine the two methods [34].

3.5 Applications of Visual Displays in Medical VR

The importance of radiological imaging for the diagnosis of diseases has increased dramatically in recent decades. This development is mainly fostered by the growing fidelity of medical imaging devices. However, these leaps in the area of image acquisition are not reflected in the process of medical image analysis and visualization. A paradigm shift from 2D slice-by-slice to efficient 3D approaches appears beneficial to cope with the accruing flood of image data in clinical practice.

Methods stemming from computer graphics have found an increasing application in the field of medicine in recent years. Visual rendering is utilized at various stages of the treatment process, including screening, diagnosis, therapy planning, intra-operative support, or outcome evaluation. Medical visualization is also applied for patient education as well as training of medical personnel such as in the area of surgical training simulation. Numerous examples of visual feedback in medical applications are provided throughout this book, for instance in Chap. 8. More details on generating triangle meshes of anatomical objects needed for the visual rendering will be provided in Chap. 10.

References

1. Agrawala, M., Beers, A., McDowall, I., Fröhlich, B., Bolas, M., Hanrahan, P.: The two-user responsive workbench: support for collaboration through individual views of a shared space. In: Proceedings of the 24th Annual Conference on Computer Graphics and Interactive Techniques, pp. 327–332 (1997)
2. Anttila, T.: A haptic rendering system for virtual handheld electronic products. Technical Report 347, Technical Research Centre of Finland, Espoo (1998). ISBN 951-38-5232-6; 951-38-5233-4
3. Appel, A.: Some techniques for shading machine renderings of solids. In: Proceedings of the Spring Joint Computer Conference. AFIPS '68, pp. 37–45 (1968)
4. Blinn, J.: Models of light reflection for computer synthesized pictures. In: Proceedings of the 4th Annual Conference on Computer Graphics and Interactive Techniques, vol. 11, pp. 192–198 (1977)
5. Blinn, J.: Simulation of wrinkled surfaces. In: Proceedings of the 5th Annual Conference on Computer Graphics and Interactive Techniques, vol. 12, pp. 286–292 (1978)
6. Bowmaker, J.K., Dartnall, H.J.A.: Visual pigments of rods and cones in a human retina. J. Physiol. **298**, 501–511 (1980)
7. Buxton, W., Fitzmaurice, G.: Hmd's, caves and chameleon: a human-centric analysis of interaction in virtual space. Comput. Graph. **32**(4), 64–68 (1998)
8. Cruz-Neira, C., Sandin, D., DeFanti, T., Kenyon, R., Hart, J.: The CAVE: audio visual experience automatic virtual environment. Commun. ACM **35**, 64–72 (1992)
9. de Boor, C.: A Practical Guide to Splines. Springer, New York (1978)
10. Duh, H., Lin, J., Kenyon, R., Parker, D., Furness, T.: Effects of characteristics of image quality in an immersive environment. Presence **11**(3), 324–332 (2002)
11. Euler, L.: Formulae generales pro translatione quacunque corporum rigidorum. Novi Comment. Acad. Sci. Petropolitanae **20**, 189–207 (1776)
12. Goral, C., Torrance, K., Greenberg, D., Battaile, B.: Modeling the interaction of light between diffuse surfaces. In: Proceedings of the 11th Annual Conference on Computer Graphics and Interactive Techniques, vol. 18, pp. 213–222 (1984)
13. Gouraud, H.: Continuous shading of curved surfaces. IEEE Trans. Comput. **20**(6), 623–629 (1971)
14. Hand, C.: A survey of 3D interaction techniques. Comput. Graph. Forum **16**(5), 269–281 (1997)
15. Kaufman, A., Mueller, K.: Overview of volume rendering. In: Hansen, C.D., Johnson, C.R. (eds.) The Visualization Handbook, pp. 127–174. Academic Press, New York (2005)
16. Kircher, A.: Ars magna lucis et umbrae, vol. 10. Rome, Italy (1646)

17. Krueger, W., Froehlich, B.: The responsive workbench. IEEE Comput. Graph. Appl. **14**(3), 12–15 (1994)
18. Möbius, A.: Der Barycentrische Calcul – Ein Neues Hülfsmittel zur Analytischen Behandlung der Geometrie. Verlag von J.A. Barth, Leipzig (1827)
19. Nicodemus, F.: Directional reflectance and emissivity of an opaque surface. Appl. Opt. **4**(7), 767–775 (1965)
20. Osterberg, G.: Topography of the layer of rods and cones in the human retina. Acta Ophthalmol. **6**, 1–103 (1935)
21. Phong, B.-T.: Illumination for computer generated pictures. Commun. ACM **18**(6), 311–317 (1975)
22. Randi, J., Licea-Kane, B., Ginsburg, D., Kessenich, J., Lichtenbelt, B., Malan, H., Weiblen, M.: OpenGL Shading Language, 3rd edn. Addison-Wesley, Reading (2009)
23. Regan, E., Price, K.: The frequency of occurrence and severity of side-effects of immersion virtual reality. Aviat. Space Environ. Med. **65**(6), 527–530 (1994)
24. Shoemake, K.: Animating rotation with quaternion curves. Comput. Graph. **19**(3), 245–254 (1985)
25. Shreiner, D.: OpenGL Programming Guide: The Official Guide to Learning OpenGL. Addison-Wesley, Reading (2009)
26. Slater, M., Usoh, M.: Body centred interaction in immersive virtual environments. In: Artificial Life and Virtual Reality, pp. 125–148 (1994)
27. Slater, M., Usoh, M., Steed, A.: Taking steps: the influence of a walking technique on presence in virtual reality. ACM Trans. Comput.-Hum. Interact. **2**(3), 201–219 (1995)
28. Smith, T., Guild, J.: The C.I.E. colorimetric standards and their use. Trans. Opt. Soc. **33**(3), 73–134 (1931)
29. Souman, J., Robuffo, P., Schwaiger, M., Frissen, I., Thümmel, T., Ulbrich, H., Di Luca, A., Bülthoff, H., Ernst, M.: Cyberwalk: enabling unconstrained omnidirectional walking through virtual environments. Trans. Appl. Percept. (2011)
30. Sutherland, I.E.: A head-mounted three dimensional display. In: Proceedings of the December 9–11, 1968, Fall Joint Computer Conference, Part I, AFIPS '68, pp. 757–764. ACM, New York (1968). doi:10.1145/1476589.1476686
31. Templeman, J., Denbrook, P., Sibert, L.: Virtual locomotion: walking in place through virtual environments. Presence **8**, 598–617 (1999)
32. Terzopoulos, D., Platt, J., Barr, A., Fleischer, K.: Elastically deformable models. In: Proceedings of the 14th Annual Conference on Computer Graphics and Interactive Techniques, vol. 21, pp. 205–214 (1987)
33. Wald, I., Mark, W., Günther, J., Boulos, S., Ize, T., Hunt, W., Parker, S., Shírley, P.: State of the art in ray tracing animated scenes. Comput. Graph. **6**(28), 1691–1722 (2009)
34. Wallace, J., Cohen, M., Greenberg, D.: A two-pass solution to the rendering equation: a synthesis of ray tracing and radiosity methods. In: Proceedings of the 14th Annual Conference on Computer Graphics and Interactive Techniques, vol. 21, pp. 311–320 (1987)
35. Walls, G.: The filling-in process. Am. J. Optom. Arch. Am. Acad. Optom. **31**(7), 329–341 (1954)
36. Ware, C., Arthur, K., Booth, K.: Fish tank virtual reality. In: Proceedings of the INTERACT '93 and CHI '93 Conference on Human Factors in Computing Systems, pp. 37–42 (1993)
37. Whitted, T.: An improved illumination model for shaded display. Commun. ACM **23**(6), 343–349 (1980)

Chapter 4
Haptic Aspects

4.1 What Is Haptics?

The term *haptics* originates from the 19th century, where it was used mainly in relation to psychophysics research. It is derived from the Greek word *haptikos*, which means "able to touch/grasp". Today it is used to describe all *tactile* (related to skin deformation), *kinesthetic* (related to muscle forces) and *proprioceptive* (related to joint positions) sensations in the body. An important aspect to note about haptics is that it involves both a passive receptive and an active explorative component, thus, requiring bi-directional input and output.

Tactile perception is related to the sense of touch, which includes the feeling of pressure, vibration, temperature, and pain. The tactile cues are perceived by a variety of receptors located under the surface of the human skin. Each kind of receptor responds to different stimuli. For example, mechanoreceptors sense pressure and vibration, thermoreceptors detect changes in skin temperature, and nociceptors sense pain.

Many haptic devices have been built to date, most of them at various research institutes around the world. A few of these devices have made it to the mass production stage and can be bought on the market. The majority incorporate only the force feedback component of touch, thus, providing mainly kinesthetic and proprioceptive sensations [14]. Without doubt the most famous of these interfaces is the PHANTOM device from Sensable Technologies (Fig. 4.1(a)). Originally developed at MIT, it can now be found in many research labs working with haptics. The device can provide haptic interaction only for a single point (usually in the form of a pen or finger gimbal), but has a large range of motion and a wide range of applications. The CyberGrasp, CyberGlove Systems LLC, (Fig. 4.1(b)) with its 22 sensors is another commercial device [1]. Actuators attached to each finger allow the user to grip and feel a virtual object with four fingers. Furthermore it can be attached to the CyberGrasp exoskeleton. The exoskeletal device MAHI of Sledd and O'Malley [74] provides force feedback mainly to the palm of the user as well as the elbow (Fig. 4.1(c)). It can be used in combination with the cyberglove to add haptic

R. Riener, M. Harders, *Virtual Reality in Medicine*,
DOI 10.1007/978-1-4471-4011-5_4, © Springer-Verlag London 2012

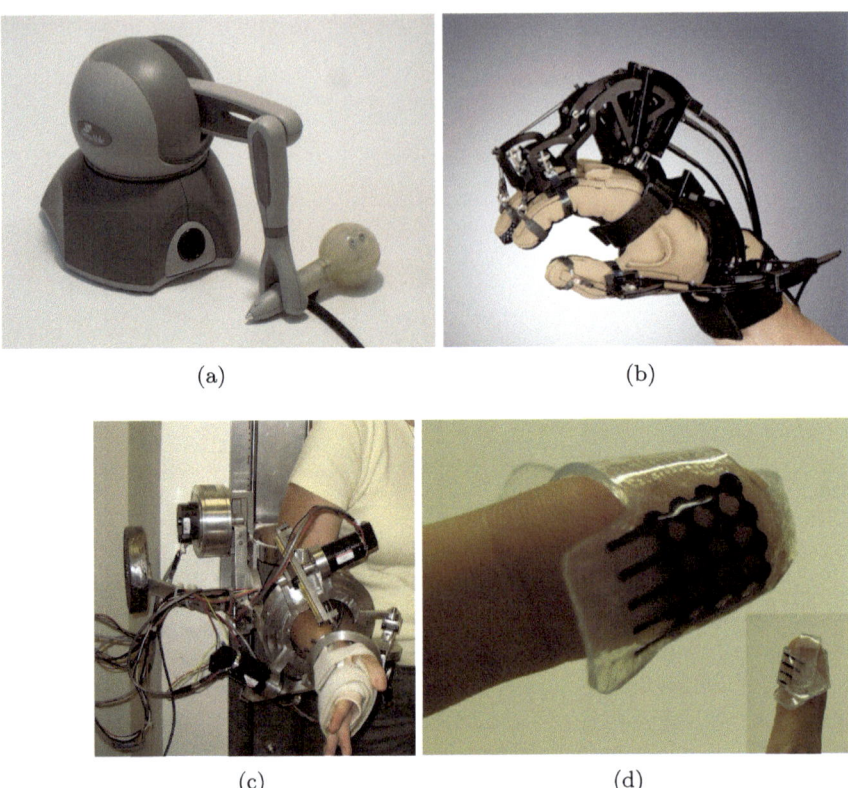

Fig. 4.1 Variety of different haptic display devices: (**a**) PHANTOM, by courtesy of RE-Lab [26, 30], ETH Zurich, Switzerland; (**b**) CyberGrasp, by courtesy of CyberGlove Systems LLC; (**c**) MAHI Exoskeleton, by courtesy of Marcia O'Malley [74]; (**d**) Example of a tactile display, by courtesy of Ig-Mo Koo [48]

feeback to the fingers, as has been shown, for instance, with the display device developed by Koo [48]. Only a few solutions support tactile feedback, which is harder to generate as the biological process of tactile receptors is not fully understood [14], and as there are greater design challenges to meet the spatial and temporal requirements of tactile perception (see Sect. 4.2). Tactile displays can be used to provide tactile perception to the finger tips (Fig. 4.1(d), see also Sect. 4.3.4).

4.2 Haptic Sense and Perception

The human haptic sense can be divided into two main parts: tactile perception and kinesthetic perception. In the following sections, anatomical, physiological, and perception-related characteristics of the haptic sense will be outlined.

4.2.1 Anatomy and Physiology

4.2.1.1 The Human Skin

The human skin has several different functions such as protection, thermoregulation, water balance, immune defense, communication, and sensing. This last function, the sensory function of the skin, is illuminated in this section. The skin consists of different layers. The epidermis builds the most superficial layer of the human body. The epidermis is thicker at the palm of the hand and the sole of the foot (0.8–1.5 mm) than at most of the other parts of the body (0.1–0.2 mm). The dermis, which is beneath the epidermis, contains blood vessels and lymphatic vessels. The dermis consists of collagen and elastic fibers which guarantee tear strength and plasticity. Below the dermis, the subcutis acts as a fat storage [28].

Skin characteristics vary among the many parts of the human body. However, current research focuses mainly on the glabrous (hairless) skin. Applications have been developed for the palm and finger, but also other parts of the body, such as the abdomen or the arm. The skin can sense positive or negative pressure, vibration, texture, normal and tangential forces, temperature, electric voltage and current. In order to facilitate the sense of touch, the skin includes mechanoreceptors, thermoreceptors, nociceptors, and proprioceptors [11].

4.2.1.2 Tactile Receptors

Four mechanoreceptors with specific functional properties can be found in the tissue of the glabrous skin, each at specific depths (Fig. 4.2). Among the different classes of mechanoreceptors, the most commonly exploited in tactile display applications are the Merkel cells, the Meissner corpuscles, and the Pacinian corpuscles (Table 4.1) [11, 45]. Merkel cells are located right below the skin surface in the epidermis. Merkel cells have the highest spatial resolution of all mechanoreceptors. However, the spatial resolution is highly dependent on the location on the body. Merkel cells with a temporal resolution of about 10 Hz are most sensitive to surface texture of objects, especially for moving mechanical stimuli (Table 4.2). Meissner corpuscles are found in the shallow dermis. Meissner corpuscles are able to detect relative movements of objects on the skin and are most sensitive to low-frequency vibrations around 30 Hz. They are needed to regulate grip forces, e.g. for holding an object with the fingers. Pacinian corpuscles are placed in the deep dermis and subcutaneous adipose tissue and are most sensitive to high-frequency vibrations around 250 Hz. Ruffini nerve endings are located in the dermis, register skin deformation and are involved in finger position control. On the hairy skin, hair follicle receptors can additionally sense skin contact and touch [20]. The threshold of perception of vibration depends not only on the frequency of vibration but also on the location on the body, contactor surface area, and the kind of probe used in the experiments. Lowest vibrotactile thresholds were found at the fingertips, compared to the large toe, the heel, and the volar forearm [60].

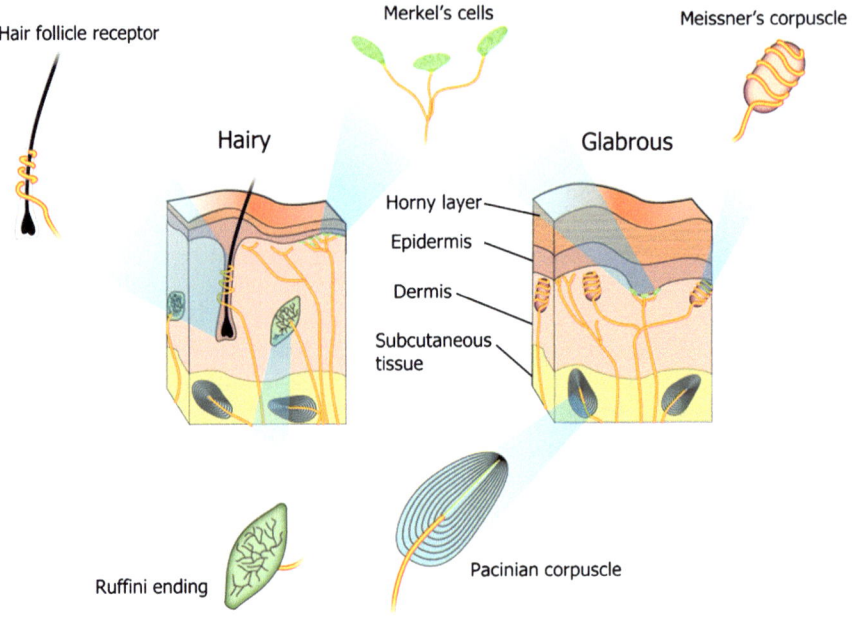

Fig. 4.2 Skin and its receptors; © ADInstruments Pty Ltd. Reproduced with permission

Table 4.1 Mechanoreceptors [18, 32]

	Meissner	Merkel	Ruffini	Pacinian
Sensory function	Low frequency vibration and motion detection; grip control; tactile flow perception	Pattern/form detection; texture perception; tactile flow perception	Finger position; stable grasp; tangential force; motion detection	High frequency vibration detection; tool use
Adaption rate	Fast	Slow	Slow	Fast
Spatial acuity (mm)	3–4	0.5	7+	10+
Frequency range (Hz)	3–40	0.3–3	15–400	10–500
Effective stimuli	Temporal changes in skin deformation	Spatial deformation; sustained pressure; curvature, edge, corners	Sustained downward pressure; Lateral skin stretch; skin slip	Temporal changes in the deformation

Further, free nerve endings in the skin sense temperature and pain and contribute to the tactile sense. Thermoreceptors are divided into two classes, cold thermoceptors (sensitivity between 8–38°C) and warm thermoreceptors (29–44°C). Although it seems that the skin is sensitive to temperature, our receptors cannot detect the

Table 4.2 Tactile perception ranges

Temporal resolution	300 Hz	[10]
Two point discrimination	finger: 3–4 mm; belly: 37 mm; shank: 47 mm	[32]
Force threshold	> 0.01 N	[88, 91]
Pressure resolution	> 3%	[19]
Temperature range	17–44°C	[92]
Temperature resolution	> 0.2°C	[69]

Table 4.3 Kinesthetic perception

Joint angle resolution	0.8–2.5°	[79]
Perception threshold	0.2–1.3°	[69]
Joint angle bandwidth	20–30 Hz	[69, 79]
Torque differences (fingers)	13%	[43]
Force differences	5–15%	[24]

exact temperature of the surface but rather sense the thermal energy flow [11]. Note that temperature adds quality characteristics to the tactile sense. Nociceptors register pain and can be found in skin, muscles, joints and organs. Nociceptors are activated by strong mechanical stimuli, very cold or hot temperatures but also by inflammation of tissue [20].

4.2.1.3 Kinesthetic Receptors

Kinesthetic receptors are located in the joints and muscles of the body. They mainly detect position and movement of the limbs, and the amount of force exerted by the muscles or movement and gravitation. Therefore, these receptors are relevant for haptic interaction with the environment. Kinesthetic receptors are located in the tendons and sense muscle forces, which can be mapped to joint torques. Kinesthetic receptors are a collection of sensors that give information related to the current joint positions (Table 4.3). Muscle length is sensed by receptors in the muscle spindle, the so-called intrafusal muscle fibers. The intrafusal muscle fibres are arranged in parallel to the extrafusal muscle fibers (standard muscle fibers outside the muscle spindle) in the center of the muscle. Muscle spindles are located in the center of the muscle. The Golgi tendon organ senses the tension of the muscle, for example if the antagonist (i.e. muscle that counteracts the agonist) is contracting. The Golgi tendon organ is arranged serially to the extrafusal muscle fibers at the transition of the muscle and the tendon. Mechanoreceptors located in the joint capsule provide information about joint position and joint movement [20] and are also referred to as joint receptors.

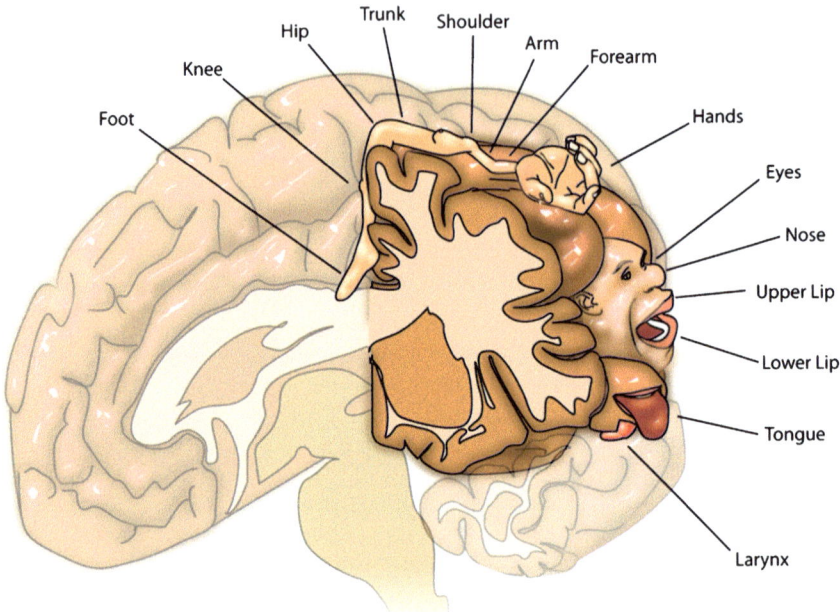

Fig. 4.3 The sensory homunculus resembles those proportions of the brain that are required by the respective body parts for sensory perception; © ADInstruments Pty Ltd. Reproduced with permission

4.2.1.4 Cortical Representation

Once a haptic stimulus is detected by either a tactile or a kinesthetic receptor, the signal has to be interpreted by the brain. The regions in the brain responsible for processing of haptic stimuli are the pre and post central gyrus. These regions can be divided into smaller areas, of which each one is responsible for a specific sensation (Fig. 4.3) or generation of movement of a certain part of the body. A more than proportional part of the somato-sensory gyrus is allocated for the hands and fingers as well as for the mouth area. This matches the increased sensitivity of these body parts compared to the rest of the body.

4.2.2 Psychophysics

Psychophysics research examines the relation of physical stimuli to perception, and it focuses on how sensory cues are interpreted by the human. In the field of haptic psychophysics, the goal is to study the quantitative relationship between the haptic stimulus in the physical domain and the associated sensation in the psychological domain.

Table 4.4 Typical kinematic and kinetic musculoskeletal values

Movement	Angular velocity (knee)	250°/s	[65]
	Frequency	12 Hz	[89]
Mechanical loads	Compression force index finger	50 N	[77]
	Grip strength fist	400 N	[2]
	Holding force shoulder	102 N	[79]
	Holding weight arm	<300 N	[39]
	Maximal joint torque (knee)	220 Nm	[84]

Psychophysics plays an important role in haptic systems design, because it gives estimates of what the limits of the human haptic perception are. The so-called *sensory threshold* denotes the threshold above which mental events are registered consciously, for example, with regard to cues such as velocity, forces and displacements. The sensory threshold is classified in absolute and difference thresholds. Absolute threshold is defined as the minimum amount of stimulation intensity that is necessary to produce a sensation, also known as *stimulus threshold*. Difference threshold is the smallest necessary amount of change in physical stimulation that is perceived, which is defined as just noticeable difference (JND). The JND is not constant, but it increases with background intensity [78]. This is captured in the constant Weber fraction, the relationship between JND and background intensity.

The knowledge of these thresholds simplifies the design of haptic devices, because it gives a lower bound on required device accuracy. Tables 4.2, 4.3, and 4.4 give an overview of tactile and kinesthetic perception thresholds and resolutions as well as physiological ranges. Another useful outcome of psychophysical research is knowledge on haptic illusions, which can be used for a similar purpose.

4.2.3 Haptic Exploration

Haptic interaction can either be active or passive. Passive interaction happens without voluntary movement generated by the user and focuses mainly on the sensory experience. Active interaction, on the other hand, is more focused on the object, which is explored by voluntarily moving the hand. In order to actively determine the properties of an object, subjects have been observed how they use different techniques while exploring different object properties (Fig. 4.4) [50].

4.3 Haptic Display Technology

Haptic displays can be classified into sub-categories based on different criteria, for example, according to the kinematic design, into serial kinematics and parallel kinematics. Alternatively, they can be classified according to the actuation principle,

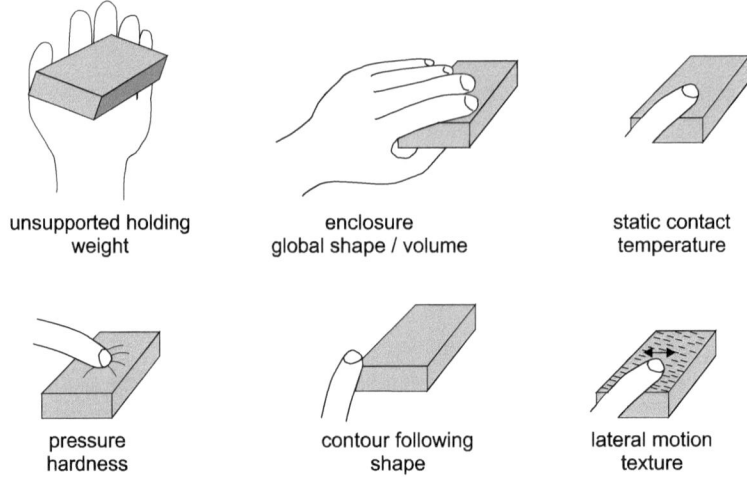

Fig. 4.4 Common ways of haptic exploration; adapted from [50]

referring to how the force is generated. Possible actuation principles are electromagnetic, pneumatic or hydraulic, electrorheological, magnetorheological, shape memory alloys, electroactive polymers, or piezoelectric.

Another classification could be done according to which sensory pathway is addressed, either tactile (thermal), kinesthetic, or pain receptors. Furthermore, haptic devices can be distinguished according to the chosen control strategy, which determines how the system interacts with the user. Fundamental building blocks are compliant control strategies such as admittance or impedance control.

4.3.1 Kinematic Principles of Haptic Displays

In general, a haptic display generates forces and movements while interacting with the human operator. One can distinguish two main kinematic structures, characterized by a parallel kinematic or serial kinematic design (Fig. 4.5). The workspace, amount of force/torque, and other performance criteria of haptic displays depend on the type of the kinematic structure.

4.3.1.1 Serial Kinematics

In a serial kinematic structure actuators and links are arranged in a chain, one after the other. Thus, each actuator generates motions relative to the preceding one. In general, one can distinguish (Fig. 4.6):

- *Linear axes:* This type of kinematics produces movements along translational axes driven by linear actuators.

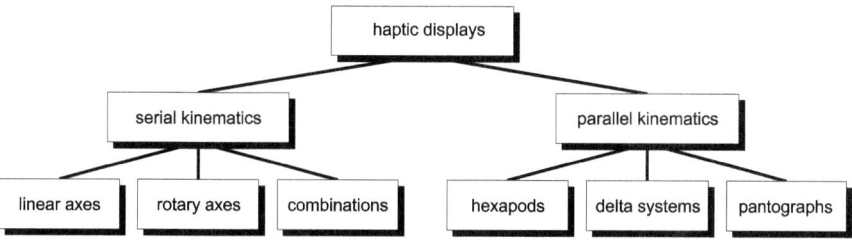

Fig. 4.5 Haptic displays: kinematics design principles

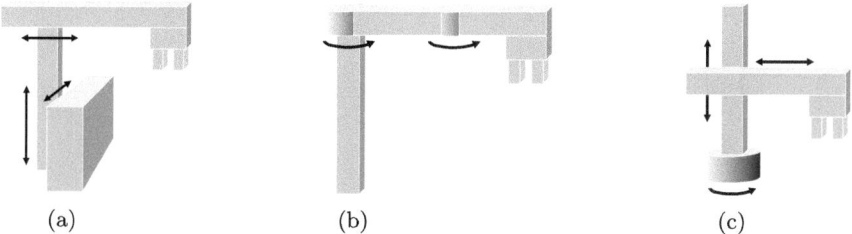

Fig. 4.6 Different serial kinematic structures. (**a**) Linear axes; (**b**) Rotary axes (SCARA-type); (**c**) Combination of linear and rotary axes

- *Rotary axes:* The movements are obtained by rotary joints (e.g., SCARA[1]-type robot)
- *Combination of linear and rotary axes:* The movement of the end-effector is produced by the combination of both linear and rotary actuators.

4.3.1.2 Parallel Kinematics

In parallel kinematic structures two or more linear or rotary actuated links are arranged in a parallel way, such that they form at least one closed kinematic chain. These links connect the base to a moving platform. The position and/or orientation of this platform depend on the positions and angles of the parallel links.

A survey on parallel mechanisms can be found in [55]. To select a parallel structure that suits the necessary degrees of freedom, workspace and force requirements, a systematic approach of "type synthesis" can be used [46]. In general, a parallel structure ensures very good positioning accuracy (because the legs are not subjected to bending, only to compression and tension). It exhibits high stiffness, high accuracy, and low moving inertia. Problems are the small workspace and singularities.

---

[1] A SCARA (Selective Compliance Assembly Robot Arm) is a type of robot that is frequently used in industrial applications, it resembles the human arm in terms of kinematics, and its most frequent realization has four degrees of freedom in serial configuration.

Fig. 4.7 Hexapod (Steward Platform)

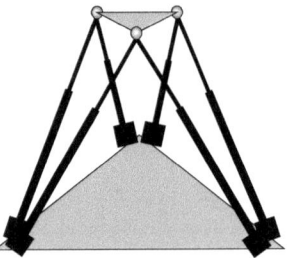

Fig. 4.8 Delta mechanism [12, 85]

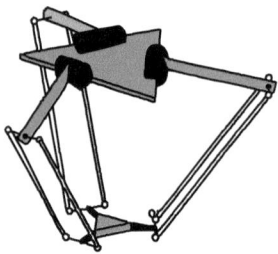

Control is less straightforward than in serial robots due to a complex input-output relationship. Therefore, careful design is needed and optimizing geometrical parameters remains a major field of research.

Prominent examples of parallel robots are the Hexapod with six degrees of freedom [33], the Delta robot [12], and parallel mechanisms based on the pantograph principle [40].

A *Hexapod* contains six linear actuators, which connect a lower and upper platform via passive low-friction ball-and-socket joints (Fig. 4.7). Such a structure can produce motions of the upper platform in six degrees of freedom (three translations and three rotations). It was originally suggested by Gough [33] for a tyre-testing machine. Stewart later suggested to use a six degrees of freedom platform (not identical to the Hexapod) for a flight simulator [75].

The *Delta* [12] uses three linkages to constrain a platform to purely translatory movements (Fig. 4.8). It can be extended by an independent central cardanic joint to allow also rotations about the vertical axis. This type of structure is frequently used in packaging machines.

The *pantograph* is a historical mechanical device used to copy and scale drawings; it was invented in 1603 by Christoph Scheiner. A parallel manipulator based on this type of linkages was first suggested in [40]. A whole family of possible kinematics based on the pantograph mechanism is described in [7]. The interesting fact about the pantograph mechanism (Fig. 4.9) is that the actuation can be placed quite close to the center base of the system. If devices with spatial range of motions are used, movement in vertical and horizontal directions can be decoupled [7]: A linear actuator moves the platform in horizontal direction, and another linear actuator attached moves the platform exclusively up and down. In this way, strong actuators can be used for vertical displacements, if heavy masses need to be lifted,

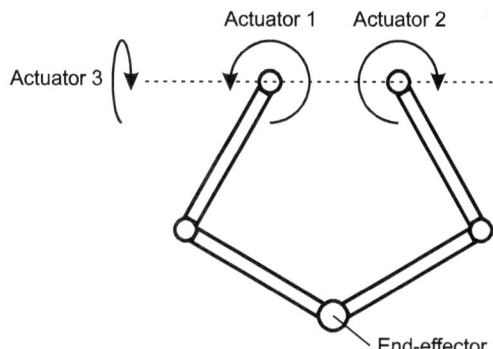

Fig. 4.9 Pantograph mechanism

and less powerful actuators can generate horizontal movement. A set of three pantograph mechanisms provides a larger range of motion of the end-effector compared to a Stewart platform. Furthermore, the heavy load of motors and drives can be integrated closer to the base, which improves the dynamics of the system as lower inertia allows faster movements.

4.3.2 Actuation Principles of Haptic Displays

Most haptic devices available today make use of electrical motors or fluidic actuation systems based on pneumatic or hydraulic pressure. However, since these technologies are often too heavy, slow, space consuming, or restricted to certain interactions and environments, many new actuator technologies are emerging. The most important of these are electroactive polymers, shape memory alloys, rheological fluids, and piezoelectric actuators.

4.3.2.1 Electromagnetic Actuators

Electromagnetic actuators come mainly in the form of brushless DC[2] motors, brush-commutator permanent magnet DC motors, linear motors, and stepper motors.

The basic principle is to exploit the *Lorenz force*, which is produced when a current $\mathbf{I}$ flows through a conductor of length L in a magnetic field $\mathbf{B}$ (Fig. 4.10). The Lorenz force $\mathbf{F}$ can be calculated as:

$$\mathbf{F} = L\mathbf{I} \times \mathbf{B}. \tag{4.1}$$

---

[2]A DC motor runs on Direct Current (DC), whereas an AC motor runs on Alternating Current (AC). Both types of motors generate torque by exploiting the interaction of magnetic and electric fields.

Fig. 4.10 Working principle
of electromagnetic actuators

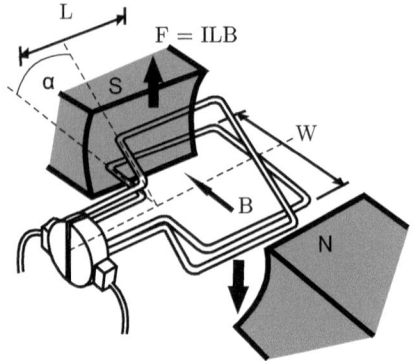

The resulting motor torque τ depends on the rotor angle α and on the angular velocity ω:

$$\tau = |\mathbf{F}|\omega \cos\alpha = \mathbf{IB}A\cos\alpha. \qquad (4.2)$$

Electromagnetic actuators have the advantage of being quiet, clean and easy to design, control and install. However, the power to weight ratio is not optimal, and these kinds of actuators sometimes may take up too much space to integrate with a haptic device.

4.3.2.2 Pneumatic Actuators

Pneumatic actuators transfer energy from a power source to the haptic interface via air pressure. This has the advantage that the actuator needs less space and weight on the moving parts of the device. Furthermore, pneumatic actuators are not expensive and relatively easy to maintain. On the other hand, pneumatic actuators require a large power source, and also have a large compliance, which makes them difficult to control with high position accuracy (Table 4.5).

4.3.2.3 Hydraulic Actuators

Hydraulic actuators are controlled by pressurized fluid (oil or water) from a compressor. They have a high power to weight ratio and a higher stiffness than pneumatic actuators. However, there can be problems with leakage. Furthermore, they are rather expensive. In contrast to pneumatic actuation, an additional reservoir must be arranged for the pressurized fluid (Table 4.5).

4.3.2.4 Rheological Fluids

Rheological fluids are suspensions of fine non-conducting particles in an electrically insulating fluid. The particles range from between 0.1–100 μm. The fluids can

Table 4.5 Summary of actuator properties: hydraulic and pneumatic

Actuation Type	Hydraulic	Pneumatic
Working Principle	Hydraulic fluid (oil or water) is pressurized by a compressor, controlled by valves, and delivered to linear actuators (cylinder) or rotary actuators (motor)	Compressed air is controlled by valves to drive linear actuators (pneumatic muscle) or rotary actuators (motor)
Linearity	Rather linear	Nonlinear
Amount of Force	Large	Medium
Power	Large	Medium
Power to weight ratio	High	High
Bandwidth	Medium	Medium
Efficiency	Low efficiency; very high mechanical coupling efficiency	Low efficiency; high mechanical coupling efficiency
Backdrivability	No	Yes
Speed	Slow	Medium
Advantages	High power to weight ratio; high output stiffness; large payload	Simple and easy to maintain; high power to weight ration; light weight; cheap, air is always available
Limitations	Risk of leakage problems; noisy; complex system; expensive; can be dangerous; difficult force control	Possible air leakage; compliant due to compressability; friction; time delays; can be noisy; limited accuracy

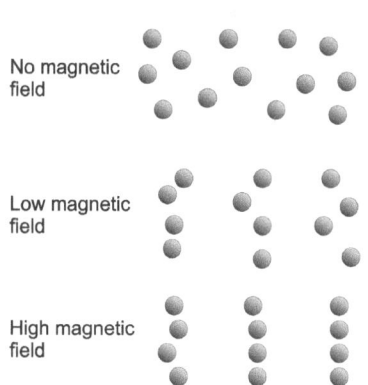

Fig. 4.11 Working principle of rheological fluids showing magnetic particles of a fluid that get in alignment with increasing magnetic field strength

No magnetic field

Low magnetic field

High magnetic field

change their rheological properties dramatically, such as viscosity and yield stress, in response to a changing electric field, at switching rate of milliseconds (Fig. 4.11) [52, 63].

A prototype device using a magneto-rheological fluid has been developed at the University of Pisa (Fig. 4.12) [4, 66, 71]. A vat is filled with the rheological fluid. Magnetic coils placed around the vat can be turned on and off to generate a magnetic

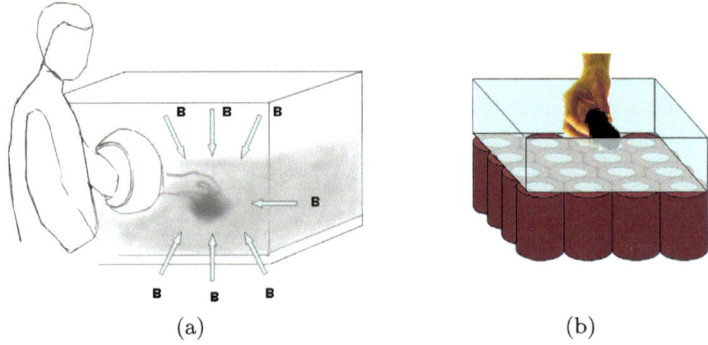

Fig. 4.12 Haptic displays based on rheological fluid actuation [4, 66, 71]: (**a**): Prototype haptic display using rheological fluids, by courtesy of Antonio Bicchi, University of Pisa, Italy; (**b**): Coil arrangement, by courtesy of Antonio Bicchi, University of Pisa, Italy

field in particular spots of the fluid within the vat. Theoretically, this approach allows to render regions exhibiting different tactile properties to be explored by the user. However, the device is not particularly suited for rendering sharp edges and also as compared to other haptic devices, it creates only dissipative effects, such as passive compliant behaviors rather than active forces and movements.

4.3.2.5 Shape Memory Alloys

Shape memory alloys are examples of thermo-mechanical material actuation. They are characterized by two material states: In one state, the alloy can be freely deformed. When switched to the other state, the alloy returns to its original shape. The two states are switched by temperature: at low temperature, the alloy is in martensitic state and can be deformed, while at high temperature, the alloy is in austenitic state, where it "remembers" its predefined shape (one-way memory effect). The advantage of these alloys for a haptic device is the excellent power-to-weight ratio. However, the bandwidth, i.e. rate of change from one state to another, is quite low due to the needed temperature change. Table 4.6 compares properties of thermo-mechanical materials and rheological fluids.

4.3.2.6 Electroactive Polymers

Electroactive polymers are increasingly finding their place in various haptic displays. These polymers experience a significant change in size or shape when a voltage is applied in a movement reminiscent of a muscle (Fig. 4.13).

Compared to shape memory alloys, electroactive polymers have a higher response speed as well as better resilience. Until recently, however, electroactive polymers have presented practical problems. They required too high voltages, could not

Table 4.6 Rheological fluids and thermo-mechanical materials actuation

Actuation Type	Rheological Fluids	Thermo-Mechanical Materials
Working Principle	Viscosity changes due to electric/magnetic field acting on micron-sized electric or magnetic particles; change from liquid into solid state within milliseconds	Shape memory alloy (SMA) is stable in two phases: austenite (high temperature) and martensite (low temperature) State changes due to temperature change.
Linearity	Nonlinear	Nonlinear
Amount of Force	Only resistive force, can be large	Low
Power	No power is generated	Low
Power to weight ratio	N/A	High
Bandwidth	Low	Very low
Efficiency	High	Low efficiency; very low mechanical coupling efficiency
Backdrivability	Yes	No
Speed	Medium	Slow
Advantages	Can be used for various damping applications	Can be manufactured to almost any shape and size; high level of recoverable plastic strain can be induced
Limitations	High-quality fluids are expensive; fluids get thicker after prolonged use and need replacing; only dissipative (no kinetic energy generated, therefore often used with active components)	Cooling is difficult; no position between two states; difficult to adjust force; large hysteresis

Fig. 4.13 Working principle of electroactive polymers

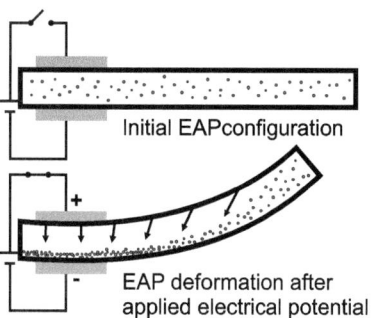

generate enough force, and did not last long enough. Recently, ways have been found to make the polymers stronger, more robust, and more efficient. Table 4.7 compares electroactive polymers to human muscles.

Table 4.7   Electroactive polymer actuators compared to human muscle actuation

Actuation Type	Electroactive Polymers (EAP)	Human Muscle
Working Principle	Significant change of shape or size in response to electrical currents or voltages	Human muscle contraction and relaxation
Linearity	Nonlinear	Highly nonlinear
Amount of Force	Low	Medium
Power	Low	Medium
Power to weight ratio	High	Medium
Bandwidth	Very Low	Low
Efficiency	Low efficiency; low mechanical coupling efficiency	Metabolic "waste" for healing; low mechanical coupling efficiency
Backdrivability	No	Yes
Speed	Slow, but higher than SMA	Medium
Advantages	Faster response, lower densities and improved resilience than SMAs; undergo large deformation while sustaining large forces; behavior similar to that of biological muscles	
Limitations	Dielectric EAPs need a large actuation voltage; for ionic EAPs, energy is needed to keep it at a given position	

Fig. 4.14   Working principle of piezoelectric actuators

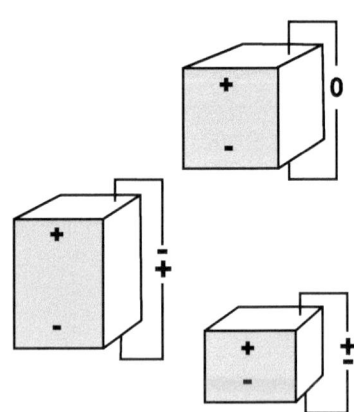

4.3.2.7   Piezoelectric Actuators

Piezoelectric crystals can be used both for force sensing and for actuation. Forces applied to piezoelectric materials generate a charge which is roughly proportional

Table 4.8 Electromagnetic compared to piezoelectric actuators

Actuation Type	Electromagnetic	Piezoelectric (ceramic)
Working Principle	Force/torque is produced when current passes through the magnetic field	Applying voltage on piezoelectric materials generates deformation, which can be used for actuation
Linearity	Rather linear	Linear
Amount of Force	From very small to very large	Medium
Power	Low	Medium
Power to weight ratio	From very small to very large	Small
Bandwidth	High	Low
Efficiency	High efficiency at high speed and small torque; very high mechanical coupling efficiency	High efficiency; medium mechanical coupling efficiency
Backdrivability	Yes	No
Speed	Slow to fast, big range	Slow
Advantages	Quiet; clean; simple design; widely available and cheap; easy to use and control	Suitable for miniaturization; produce no electromagnetic noise
Limitations	To produce large torque; the motor has to work at low speed and low efficiency and can heat up	Piezoelectric ceramics show substantial hysteresis and friction. Hence, piezoelectric actuation cannot be driven open-loop

to the applied mechanical force or stress (Fig. 4.14). Conversely, an applied voltage generates deformation of the piezoelectric material, which can be used for actuation.

Strains from piezoelectric materials are often too small to be directly useful. To amplify these strains, various mechanism have been created, such as piezo-ultrasonic motors.

Piezoelectric ceramics show substantial hysteresis. Hence, piezoelectric actuation cannot be driven open-loop and requires accurate positioning. Table 4.8 gives an overview of piezoelectric actuator properties compared to electromagnetic actuators.

4.3.3 Control Principles of Haptic Displays

4.3.3.1 Terminology

There are two technical terms that are important for understanding the basic control strategies of haptic displays. These terms are *impedance* $\mathbf{Z}$ and *admittance* $\mathbf{Y}$. The terminology comes from electrical-mechanical equivalence (voltage $\sim$ force, current $\sim$ velocity).

Mechanical impedance $\mathbf{Z}$ represents the force response to mechanical interactions between a user and an object. It relates motions (given as positions $\mathbf{x}$ and their first and higher derivatives) to forces $\mathbf{F}$ acting on the system. As the definition of impedance relating *velocity* to force will be useful for stability analysis later, this will be employed here:

$$\mathbf{F}(t) = \mathbf{Z}\big(\dot{\mathbf{x}}(t)\big). \tag{4.3}$$

An analog formulation can be used for a rotary system with angular velocity $\dot{\varphi}$ and torque $\mathbf{M}$. The impedance comprises mechanical properties such as elastic effects, viscous effects, inertial forces as well as active forces generated by an artificial drive or a living organism.

Mechanical admittance $\mathbf{Y}$ is the inverse of the mechanical impedance. It translates forces to motions (positions and their derivatives):

$$\mathbf{Y} = \mathbf{Z}^{-1}, \qquad \dot{\mathbf{x}}(t) = \mathbf{Y}\big(\mathbf{F}(t)\big). \tag{4.4}$$

These technical terms can be used to describe force reaction behaviors of the simulated objects in the virtual environment. For example, when the system simulates a rigid wall situation, the impedance approaches infinity ($\mathbf{Z} \to \infty$) while the mechanical admittance value is equal to zero ($\mathbf{Y} = 0$).

In general, VR users can interact with and feel the haptic feedback from the virtual objects through haptic display hardware such as the commercial PHANTOM device. The ideal haptic device must produce an impedance that is identical to the impedance of the virtual objects the user interacts with. This means, the haptic display must be *transparent*. There are two haptic control strategies that are commonly used to produce haptic feedback, i.e. an impedance architecture and an admittance architecture (see e.g. [36, 73]).

In the impedance control architecture (Fig. 4.15(a)), the position of the user is measured when the user applies actions (i.e. movements) on the haptic device, and a response force is calculated and displayed to the user via the haptic device. After perceiving the displayed force, the user reacts to it by his or her muscles.

In the admittance architecture (Fig. 4.15(b)), input force information is measured from the user's actions to compute the new position, which is displayed to the user via the haptic device (Fig. 4.16). Position is then transformed into response force according to the impedance of the user.

Transparency is a parameter to quantify the fidelity of the haptic display. The goal of a good haptic display is to obtain maximum transparency. That means

$$\mathbf{x}_U \equiv \mathbf{x}_V, \qquad \mathbf{F}_U \equiv \mathbf{F}_V. \tag{4.5}$$

4.3.3.2 Implementation of Admittance and Impedance Control Architectures

In an admittance controller, a force–torque sensor records the interaction forces between user and haptic device. The force information is used to compute the desired motion on the basis of a virtual admittance law. The desired motion is then fed into a

Fig. 4.15 Control aspects of
haptic displays drawn as
two-port system:
(**a**) impedance architecture,
(**b**) admittance architecture.
The index U refers to the
user, the index V to the
virtual impedance or
admittance. User and device
exchange forces **F** and
positions **x**, and they are
represented by either
impedance **Z** or admittance **Y**

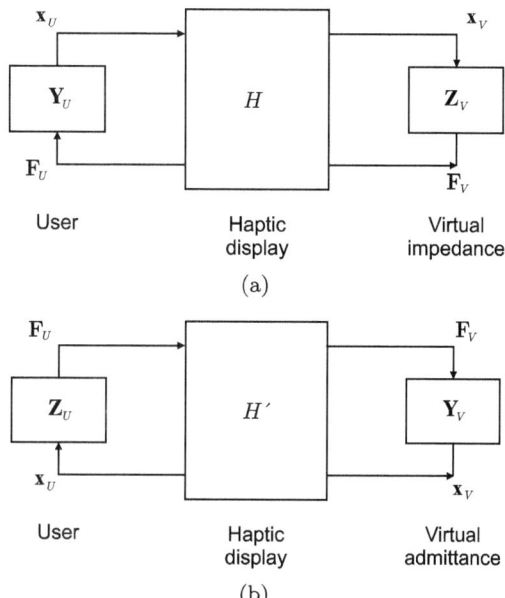

standard position controller to change the position of the haptic display end-effector
(Fig. 4.16).

In an impedance controller, a position sensor is implemented to measure the real
position of the end-effector. This information is used to calculate the interaction
forces in the virtual environment according to the impedance law. The force is then
fed into an inner force controller to display the force on the haptic display end-
effector (Fig. 4.17). If there is no force sensor available at the end-effector, force
can only be controlled in a feedforward manner through motor currents, which is
called open-loop impedance control (Fig. 4.18). This strategy is inferior in terms of
transparency.

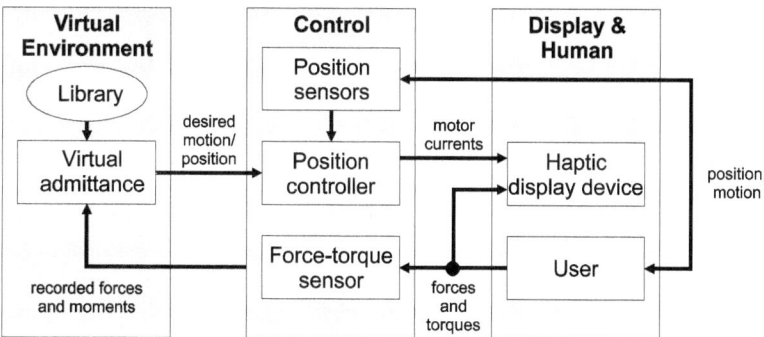

Fig. 4.16 Admittance control architecture

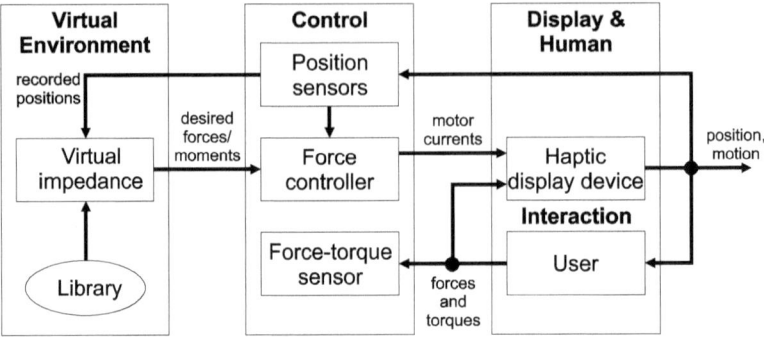

Fig. 4.17   Impedance control architecture

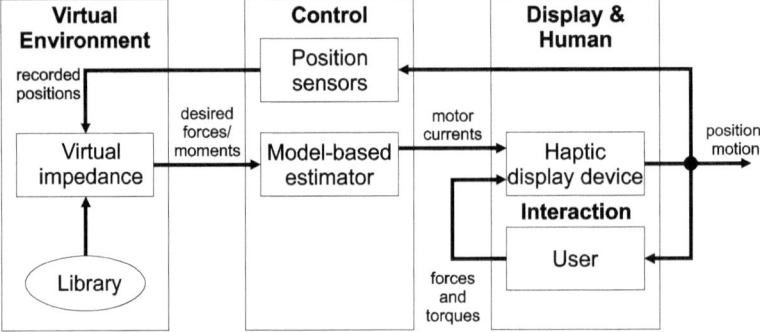

Fig. 4.18   Open-loop impedance control

4.3.3.3 Stability and Passivity of Haptic Displays

An analysis of its impedance $\mathbf{Z}$, introduced in Sect. 4.3.3.1, allows to assess stability of a haptic device when coupled to a user in terms of *passivity*. The power that is transferred to the robot is equal to the product of force $\mathbf{F}$ and velocity $\mathbf{v}$, and the accumulated energy is equal to the integral of this product over time. In order for the robot to behave like a passive system (i.e. equivalent to a combination of springs, dampers, and masses), it has to be either conservative or dissipative, meaning that at any time instant t, the energy supplied by the robot must be zero or negative:

$$\int_0^t \mathbf{F}(\tau)\dot{\mathbf{x}}(\tau)\mathrm{d}\tau \leq 0 \quad \forall t \geq 0. \tag{4.6}$$

There is a strong relationship between Lyapunov stability analysis for autonomous systems and input-output passivity analysis. However, as opposed to only analyzing stability, an important advantage of looking at systems in terms of passivity is that this description allows analyzing *stability of coupled systems* in a simple manner: Two passive systems coupled either in parallel or in feedback manner are again passive, which is not necessarily true for systems that are only stable in the autonomous case. Under the assumption that the human would behave like a passive system during interaction with a haptic device, stability of the coupled human-robot system can be guaranteed *without an explicit model of the human*. This gives a very useful basic requirement for designing safe haptic systems.

For linear systems, the general formulation of Eq. (4.6) can be simplified considerably: There, passivity is ensured if the impedance transfer function $\mathbf{Z}(s)$ as a function of the complex variable $s = \sigma + j\omega$ is positive real [16]. Necessary and sufficient conditions for this are:

- $\mathbf{Z}(s) = \frac{\mathbf{F}(s)}{s\mathbf{x}(s)}$ must be stable,
- the real part of $\mathbf{Z}(j\omega)$ must be non-negative for all ω for which $j\omega$ is not a pole of $\mathbf{Z}(s)$.

Using this formulation, it has been shown that a haptic device with linear force feedback is only passive for a limited range of feedback gains [15]. For too high gains, the system is not passive anymore, which means that it is only stable when interacting with a certain range of mechanical environments (like for example a mass). When interacting with a spring, the system gets unstable.

4.3.3.4 Safety Features of Haptic Displays

As a haptic display provides the user with force feedback, the device must always have physical contact with the user's body. Therefore, safety is an important issue for the design and development of haptic displays to avoid harming the user. There are many safety features possible such as, passive mechanical stops, barriers at the boundary of the haptic device workspace, magnetic or pneumatic overload protection at the end-effector, hardware and software control of positions, velocities, forces, generation of reduced forces to limit acceleration and fatigue, and emergency stops and deadman buttons.

4.3.4 Examples of Haptic Displays

Many haptic displays have been developed over the years. These devices vary in terms of appearance, function, actuator type, etc. In this section, we classify haptic display systems into three categories: Desktop systems, ground and wall-mounted systems, and portable systems. In a fourth subsection, we add examples of tactile display devices.

4.3.4.1 Desktop Systems

The haptic devices of this category are placed on a desk or a table. They are often small devices, such that they can be placed next to a PC or monitor (Fig. 4.19).

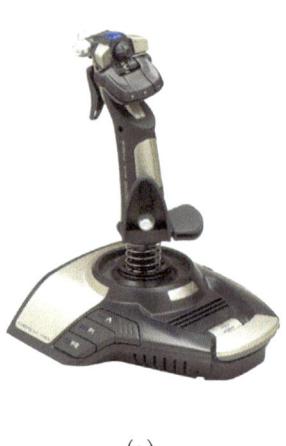

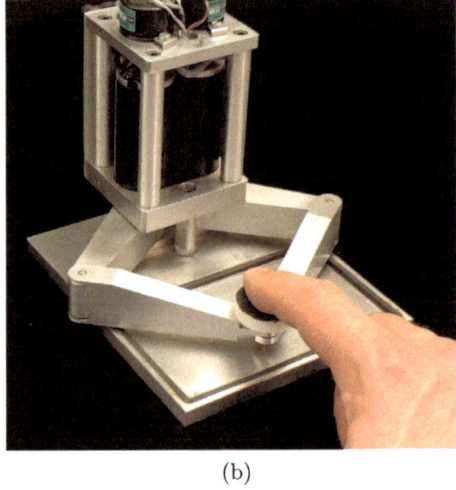

(a)   (b)

Fig. 4.19 Desktop haptic display systems: (**a**) Cyborg Evo Force Joystick, Saitek (by courtesy of MAD CATZ GMBH, Munich, Germany), (**b**) McGill Pantograph (by courtesy of Vincent Hayward)

Most desktop systems work endeffector-based, where the haptic display device induces the force only through the endeffectors of its kinematic structure. In robot-assisted surgery, these devices are frequently used as input devices for the surgeon, such as the Impulse Engine. This force-feedback joystick allows to track the movements of the user and to convey tactile sensations to the user via force feedback. A very popular desktop system is the commercially available PHANTOM haptic device (Fig. 4.1(a)), which provides motions of the end-effector in three or more degrees of freedom. The control of the PHANTOM is based on a simplified impedance control. The device does not use any force sensor to measure the applied forces, so it is controlled using an open-loop impedance strategy (Sect. 4.3.3.2). Table 4.9 shows some technical data of the aforementioned desktop-type haptic displays. Here, it can be appreciated that a parallel design as in the Haptic Master allows for higher loads (compare Sect. 4.3.1), but at the cost of a smaller workspace in comparison to a serial design as in the PER-force or PHANTOM.

Joysticks are generally used in their main function as position input devices, e.g. for navigation in surgical VR systems (see Sect. 4.5), and force feedback can be added to inform the operator about collisions with soft or hard objects. For such navigation tasks, only a limited number of degrees of freedom and a low force range are usually required.

4.3.4.2 Ground- and Wall-Mounted Systems

Haptic displays can also be fixed to the ground or a wall (Fig. 4.20). Also most ground and wall-mounted systems work as endeffector-based systems, (Table 4.10).

Table 4.9 Technical data of representative desktop haptic display systems (DoF: degrees of freedom)

Display	DoF	Maximum load	Work space	Band width[a]
Sidewinder 2 Joystick, Microsoft	2	10 N	$36° \times 36°$	about 50 Hz
PER-Force, Cybernet Systems	2–6	53 N	10 cm; 90–180° per joint	100 Hz
PHANTOM 1.0, Sensable Tech.	3	10 N	$8 \times 17 \times 25$ cm^3	about 200 Hz
PHANTOM 3.0, Sensable Tech.	6	22 N	$42 \times 59 \times 82$ cm^3	about 200 Hz
Haptic Master, Nisho Electronics	6	69 N	$20 \times 40 \times 40$ cm^3	< 50 Hz

[a]at zero load, i.e. without user interaction

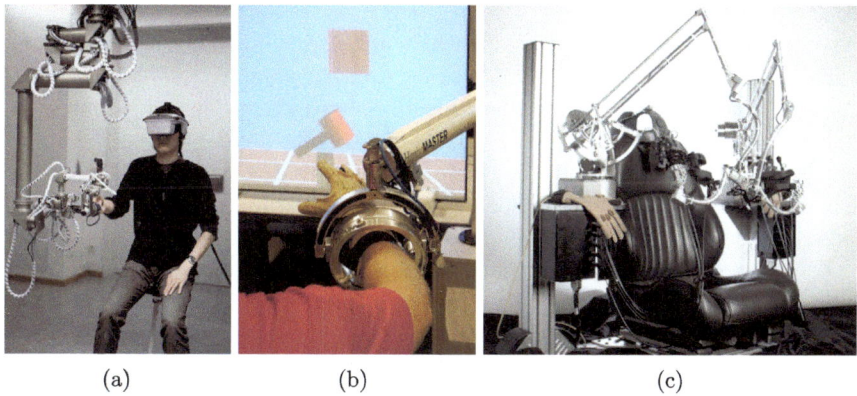

(a)   (b)   (c)

Fig. 4.20 Ground and wall-mounted haptic display systems: (**a**) Hyper-redundant haptic interface ViSHaRD10 (by courtesy of LSR, Technical University of Munich [31, 82] and SPRINGER), (**b**) HapticMASTER, Fokker Control Systems (by courtesy of S.V. Adamovich), (**c**) Haptic Workstation (by courtesy of CyberGlove Systems LLC)

Compared to desktop systems, these devices allow for a considerably heavier structure, and the transmission of larger forces. For example, the hyper-redundant display ViSHaRD10 (Fig. 4.20(a)) uses ten degrees of freedom to cover a very large workspace while avoiding singular configurations [82]. The Haptic Master (Fig. 4.20(b)) has a simpler kinematic design, but it covers a large workspace for the arm with high applicable force [83]. These properties make it a frequently employed device for studies in human motor learning or rehabilitation [54]. The Haptic Workstation is a 2-handed grounded force feedback systems designed for seating buck applications (Fig. 4.20(c)).

Table 4.10 Technical data of representative ground- and wall-mounted haptic display systems (DoF: degrees of freedom)

Display	DoF	Maximum load	Work space	Band width[a]
ViSHaRD10, TUM	10	100 N	$30 \times 30 \times 80$ cm^3	10–15 Hz
HapticMASTER, FCS	3	250 N	$36 \times 40 \times 46$ cm^3	–
PemRAM 303, Denne	3	5,000 N	36 cm, 40°	50 Hz
PemRAM 306, Denne	6	10,000 N	40 cm, 40°	50 Hz
SARCOS Master exoskeleton	10	97 Nm shoulder, 50 Nm elbow/hand, 5.5 Nm finger	180° shoulder, 105° elbow, >105° hand, 80°	10–100 Hz
FREFLEX Master exoskeleton, Odetics	7	25 N fist force	$125 \times 100 \times 75$ cm^3	20 Hz

[a]at zero load, i.e. without user interaction

4.3.4.3 Portable Systems

In contrast to desktop and ground-mounted haptic displays, portable systems can be worn by the user. With a portable device the user has more freedom to move, and it can by applied in different environments. In contrast to desktop and ground/wall-mounted systems, these devices are mostly of exoskeletal type, and the haptic interaction forces are usually induced via cuffs from the exoskeletal structure to the human limb. A drawback is that the user has to support the weight of the device. Thus, such devices should be small and lightweight.

Various portable systems have been developed for the hand, allowing to interact with and to assist human fine manipulation. Examples are the Rutgers Master II (Fig. 4.21) [5, 35, 42] that uses a sensing/feedback exoskeleton producing 16 N per finger, or the CyberGrasp (Fig. 4.1(b)). Heavier constructions are needed for the arms or in exoskeletons for the whole body, making portability a challenge for hardware design. Table 4.11 presents some technical data for this category.

4.3.4.4 Tactile Displays

Tactile displays are, for instance, applied in the area of sensory substitution for the disabled [37]. This includes, for example, tactile pin arrays to convey visual information to blind persons, and vibrotactile displays to transfer auditory information to hearing-impaired persons. Rather than mapping phenomena from one modality to another, tactile displays for teleoperation and virtual environments aim to replicate stimuli in the original sensory modality. Exploiting the modalities of the skin receptors, systems can be classified into pressure displays, vibration interfaces, pin arrays, electro-tactile displays, and temperature displays. Examples of such tactile displays are presented in the following.

Fig. 4.21 Rutgers Master II haptic glove was successfully used in stroke rehabilitation and in hand rehabilitation post Carpal Tunnel release surgery. Copyright Rutgers University. Reprinted by permission

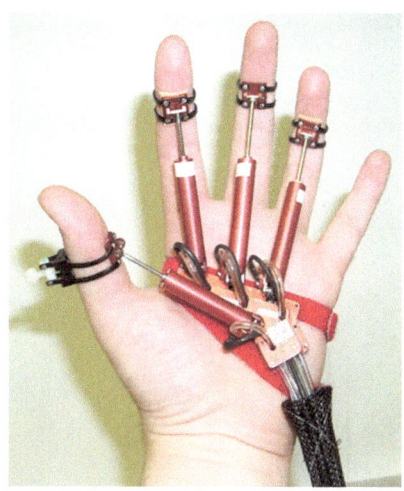

- **Pressure displays** The Teletact II glove displays tactile feedback through 30 air pockets located under the user's palm and fingers. The glove is controlled by a pneumatic actuator. The air pockets are fed by micro capillary tubes and can be inflated or deflated conveying the feeling of the simulated object. The glove displays two pressure ranges. The palm feedback pocket provides a maximum pressure of 30 psi, the other 29 pockets are limited to 15 psi.
- **Vibration interfaces** Vibrations can relay information about phenomena like surface texture, slip, impact, and puncture when sweeping over the objects [47]. In many situations, vibrations are experienced as diffuse and unlocalized, so a single vibrator for each finger or region of skin may be sufficient. The frequency range of interest is roughly a few Hertz to a few hundred Hertz, and effective single-channel devices are relatively easy to build. Kensington developed a computer

Table 4.11 Characteristics of the examples of portable haptic display systems (DoF: degrees of freedom)

Display	DoF	Maximum load	Work space	Band width[a]
Univ. of Salford Arm Master	7	1,000 N shoulder, 200 N hand	90% of physiol. range	1–2 Hz
EXOS ArmMaster	5	40 Nm shoulder, 13.4 Nm elbow	120° shoulder and elbow	30 Hz
GLAD-IN-ART Arm Exoskeleton	5	20 Nm shoulder, 10 Nm elbow	–	–
CyberGrasp Sensable Tech.	5 × 1	12 N per finger	physiological (only flexion)	–
LRP Hand Master	14	11 Nm	physiological	–
Rutgers Master II	4 × 1	16.4 N per finger	50–90°	15 Hz

[a]at zero load, i.e. without user interaction

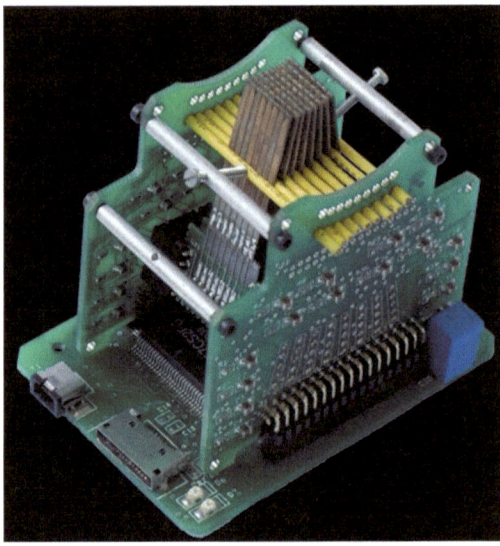

Fig. 4.22 Latero-tactile display, previously presented as $STReSS^2$; by courtesy of Vincent Hayward, www.tactilelabs.com

mouse that can produce vibrations in order to transfer some tactile information, when a user explores any image on a computer screen.

Merret et al. (2011) developed a mobile device that can produce tactile perception through vibration [56]. Two miniature vibration motors, as can be found in mobile phones and pagers, were attached to the digit finger and thumb. They had a nominal speed of 12,000 rpm (200 Hz). Merret et al. suggested to use their device for stroke rehabilitation.

TactaBelt uses vibrotactile cues on the torso, as a means of improving user performance in a spatial task. The vibrotactile stimuli are delivered using tactors placed at eight, evenly spaced compass points around the torso of the subject. The tactors are held in place by pressure using a neoprene belt. The tactors vibrate at a frequency of 142 Hz [11].

Another type of tactile glove is the CyberTouch, CyberGlove Systems LLC. CyberTouch^{TM} places small vibrotactile actuators on each fingertip and palm. The array of the actuators can generate pulses, vibrations, and even textures.

- **Pin and bar arrays** One of the most common design approaches is an array of closely-spaced pins that can be individually raised and lowered against the finger tip (or other regions of the body) to approximate the desired shape or texture. To match human finger movement speeds, bandwidths up to several ten Hertz may be required, and to match human perceptual resolution pin spacings of less than a few millimeters are required [37]. The pins are moved by piezoelectric, pneumatic, hydraulic, or electromagnetic actuators [61] (see Fig. 4.23). In addition, the display often must be small and light weight so that it can be mounted on a force-interface or carried by the user [72].

The STReSS tactile display can produce rapid sequences of tactile images at an update rate of 700 Hz, so called "tactile movies" (Fig. 4.22). An array of one hundred laterally moving skin contactors can create a time-varying programmable

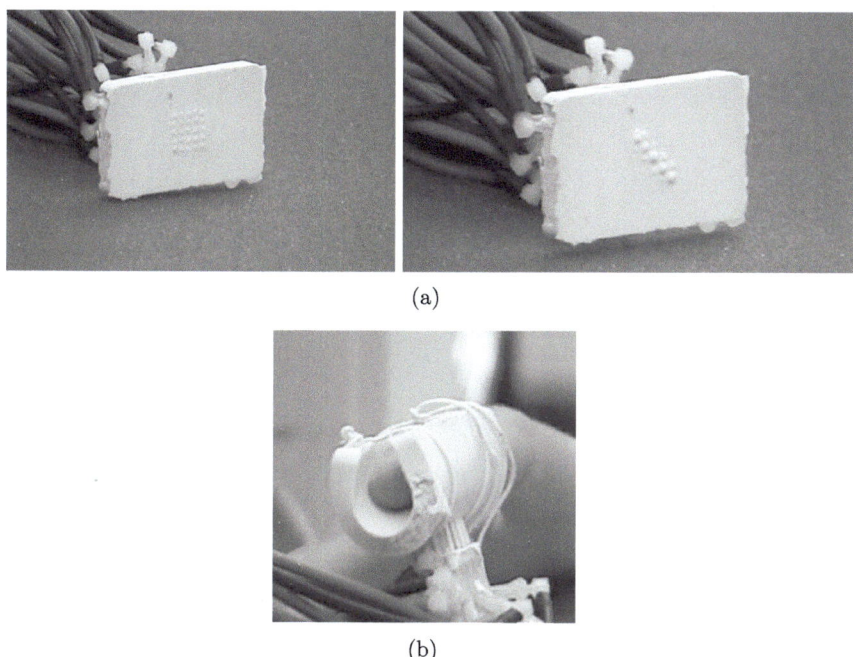

Fig. 4.23 Pneumatic pin array; © 2004 IEEE. Reprinted, with permission, from [61]

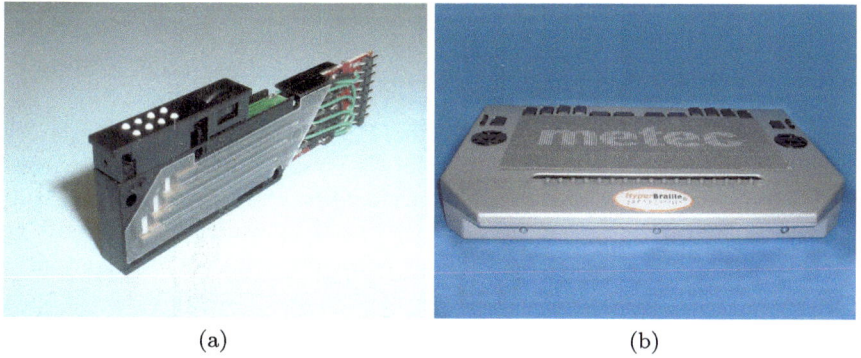

Fig. 4.24 Examples of tactile braille displays: (a) Braille cell, (b) Tactile tablet display; by courtesy of metec AG, Stuttgart, Germany

strain field at the skin surface. With one contactor per millimeter square, the device has a high spatial and temporal resolution [86, 87].

Braille modules are often realized by pin arrays in order to present tactile information to blind people. Such modules can be integrated into computer mice and keyboards to generate a tactile image of any screen picture and text (Fig. 4.24).

Fig. 4.25 FEELEX 2 can
deform a plane surface, e.g. to
simulate palpation of patients;
by courtesy of Hiroo Iwata

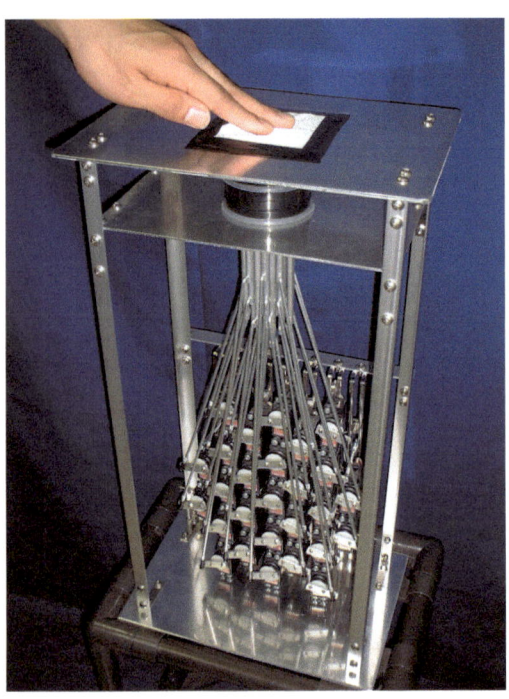

FEELEX 2 considers the situation of a medical doctor, who palpates a patient. It is composed of linear actuators, which deform a plane surface of 50 mm^2 (Fig. 4.25). The rods are 6 mm in diameter and 8 mm apart, arranged in a quadratic array. The stroke of the rod is 18 mm and can reach a speed of 250 mm/s. At the top of each rod, a force of 11 N can be applied by the maximum torque of 3.2 Nm of the servo-motor [41].

- **Electro-tactile displays** An electro-tactile display (also called electrocutaneous display) is a tactile device that activates nerve fibers directly within the skin with electrical current. Surface electrodes deliver electrical current, thus, sensations of pressure or vibration can be generated without the need of any mechanical actuator [11]. In the SmartTouch System, stainless steel electrodes, each 1 mm in diameter, are arranged as a 4×4 matrix. Using short pulses, selective stimulation of the Merkel cells (pressure sensation) and the Meissner corpuscles (vibratory sensation) was possible [45].
- **Thermal displays** Temperature changes can be produced by Peltier elements, which utilize the Peltier effect converting an electric voltage to a heat difference. Such temperature actuators typically have a small size and they can produce large temperature ranges and temperature gradients of 20°/s for heating. The cooling performance depends on the thermal mass of the device, i.e. its passive temperature conduction/convection properties. Other systems use cold and hot air or liquid, which is transported to the region of interest via little pumps and pipes. Climatic chambers can also be considered as temperature displays, where the im-

Table 4.12 Technical data of representative tactile displays

Displays	Channels	Mechanical Impedance	Temporal Resolution	Spatial Resolution
Teleact Glove II, pneumatic	30 air pockets	high	low	30 channels per hand
Kensington Orbit Mouse	1 vibrator	low	high	1 channel per hand
Pin array, Shinohara, motors	4096 pins	high	low	3 mm per distance
Braille module, electromagnetic	8 pins per module	low	> 10 Hz	2.5 mm per distance
STReSS, tactile labs	100 contactors	–	> 700 Hz	1 mm per distance
FEELEX 2	23 rods	–	7 Hz	8 mm between rods

pression of hot and humid or cold and wet air can be displayed to the entire human body.

A general overview of the properties of each tactile display device is given in Table 4.12.

4.4 Haptic Rendering

Haptic rendering refers to the process of creating haptic impressions or force feed-back from a virtual environment through haptic displays. The process consists of two main steps: collision detection and contact force computation.

Collision detection is a process to detect the intersection occurring between the user (in the virtual environment) and the virtual object the user is interacting with. As soon as the interacting body part of the user (e.g. the user's fingertip) penetrates the virtual object, a collision between the user and the object takes place, which implies that the user touches the virtual object. Haptic devices must then render reaction forces that prevent the user from penetrating too deep into the virtual object. The rendered force should resemble the contact force when touching an equivalent object in a real scenario. Some basic haptic rendering techniques for rigid objects of simple geometry are explained in the following sections.

4.4.1 Penalty Method

When a user interacts with a virtual rigid wall (Fig. 4.26), the penalty method can be used to compute the appropriate contact force (Fig. 4.27). The position of the user's fingertip in the virtual environment is described by the point **P**, which also

Fig. 4.26 PHANTOM device used to render contact forces in a virtual Nine Hole Peg Test (NHPT) to assess grasping and placing abilities of patients suffering from different neurological pathologies [26, 30], by courtesy of RELab, ETH Zurich, Switzerland. (**a**) before collision; (**b**) during collision

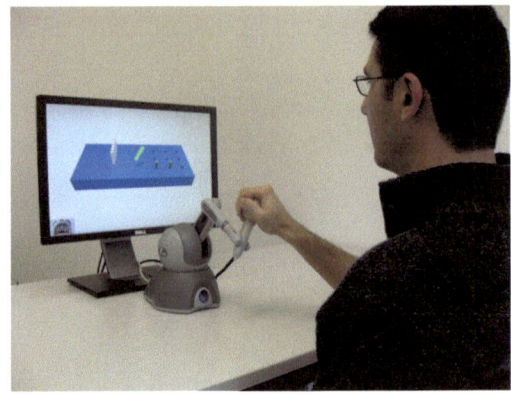

represents the user as *avatar*[3] in this example (Fig. 4.27(a)). This (finger) avatar can also be called *haptic point*. The position of the avatar in the virtual environment is updated according to the actual position of the user's fingertip.

As soon as the collision is detected (the avatar is inside the virtual wall), a repulsive force will be computed that acts against the user's motion, in order to prevent the user from penetrating further into the virtual wall. The force is determined as a function of the penetration depth, velocity, and the impedance of the virtual wall (Fig. 4.27(b)).

It is important that the sampling rate be as high as possible. If the rate is too low, the avatar may penetrate too deep into the wall, resulting in unreasonably high repulsive forces. If the wall is thin, the avatar may pass through it. As a rule of thumb, the sampling rate for haptic displays should be around 1,000 Hz in order to ensure stability and to avoid vibrations. The exact required minimum frequency depends on the virtual scenario (impedances of objects the user interacts with) and physical damping properties of the haptic display.

The force response can be described by viscoelastic properties of the virtual wall and be computed from:

$$\mathbf{F} = C(\mathbf{x} - \mathbf{x}_w)^n - B(\mathbf{x} - \mathbf{x}_w)^n \dot{\mathbf{x}}, \tag{4.7}$$

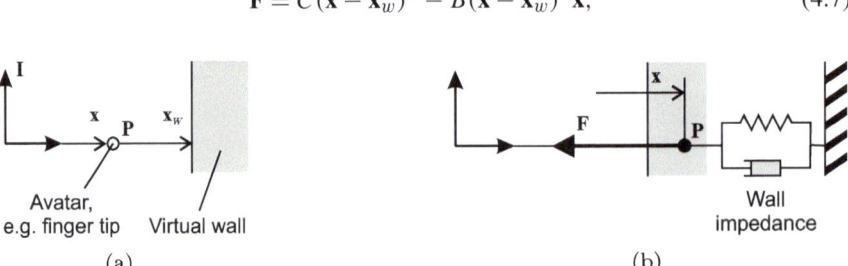

Fig. 4.27 Haptic rendering of a rigid wall applying the penalty method. (**a**) before collision; (**b**) during collision

---

[3]The word avatar is normally used in the context of full embodiment in virtual worlds.

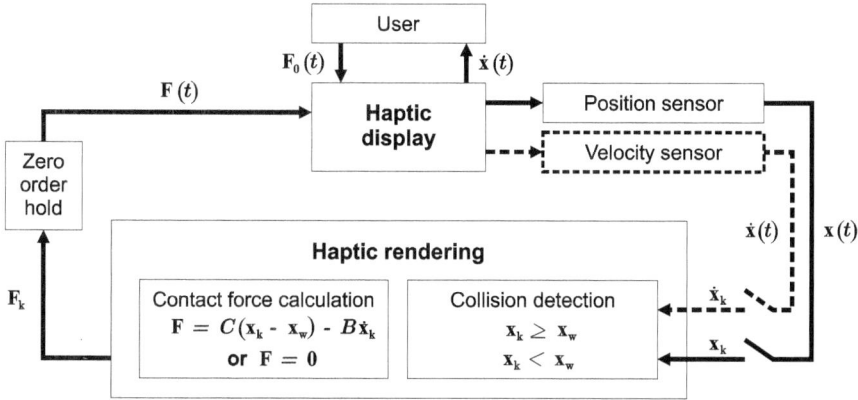

Fig. 4.28 Haptic rendering: Implementation of the impedance architecture

or in a simpler, linearised way from:

$$F = C(x - x_w) - B\dot{x}, \tag{4.8}$$

where x is the avatar's position, x_w is the wall's position, C is the virtual stiffness coefficient, and B is the virtual viscous coefficient. In this one-dimensional example, all variables are scalars. Such a haptic rendering algorithm can be implemented in an impedance architecture (Fig. 4.28). There, the continuous variable x is sampled to the discrete variable x_k, which is then used for control.

4.4.1.1 Numerical Problems

There are two main problems related to haptic rendering. The first problem is the *sampling time* problem. As mentioned earlier, too low sampling rates (large sampling time T_s) can result in high forces:

$$F = Cv T_s \tag{4.9}$$

where C is the stiffness of the object, and v is the penetration velocity (see also Fig. 4.29(a)). Viscous effects are neglected in this consideration. Too high forces F may cause vibrations, when the avatar jumps between contact and contact-free states.

The second problem is called the *active wall* problem. In theory, the stiffness of a spring can be approximated by a linear function between the force and the length of the spring (i.e. the depth of penetration). Due to discretization effects, the stiffness of the virtual spring is not a linear function anymore, but a staircase function (Fig. 4.29(b)). This causes an energy imbalance between the stretching and relaxing process. Thus, energy is accumulated, which can result in vibration. To avoid this situation, it is recommended to employ a high sampling rate T_s, a high

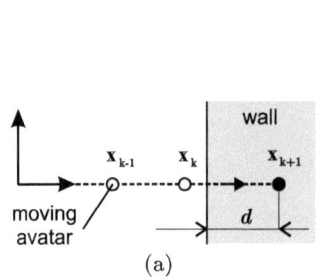

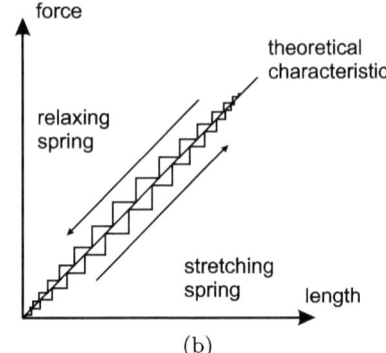

(a)   (b)

Fig. 4.29 Numerical problems of haptic rendering: (**a**) Sampling time problem, and (**b**) active wall problem

Fig. 4.30 Vector Field
Method: (**a**) Problem that can
appear in the penalty method.
When the avatar is near the
corner of the square, the
direction of the force is not
clear. (**b**) The Vector Field
Method divides the volume
into small regions. Each
region is assigned to a
particular direction (edge) in
order to avoid ambiguity

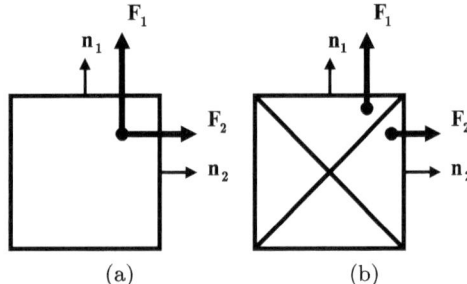

viscosity B of the virtual object, and high physical damping b of the haptic display.
To render a certain stiffness K, the necessary physical damping b is given by [17]:

$$b > \frac{K T_s}{2} + B. \tag{4.10}$$

4.4.2 Vector Field Method

Since a virtual wall represents an infinite planar boundary, the repulsive force can
be simply computed by the penalty method. However, for 3D objects with complex surface geometries, a number of difficulties arise when applying the penalty
method. For example, when the avatar is located inside the object and near a corner,
the direction of the reaction force may become ambiguous (there are two possible
directions, see Fig. 4.30(a)).

The Vector Field Method (also called Volume Method) [90] is used to solve this
ambiguity. The method divides the object into small sub-regions. A certain force

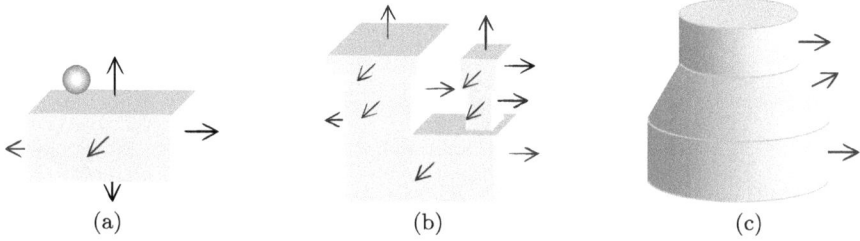

Fig. 4.31 Vector field methods for 3D objects

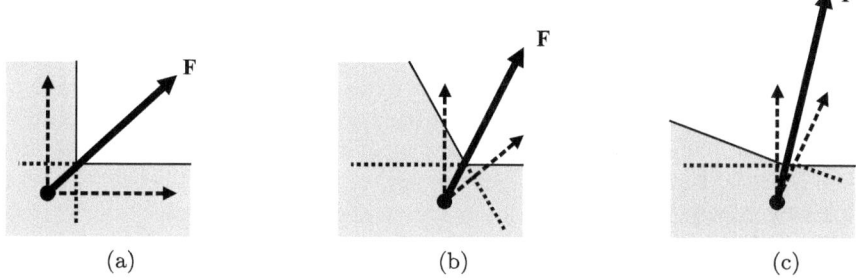

Fig. 4.32 Problem with concave corners and edges

direction is assigned to each region, and it is displayed when the avatar is inside the region (Fig. 4.30(b)). This method can convey the feeling of sharpness at the corner of a virtual object. This feeling is generated by a sudden discontinuity of the simulated force when the avatar is moving from one region to another one when passing the corner.

This method can be expanded to three-dimensional objects (Fig. 4.31). They can be considered as a combination of simpler object volumes, e.g. cubes, cones, and cylinders.

4.4.2.1 Concave Corners and Edges

When the avatar approaches concave corners, the net reaction force could be computed from the summation of the force vectors contributed from each single surface patch. However, this method will not always give the correct reaction force. When the corner has a right angle, the vector field method gives an appropriate reaction force from the summation of the two force vectors (Fig. 4.32(a)). However, at obtuse (or acute) corners, the reaction force becomes larger (smaller) than expected. For instance, if the angle is close to 180°, the force equals almost twice the desired reaction force (Fig. 4.32(c)). Therefore, model extensions are necessary to achieve acceptable rendering results with the Vector Field Method.

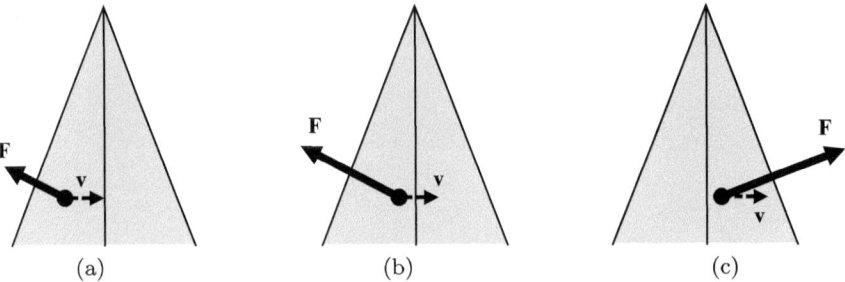

Fig. 4.33 Problems with the Vector Field Method at convex corners and edges

4.4.2.2 Convex Corners and Edges

Applying a linear model, the depth of penetration of the avatar is proportional to the force applied by the user. The deeper the avatar penetrates into the object, the higher is the force. In some cases, if the object is too soft or the user applies too high forces, the avatar may go to another region, which is not associated with the originally penetrated surface patch. As a result, the system may render an incorrect haptic feedback resulting in forces pulling the avatar out of the virtual object instead of resisting the user's action. This problem is often found at sharp convex corners (Fig. 4.33).

The Vector Field Method is an attractive solution to render simple objects, which have a limited number of corners and edges or geometries that can be expressed by analytical functions. However, with complex geometries, such as anatomical objects (organs, bones, etc.), which need to be described by a high number of polygons, the Vector Field Method becomes very inconvenient and is, therefore, not recommended.

4.4.3 God-Object Method

The God-Object method can be used to render rigid objects with complex geometries and particular surface properties (friction, texture). Therefore, it is well suited for medical scenarios, especially, when dealing with non-deformable objects such as bone. The God-Object represents a projection of the avatar's position onto the surface of the virtual object (Fig. 4.34), and it always remains on the surface of the virtual object [25, 90]. This provides a kind of memory about the side, where the object has been entered. The God-Object can also be called (virtual) proxy. When the user pushes the avatar into the object, the response force can be computed as a function of the distance between the God-Object and the avatar. Because the God-Object remains on the surface of the object, the direction of the force can be determined without ambiguity. This method provides steady forces and is suitable for arbitrary polygonal and thin objects. The God-Object can be considered equivalently as an ideal location of the avatar if the virtual object had infinite stiffness.

Fig. 4.34 God-Object
derived from the avatar
location, when approaching
and touching a virtual wall

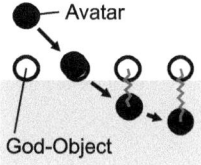

4.4.3.1 Transitions Between Surfaces

When the user interacts with a convex geometry (Fig. 4.35(a)), the transition of
the God-Object between two surfaces sharing a common edge can be done in two
steps [90]. Firstly, the method checks in each time step whether the position of the
God-Object is on the active surface (left surface). As soon as it leaves the active
surface, the projection of the avatar on the new surface must be computed and used
as a new God-Object. Thus, the new surface becomes the active surface for the
current time step.

When the user interacts with a concave geometry, both surfaces are active surfaces (Fig. 4.35(b)). Therefore, the God-Object is restricted to the corner between
the two surfaces. The force direction is determined by the connecting line between
avatar and God-Object.

4.4.3.2 Rendering Texture

Additional effects that can be displayed by haptic displays are friction and texture
of the surface. Friction can be added as a tangential force, F_t, to the surface of the
object resisting the movement of the avatar. The friction force can be either static,

Fig. 4.35 God-Object
method (**a**) Convex corners
and edges, (**b**) concave
corners and edges

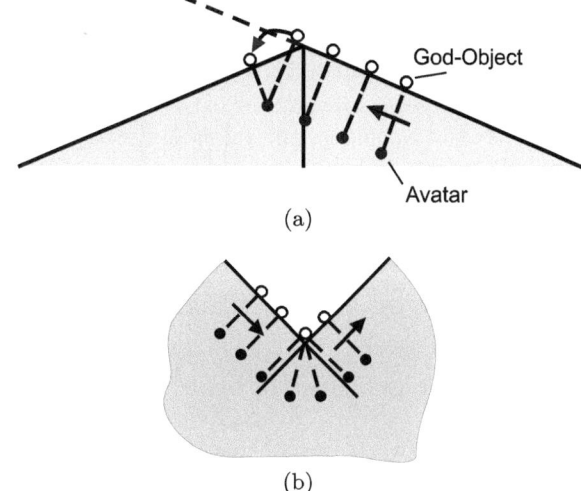

F_t, or dynamic, $F_{t,dyn}$, or a combination of both in order to simulate stick-and-slip effects.

To render static and dynamic friction, the system needs to switch between two different cases: *Static friction:* Fix God-Object as long as

$$|F_t| < \mu_s |F_n|, \tag{4.11}$$

Dynamic friction: Combination of viscous and Coulomb friction

$$F_{t,dyn} = b|v_{God}| + \mu_d |F_n|, \tag{4.12}$$

where μ_s is the static friction coefficient, μ_d is the dynamic friction coefficient, b is the damping coefficient, and v_{God} the velocity of the God-Object on the surface.

Texture effects can be simulated by introducing time and location dependent functions for the tangential and normal forces.

4.4.4 Force Shading Method

A well-known problem in haptic rendering of polygonal models is the so-called *edge effect*. When a polygonal surface is explored with the constraint-based God-Object method, one can feel the edges of the surface due to the abrupt change in the rendered force direction across adjacent polygons.

Force shading was developed to minimize undesirable edge effects during haptic rendering of smooth objects, such as a cylinder or sphere, which are approximated by polygonal meshes [59]. The idea of force shading has been taken from 3D computer graphics, where the technique is used to achieve smooth lighting on the surface of polygonal models (see Sect. 3.4.5). The force shading algorithm was built on the basis of the God-Object haptic rendering method.

Contact points and magnitude of the rendered forces caused by the penetration of the polygonal surface are initially determined by the God-Object method. Then, the force shading algorithm computes the new direction of the feedback force while retaining the force magnitude. When the force is computed, an interpolation step must be performed to calculate the local normal of the force from normal vectors at each vertex of the polygon. This interpolation step is very similar to that used in the Phong shading algorithm in computer graphics applications (compare Sect. 3.4.3).

For a polygon with three vertices, the direction of the interpolated normal vector at the point of contact can be computed by:

$$\mathbf{N}_0 = \frac{\sum_{i=1}^{3}(x_i(\sum_{j=1}^{3}\mathbf{N}_j - \mathbf{N}_i))}{\sum_{i=1}^{3}x_i}, \tag{4.13}$$

where x_i is the distance from the contact point to each vertex with associated normal $\mathbf{N}_i$ (Fig. 4.36).

The results between the God-Object force rendering method and the force shading method can be quite different (Fig. 4.37).

Fig. 4.36 Interpolated
normal at the proxy position

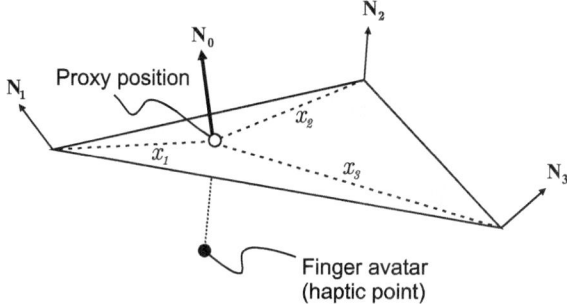

4.4.5 Two-Pass Force Shading Method

Ruspini et al. (1997) [67] proposed a two-pass force shading approach that can correctly handle multiple active surfaces and surface effects such as friction or texture, thereby improving the stability of the solutions. The algorithm results in a modification of the proxy position (God-Object position), leaving the resultant force always perpendicular to the original surface of the smooth object.

After the first pass of the force shading procedure, the interpolated normal is used to specify a new constraint plane, which contains the contact point. The algorithm proceeds forwards by, first, finding a sub-goal point using the interpolated plane instead of the original constraint planes. This sub-goal point is then treated as the user's finger position, and the second pass of the force shading procedure is performed to obtain the final goal. This second pass is performed using the actual (non-interpolated) constraint planes. While this approach is slightly more computationally expensive than the original force shading method, it properly considers the effect of all constraint surfaces in both two passes, and it produces a correct result even if multiple active surfaces exist (Fig. 4.38).

If the sub-goal position is located above all original constraint planes after the first pass, the sub-goal must be projected back onto the nearest original constraint plane. This guarantees that the new sub-goal point will always be on the object surface and that surface effects such as friction and texture will be handled correctly [67].

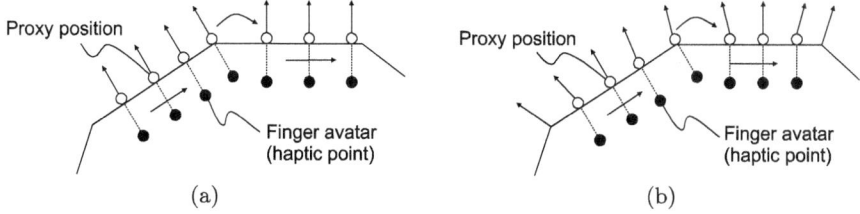

Fig. 4.37 Comparison of the proxy positions computed by (**a**) constraint-based God-Object method, and (**b**) force shading method

Fig. 4.38 Illustration of the two-pass force shading algorithm; [67], 1997 Association for Computing Machinery, Inc. Reprinted by permission

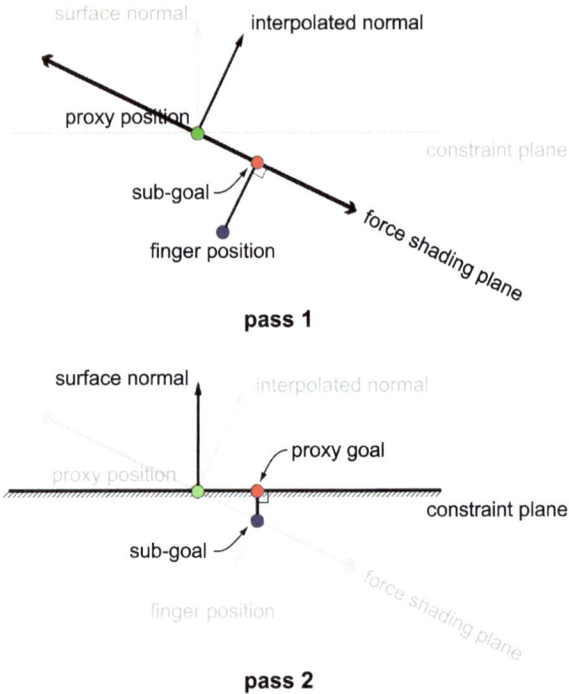

Note that force shading may increase the distance between the user's avatar position and the position of the proxy (God-Object). This increase implies that the surface is active and can transfer net energy to the user. In general, the added energy is very small and should not be noticeable by the user. In contrast to the original force shading method, the two-pass force shading method keeps the proxy on the polygonal surface (Fig. 4.39). This way, its motion is continuous, such that the resultant force feels smooth to the user (Fig. 4.39(b)) [67].

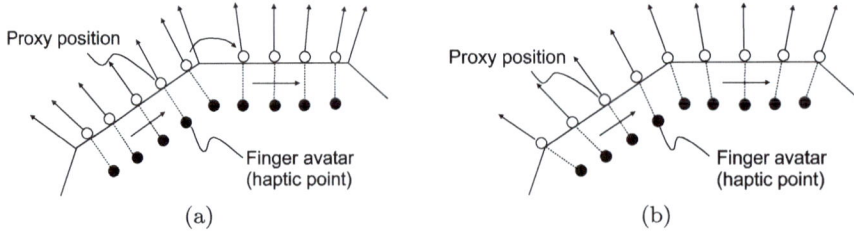

Fig. 4.39 Comparison of the proxy positions computed by (**a**) the original force shading method, and (**b**) two-pass force shading method

Fig. 4.40 Finding
subsequent contact point,
$\mathbf{P}_{1,t+1}$, by projecting $\mathbf{P}_{0,t+1}$
onto last tangent plane $\mathbf{T}_t$ to
find $\mathbf{P}'_{0,t+1}$. Then, $\mathbf{P}_{1,t+1}$ is
found on $\mathbf{S}$ as a closest point
to $\mathbf{P}'_{0,t+1}$ by gradient iteration
method

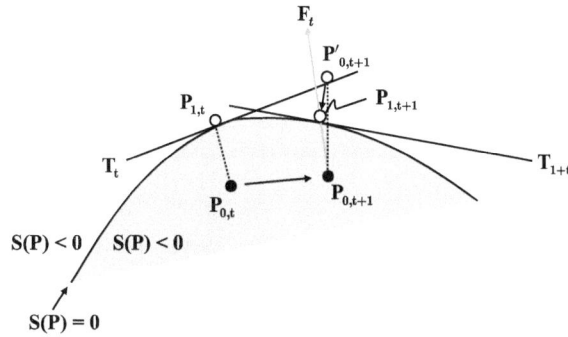

4.4.6 Haptic Rendering of Implicit Surfaces

An implicit surface is a geometric representation of a smooth curved surface, commonly used to represent simple geometrical shapes such as quadratic surfaces. Recent efforts have developed techniques to reconstruct surfaces in implicit forms from scattered points [68]. The implicit surface can be described in a compact and analytical mathematical form as $\mathbf{S}(\mathbf{P}) = 0$. This equality defines the set of points $\mathbf{P}$ on the surface of the implicit surface. Points located inside the surface satisfy $\mathbf{S}(\mathbf{P}) < 0$, while points located outside the surface satisfy $\mathbf{S}(\mathbf{P}) > 0$. For example, the surface of a sphere centered in the origin and with radius 1 is represented by the equation $x^2 + y^2 + z^2 - 1 = 0$.

When the virtual haptic point ($\mathbf{P}_0$) penetrates the surface (i.e. $\mathbf{S}(\mathbf{P}_0)$ is negative), we define the state of $\mathbf{S}$ as being touched [68]. The closest point on the implicit surface ($\mathbf{P}_1$), considered as a surface contact point (or proxy object), is tracked iteratively by using the gradient method, and it is maintained on the surface by constraining it to the local tangent plane $\mathbf{T}$ at the preceding closest point.

To determine this local closest point in each subsequent time step, the current haptic point is projected onto the constraint tangent plane (in normal direction to the plane) that has been computed at the preceding contact point, resulting in $\mathbf{P}'_0$. The new contact point $\mathbf{P}_1$ is found on $\mathbf{S}$ as the closest point to $\mathbf{P}'_0$ (Fig. 4.40).

The elastic force $\mathbf{F} = k(\mathbf{P}_1 - \mathbf{P}_0)$, as computed from the distance between the virtual probe position and the closest point, is applied to the user.

4.4.7 Direct Haptic Rendering of NURBS Models

Implicit surfaces can represent the shapes of sculpted surfaces conveniently, but they can hardly render the shape precisely. NURBS (Non-Uniform Rational B-Splines) are another choice of surface representation that allows precise control of the shape of a 3D model with parametric variables [64, 81]. NURBS are often used in 3D graphics modeling and CAD applications. Advantages of the NURBS representation include a compact mathematical representation, higher-order continuity, and exact computation of surface normals [81]. A complex sculpted model, sharp boundaries, or holes can be created from multiple NURBS surfaces. However, one disadvantage is that one may encounter difficulties generating a NURBS surface out of an unstructured point cloud taken from an existing polygonal surface model.

NURBS surfaces are piecewise-polynomial vector functions of two parametric directions (**u** and **v**). The shape of a NURBS surface is locally influenced by a set of weighted control points, polynomial order and knot vector. Each polynomial surface is entirely enclosed in the convex hull of its control points.

As computations for NURBS are more complex than for polygonal models, realtime haptic rendering using NURBS can be restricted. In general, haptic rendering methods use distance and direction from a virtual avatar (haptic point) to the global closest point found on the touched surface in order to compute the force response. An analogous technique also exists for NURBS surfaces, where we can compute a global closest point on a surface **S** to an avatar **P** by solving for the roots of:

$$(\mathbf{S} - \mathbf{P}) \times (\mathbf{S}^u \times \mathbf{S}^v) = 0. \tag{4.14}$$

The roots can be found iteratively, for instance, using gradient descent. However, the equation system may involve high-order polynomials, making the solution difficult and intensive to compute [81]. In addition, this global closest point may jump discontinuously on the surface as the avatar moves, which can produce discontinuous haptic forces. Using the closest point in the local neighborhood of the preceding time step's solution instead produces smooth haptic feedback.

Thompson [80] presented a direct haptic rendering for NURBS surfaces. The technique is broken down into four main phases: Surface proximal testing, surface tracking, contact and tracing, and transition phases. These phases will be explained in the following.

4.4.7.1 Surface Proximal Testing

Instead of using a collision detection algorithm that reacts to contacts that already took place, the surface proximal testing method approximates the distance from the avatar point to the closest points on the NURBS surfaces at the time before the contacts occurs, allowing the system to predict potential contacts that may occur in one of the next time steps [81].

Since the virtual environment may contain multiple NURBS surfaces, checking for possible contact must be done for each surface. A rough check for surface proximity uses the bounding box around individual NURBS surfaces to determine the closest surfaces, which quickly reduces the number of surface candidates. For the remaining NURBS surfaces, called active surfaces, we find the first-order approximation to the closest points on each surface by projecting the avatar position, **P**, onto the control polygon of the surface, resulting in a point **P′** [81]. Then, we compute approximate parametric values, (**u**, **v**), of **P′** on this control polygon by using an interpolation technique (barycentric coordinates). The first-order approximate closest point **P″** on the surface is obtained by evaluating the surface equation

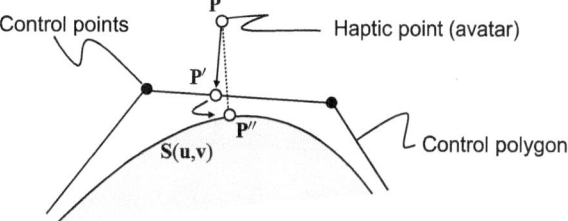

Fig. 4.41 Projection onto the control polygon and nodal mapping of the first-order approximate closest point on the control polygon to the NURBS surface

from this interpolated parameter $(\mathbf{u}, \mathbf{v})$, which leads to $\mathbf{P}'' = \mathbf{S}(\mathbf{u}, \mathbf{v})$. This process is called "nodal mapping" (Fig. 4.41). The distance between $\mathbf{P}''$ and $\mathbf{P}$ is the surface proximal distance to the virtual avatar.

4.4.7.2 Tracking Phase

Each active surface identified in the surface proximity testing phase has its local closest point. This point must be tracked until it is deactivated. The computations for determining the position of this point must be processed at the sampling rates of the haptic display, i.e. in the order of kHz. The "direct parametric tracking" method [80, 81] takes advantage of the parametric NURBS surface, making the tracking process fast enough to track these points at the force update rate.

Given the movement of an avatar point, one can track the new closest point by computing the corresponding change in the parametric space of the point on the surface ($\Delta\mathbf{u}$ and $\Delta\mathbf{v}$). However, instead of finding an exact change of the parameter space on the surface, one can use linear approximation to the surface (i.e. the tangent plane) to compute an approximate change of the parametric values. This approximation is done by projecting the new avatar point $\mathbf{P}$ on the surface tangent plane $\mathbf{T}$ at the preceding approximated closest point. The new closest point and the new tangent plane are found via parametric projection (Fig. 4.42). For further details, see [81].

4.4.7.3 Contact and Tracing

As described by Thompson II et al. (1997), contact is initiated when the penetration depth of the closest active surface is larger than zero. When a surface has been contacted, it is considered as "current" surface. During contact, the current surface's local closest point, $\mathbf{C}^*$, is updated in the same manner as during the tracking phase. However, the remaining active surface's local closest points, $\mathbf{C}_i$, are updated using $\mathbf{C}^*$ instead of $\mathbf{P}$. This allows efficient surface transition computations [81].

Once a surface has become current, it remains current until a transition either leaving the object or onto an adjacent surface occurs. This tracing method can prevent several problems including pushing through a model, force discontinuities, and inability to generate sufficient restoring forces due to lack of penetration depth [81].

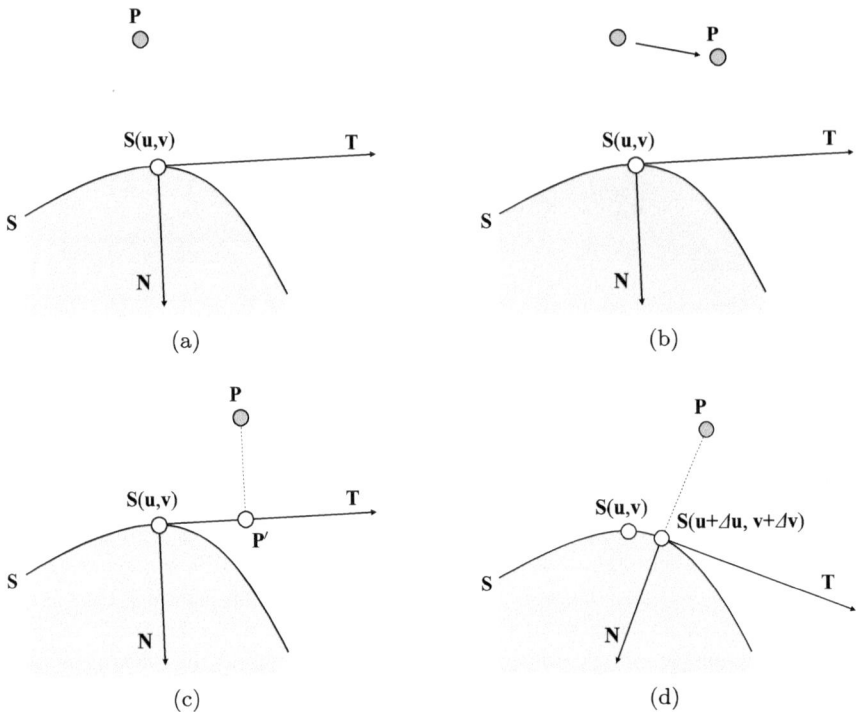

Fig. 4.42 Surface closest point tracking process: (**a**) initial state, (**b**) haptic point moves, (**c**) projection of surface haptic point onto the tangent plane, (**d**) new surface closest point and tangent plane found via parametric projection; adapted from [81]

4.4.7.4 Transitions

Most sculptured models often consist of multiple surfaces. It is necessary for the tracing algorithm to move from one surface onto another. This computation directly affects the resulting closest point, surface normal and penetration depth, and it must be performed in the haptic process. There are three main stages to the transition problem: Edge detection, selection of an appropriate surface onto which to transition, and the calculation of an appropriate normal. One special form of transition is a transition off the current surface and into free space [80, 81].

The edge detection can be performed in a parametric domain by detecting when the parametric values of C^* and (u, v), are on the boundary of the parametric domain. Once the edge has been detected, the next appropriate surface onto which to transition must be determined. Each of the active surfaces is tracked using C^* instead of P. Each C_i is, therefore, an approximation to the closest point on neighboring surfaces to C^*. When C^* lies on an edge, there will be a corresponding C_j on the adjacent surface that equals C^*. This surface is changed to current status, and the previous current surface returns to active status. The tracking algorithm is applied

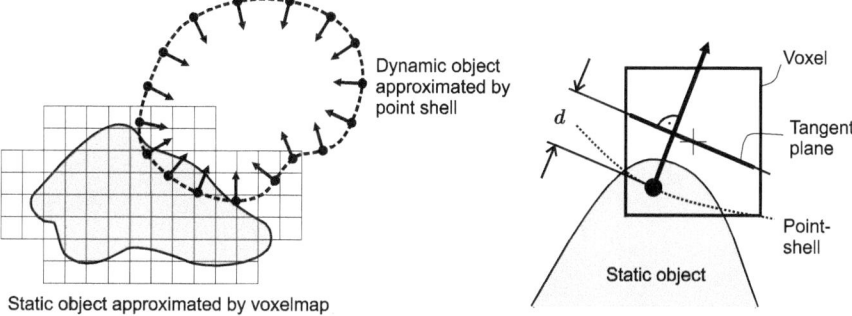

Fig. 4.43 Point-shell voxelmap method

to the new current surface using the avatar position **P**, so that this C_j represents the local closest point to **P** and can, therefore, be referred to as C^*.

If the new C^* does not lie on an edge, then the normal on the new current surface at C^* is used to compute the penetration depth and the reaction force. If it lies on the edge, special care must be taken in choosing the normal. This normal, **N**, is the normalized sum of the normals of the current and of the previously current surfaces, or a vector pointing along a line from **P** to C^* [81]. Although both choices can have undesirable side effects, these are generally not noticeable for small penetration depths.

4.4.8 Point-Shell Voxelmap Method

This method [44] is suitable for interaction between two surfaces, for example when objects collide (Fig. 4.43). The moving object (dynamic object) is represented by a set of points, which form the volume of the object (the so-called point shell). The passive object (static object) is approximated by a voxelmap representation.

As soon as one or more points of the point shell lie inside the voxels of the passive object, a collision is detected, and the contact force is computed. The contact force vector generated by each point on the point shell has a direction perpendicular to the point shell's surface. The amount of force is computed from the distance between the collision point and a plane that is normal to the force vector and passes the center of the collided voxels.

If there are more than one collision points, the net force can be determined by the sum of the force vectors computed at each collision point of the point shell.

An advantage of this method compared to the God-Object method, and further methods presented before, is that it allows the rendering of multiple-point contacts, or even of surface contacts, in a simple way. A major disadvantage is that the generated contact force can be discontinuous when sliding along the surface and transiting from one voxel to the next. This effect can be alleviated by an increase in the number of voxels.

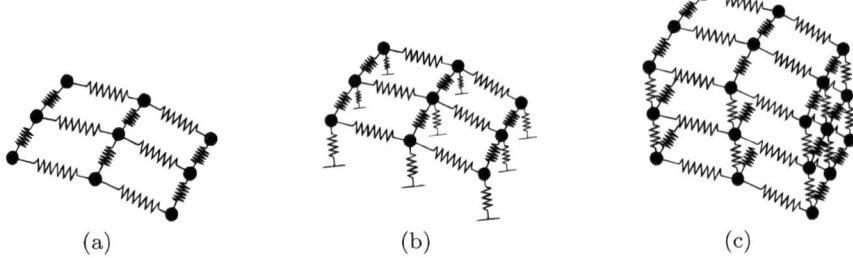

Fig. 4.44 Different spring-mass models to describe deformable objects. (**a**) Surface model; (**b**) Surface model with two layers; (**c**) Volume model

4.4.9 Rendering of Deformable Objects

Many medical applications require the haptic interaction with deformable objects, like abdominal or soft organs. To simulate deformable objects, spring-mass models are frequently employed [8, 21]. There, several mass points are connected by spring-damper elements (Fig. 4.44).

The motion of such a system can be described by a set of second-order differential equations, where the number of mass points determines the number of equations.

To geometrically represent deformable tissue, either a surface or a volume model can be generated. The choice depends on the available calculation time and the required degree of realism. The main advantage of surface models is low computational load and low demands on memory. However, they are only well-suited for hollow organs like bladder, intestine, or blood vessels. For massive organs, surface models are accurate only for small deformations. Volume models allow to simulate also large deformations of massive bodies [57]. A compromise between model complexity and achievable realism is represented by two-layer surface models [49].

Rendering of deformable objects is very challenging, because collision detection parameters must change as the surface of the soft tissue deforms. This deformation is due to the actions of various different material layers and areas of the tissue, whose properties are hardly known and too complex to be rendered in real-time [14]. Therefore, simplifications are usually required to allow a sufficiently fast response behavior. Moore and Molley present a broad overview of deformable models with a wide range of applications [58]. Other, more detailed and specific surveys are provided by Nealen et al., 2006 [62], and Meier et al., 2005 [53], who focus on visual fidelity of graphics animations and real-time surgical simulations, respectively. Recently, Famaey and Vander Sloten, 2008, published a detailed overview on continuum mechanics models applied to minimally invasive surgical simulators [29]. More details on soft tissue deformation are presented in Chap. 11.

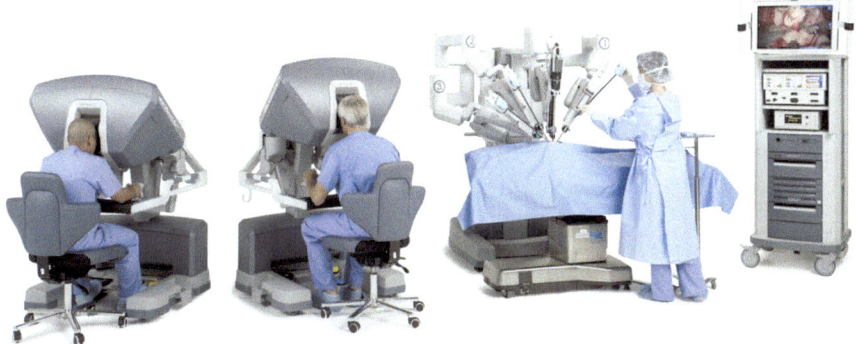

Fig. 4.45 Robotic surgery with the telemanipulation system "da Vinci", © 2011 Intuitive Surgical, Inc. [38, 76]

4.5 Applications of Haptic Displays in Medical VR

Haptic feedback is important for VR, because it substantially contributes to the user's sense of presence, targeting an additional perception channel besides vision and sound. In addition, haptic interaction is highly intuitive and can greatly simplify interaction with a virtual environment.

In medicine, haptics is currently used in a wide spectrum of different applications. For example, it can be used to provide easier manipulation in the case of robotic surgery, where a surgeon uses a computer to manipulate a robot. Haptics is used in medical simulators to provide an increased sense of immersion, such as in the endoscopy, laparoscopy, or endovascular simulator (Fig. 4.46) by the company CAE Healthcare (www.cae.com/healthcare) [9], the bone drilling simulator for surgeons [27]. Currently, the famous da Vinci Surgical System by Intuitive Surgical (Fig. 4.45) is being extended to also provide haptic feedback for minimally invasive surgical interventions. Robotic surgery provides the benefit of allowing more precise and steady handling of surgical instruments. Another example for applications of a haptic display is the Munich Knee Joint Simulator for orthopedic education (see Sect. 8.3.2). Physical rehabilitation is another area where haptics is often used (see Sect. 7). The device developed by Burdea (Fig. 7.1) applies forces to the foot of a patient and is used for rehabilitation after ankle injuries [22]. Reviews of rehabilitation robots can be found in [34] and [23].

The choice of a force feedback device depends on the requirements of the particular medical procedure or scenario to be imitated. Choosing a commercial device for specific medical applications may not work out, because the device may not fulfill the required workspace, number of degrees of freedom, accuracy, precision, etc. [14]. For example, the resolution of both position and rotation sensing need to meet the requirements of the task: if a procedure requires millimeter translational precision, a device with coarser resolution would not be suited. Even a device with too high fidelity can be a problem, as it can transfer too high frequency compo-

Fig. 4.46 Applications of haptic displays in medical training: (**a**) The CAE LaparoscopyVR surgical simulator, (**b**) the CAE EndoscopyVR simulator, (**c**) the CathLabVR simulator; photos by courtesy of CAE Healthcare

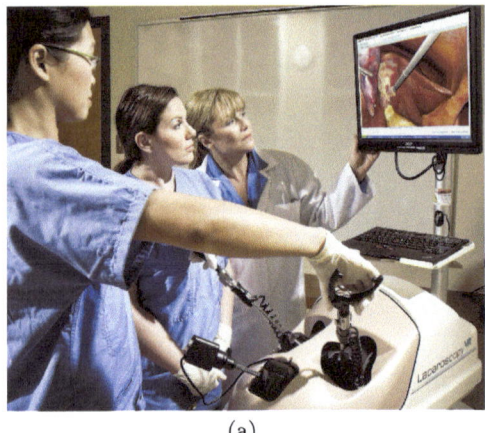

(a)

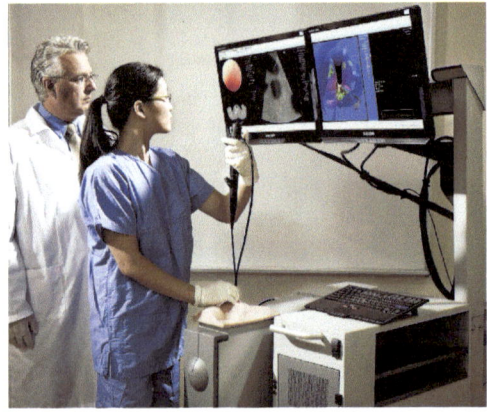

(b)

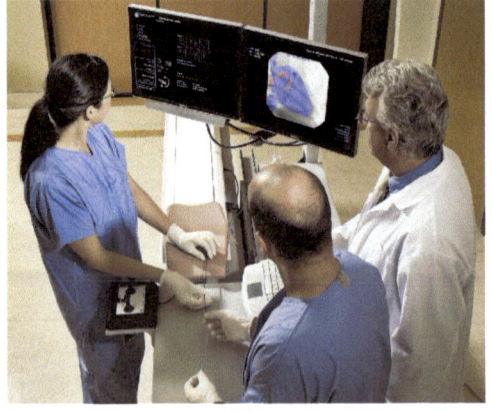

(c)

nents (resulting from collision or noise) to the operator, thus, causing an unnatural perception of the scenario.

Tactile feedback in medical applications allows medical doctors to feel the texture of tissues, to provide force feedback from medical instruments, or to display the temperature of a patient's skin, etc. Tactile feedback plays an essential role in non-invasive palpation of human skin and organs, palpation of pulse or breathing function, touch and movement of body segments, invasive palpation of pathologic tissue, e.g. tumors, invasive palpation of calcificated blood vessels, and palpation of increased body temperature (fever). A recent example of tactile display technology applied to medical simulation is presented by Coles et al., 2009, who simulated the palpation of the femoral artery in an interventional radiology procedure [13].

Not many applications exist, where pure tactile displays have been used in medical applications. Most commonly vibrating or pin-based systems have been used in the field of rehabilitation, either as a Braille display for the visually impaired (see overview in [6]), as tactile cuing device for Parkinson's disease patients [3, 51], or as training device in stroke rehabilitation [56]. In the field of laparascopic surgery, several groups suggested to instrument a laparoscopic forceps with a tactile sensor array and display the information about the tactile properties of the indented or grasped tissue via a tactile display to the surgeon's hand or fingers [see overview in [70]).

To be useful for medical training purposes, a realistic feeling of touch must be imitated that is close to the simulated medical scenario [14]. Additionally, the technology must be portable, thus, lightweight and small to be mounted on a trainee's fingertip or an end-effector of a force feedback device. These requirements have led to the evaluation and use of primarily three different tactile technologies in this context: piezoelectric pads, micro speakers, and miniaturized pin arrays.

References

1. Abu-Tair, M., Marshall, A.: An empirical model for multi-contact point haptic network traffic. In: Proceedings of the 2nd International Conference on Immersive Telecommunications, IMMERSCOM '09, pp. 15:1–15:6. ICST (Institute for Computer Sciences, Social-Informatics and Telecommunications Engineering), Brussels (2009). http://dl.acm.org/citation.cfm?id=1594108.1594127
2. An, K.N., Askew, L.J., Chao, E.Y.: Biomechanics and functional assessment of upper extremities. In: Trends in Ergonomics/Human Factors III, pp. 573–580 (1986)
3. Besio, W.G., Fasiuddin, M., Patwardhan, R.: Medical devices for the detection, prevention and/or treatment of neurological disorders, and methods related thereto, October (2005). US Patent App. 11/252,043
4. Bicchi, A., Raugi, M., Rizzo, R., Sgambelluri, N.: Analysis and design of an electromagnetic system for the characterization of magneto-rheological fluids for haptic interfaces. IEEE Trans. Magn. 41(5), 1876–1879 (2005). doi:10.1109/TMAG.2005.846280
5. Bouzit, M., Burdea, G., Popescu, G., Boian, R.: The rutgers master ii-new design force-feedback glove. IEEE/ASME Trans. Mechatron. 7(2), 256–263 (2002)
6. Brewster, S.A., Wall, S.A., Brown, L.M., Hoggan, E.E.: Tactile displays. In: The Engineering Handbook of Smart Technology for Aging, Disability, and Independence, pp. 339–352 (2008)

7. Briot, S., Arakelian, V., Guégan, S.: PAMINSA: a new family of partially decoupled parallel manipulators. Mech. Mach. Theory **44**(2), 425–444 (2009)
8. Bro-Nielsen, M.: Finite element modelling in surgery simulation. Proc. IEEE **86**(3), 490–503 (1998)
9. CAE: CAE Endoscopy VR simulator. http://www.cae.com/en/healthcare/endoscopy.asp. CAE Healtcare Inc. (2010)
10. Caldwell, D.G., Lawther, S., Wardle, A.: Multi-modal cutaneous tactile feedback. In: Intelligent Robots and Systems, Proceedings of the 1996 IEEE/RSJ International Conference on, pp. 465–472 (1996)
11. Chouvardas, V.G., Miliou, A.N., Hatalis, M.K.: Tactile displays: a short overview and recent developments. In: ICTA '05: Proceedings of Fifth International Conference on Technology and Automation, pp. 246–251 (2005)
12. Clavel, R.: Device for displacing and positioning an element in space. WIPO Patent, WO 87/03528 (1987)
13. Coles, T., John, N.W., Gould, D.A., Caldwell, D.G.: Haptic palpation for the femoral pulse in virtual interventional radiology. In: Advances in Computer-Human Interactions, 2009. ACHI '09. Second International Conferences on, pp. 193–198 (2009). doi:10.1109/ACHI.2009.61
14. Coles, T.R., Meglan, D., John, N.W.: The role of haptics in medical training simulators: a survey of the state of the art. IEEE Trans. Haptics **4**(1), 51–66 (2011). doi:10.1109/TOH.2010.19
15. Colgate, E., Hogan, N.: An analysis of contact instability in terms of passive physical equivalents. In: Proceedings of the IEEE International Conference on Robotics and Automation (ICRA), Scottsdale, AZ, USA, pp. 404–409 (1989)
16. Colgate, J.E.: The control of dynamically interacting systems. PhD thesis, MIT Department of Mechanical Engineering (1988)
17. Colgate, J.E., Schenkel, G.: Passivity of a class of sampled-data systems: application to haptic interfaces. J. Robot. Syst. **14**(1), 37–47 (1997)
18. Dahiya, R.S., Metta, G., Valle, M., Sandini, G.: Tactile sensing: from humans to humanoids. IEEE Trans. Robot. **26**(1), 1–20 (2010)
19. Deetjen, P., Speckmann, E.-J.: Physiologie. Urban und Schwarz, München (1994)
20. Deetjen, P., Speckmann, E.J., Hescheler, J.: Physiologie, 4th edn. Elsevier, Urban und Fischer Verlag, München (2005)
21. Delingette, H.: Toward realistic soft-tissue modeling in medical simulation. Proc. IEEE **86**(3), 512–523 (1998)
22. Deutsch, J.E., Lewis, J.A., Burdea, G.: Technical and patient performance using a virtual reality-integrated telerehabilitation system: preliminary finding. IEEE Trans. Neural Syst. Rehabil. Eng. **15**(1), 30–35 (2007). doi:10.1109/TNSRE.2007.891384
23. Dollar, A.M., Herr, H.: Active orthoses for the lower-limbs: challenges and state of the art. In: Proceedings of the IEEE International Conference on Rehabilitation Robotics (ICORR), pp. 968–977 (2007). doi:10.1109/ICORR.2007.4428541
24. Durlach, N.I., Mavor, A.S.: Virtual Reality: Scientific and Technological Challenges. National Academies Press, Washington (1995)
25. Dworkin, P., Zeltzer, D.: A new model for efficient dynamic simulation. In: Proceedings of the Eurographics Workshop on Animation and Simulation, pp. 135–147 (1993)
26. Emery, C., Samur, E., Lambercy, O., Bleuler, H., Gassert, R.: Haptic/vr clinical assessment tool for fine motor control. In: Proceeding Eurohaptics 2010, pp. 186–193 (2010)
27. Esen, H., Sachsenhauser, A., Yano, K., Buss, M.: A multi-user virtual training system concept and objective assessment of trainings. In: Proceedings of the IEEE International Symposium on Robot and Human Interactive Communication (RO-MAN), pp. 1084–1089 (2007). doi:10.1109/ROMAN.2007.4415242
28. Faller, S., Schünke, M.: Der Körper des Menschen. Einführung in Bau und Funktion, 14th edn. Georg Thieme Verlag, Stuttgart (2004)
29. Famaey, N., Vander Sloten, J.: Soft tissue modelling for applications in virtual surgery and surgical robotics. Comput. Methods Biomech. Biomed. Eng. **11**(4), 351–366 (2008)

30. Fluet, M.-C., Lambercy, O., Gassert, R.: Upper limb assessment using a virtual peg inser- tion test. In: Proceeding: IEEE International Conference on Rehabilitation Robotics (ICORR) (2011)

31. Fritschi, M., Ernst, M.O., Buss, M.: Integration of kinesthetic and tactile display—a modular design concept. In: Proceedings of the EuroHaptics 2006 (2006)

32. Goldstein, E.B.: Wahrnehmungspsychologie: Der Grundkurs, 7th edn. Springer, Berlin (2008)

33. Gough, V.E.: Contribution to discussion of papers on research in automobile stability, control and tyre performance. Proc. Inst. Mech. Eng., Auto Div. **171**, 392–395 (1956–1957)

34. Hesse, S., Schmidt, H., Werner, C., Bardeleben, A.: Upper and lower extremity robotic devices for rehabilitation and for studying motor control. Curr. Opin. Neurol. **16**(6), 705–710 (2003)

35. Heuser, A., Kourtev, H., Winter, S., Fensterheim, D., Burdea, G., Hentz, V., Forducey, P.: Telerehabilitation using the rutgers master ii glove following carpal tunnel release surgery: proof-of-concept. IEEE Trans. Neural Syst. Rehabil. Eng. **15**(1), 43–49 (2007). doi:10.1109/TNSRE.2007.891393

36. Hogan, N.: Impedance control: An approach to manipulation. Part I—Theory, Part II— Implementation, Part III—Applications. ASME J. Dyn. Syst. Meas. Control **107**, 1–24 (1985)

37. Howe, R.D., Peine, W.J., Kantarinis, D.A., Son, J.S.: Remote palpation technology. IEEE Eng. Med. Biol. Mag. **14**(3), 318–323 (1995). doi:10.1109/51.391770

38. Hubens, G., Coveliers, H., Balliu, L., Ruppert, M., Vaneerdeweg, W.: A performance study comparing manual and robotically assisted laparoscopic surgery using the da Vinci system. Surg. Endosc. **17**(10), 1595–1599 (2003)

39. Hwang, S.L., Barfield, W., Chang, T.C., Salvendy, G.: Integration of humans and computers in the operation and control of flexible manufacturing systems. Int. J. Prod. Res. **22**(5), 841–856 (1984)

40. Inoue, H., Tsusaka, Y., Fukuizumi, T.: Parallel manipulator. In: Proc 3rd ISRR, Gouvieux, France (1985)

41. Iwata, H., Yano, H., Nakaizumi, F., Kawamura, R.: Project feelex: adding haptic surface to graphics. In: Proceedings of the 28th Annual Conference on Computer Graphics and Interac- tive Techniques, pp. 469–476. ACM, New York (2001)

42. Jack, D., Boian, R., Merians, A.S., Tremaine, M., Burdea, G.C., Adamovich, S.V., Recce, M., Poizner, H.: Virtual reality-enhanced stroke rehabilitation. IEEE Trans. Neural Syst. Rehabil. Eng. **9**(3), 308–318 (2001). doi:10.1109/7333.948460

43. Jandura, L., Srinivasan, M.A.: Experiments on human performance in torque discrimination and control. Dyn. Syst. Control **1**, 369 (1994)

44. Johnson, D.E., Willemsen, P., Cohen, E.: Six degree-of-freedom haptic rendering using spatialized normal cone search. IEEE Trans. Vis. Comput. Graph. **11**(6), 661–670 (2005). doi:10.1109/TVCG.2005.106

45. Kajimoto, H., Kawakami, N., Tachi, S., Inami, M.: SmartTouch: electric skin to touch the untouchable. IEEE Comput. Graph. Appl. **24**(1), 36–43 (2004)

46. Kong, X., Gosselin, C.: Type synthesis of parallel mechanisms. In: Springer Tracts in Ad- vanced Robotics, vol. 33. Springer, Berlin (2007)

47. Kontarinis, D.A., Howe, R.D.: Tactile display of vibratory information in teleoperation and virtual environments. Presence: Teleoperators and Virtual Environments **4**(4), 387–402 (1995)

48. Koo, I.M., Jung, K., Koo, J.C., Nam, J.-D., Lee, Y.K., Choi, H.R.: Development of soft- actuator-based wearable tactile display. IEEE Trans. Robot. **24**(3), 549–558 (2008)

49. Kühnapfel, U., Kuhn, C., Hubner, M., Krumm, H.G., Maass, H., Neisius, B.: The Karlsruhe endoscopic surgery trainer as an example for virtual reality in medical education. Minim. Invasive Ther. Allied Technol. **6**(2), 122–125 (1997)

50. Lederman, S.J., Klatzky, R.L.: Hand movement: a window into haptic object recognition. Cogn. Psychol. **19**(3), 342–368 (1987)

51. Lim, I., Van Wegen, E., De Goede, C., Deutekom, M., Nieuwboer, A., Willems, A., Jones, D., Rochester, L., Kwakkel, G.: Effects of external rhythmical cueing on gait in patients with Parkinson's disease: a systematic review. Clin. Rehabil. **19**(7), 695 (2005)

52. Liu, Y., Davidson, R., Taylor, P.: Touch sensitive electrorheological fluid based tactile display. Smart Mater. Struct. **14**, 1563–1568 (2005)
53. Meier, U., López, O., Monserrat, C., Juan, M.C., Alcañiz, M.: Real-time deformable models for surgery simulation: a survey. Comput. Methods Programs Biomed. **77**(3), 183–197 (2005). doi:10.1016/j.cmpb.2004.11.002
54. Merians, A.S., Fluet, G.G., Qiu, Q., Saleh, S., Lafond, I., Davidow, A., Adamovich, S.V.: Robotically facilitated virtual rehabilitation of arm transport integrated with finger movement in persons with hemiparesis. J. NeuroEng. Rehabil. **8**(1), 1–10 (2011). doi:10.1186/1743-0003-8-27
55. Merlet, J.-P., Gosselin, C.: In: Siciliano, B., Khatib, O. (eds.) Springer Handbook on Robotics, pp. 269–285. Springer, Berlin (2008)
56. Merrett, G.V., Metcalf, C.D., Zheng, D., Cunningham, S., Barrow, S., Demain, S.H.: Design and qualitative evaluation of tactile devices for stroke rehabilitation. In: IET Assisted Living (2011)
57. Miyazaki, S., Ueno, J., Yasuda, T., Yokoi, S., Torikawi, J.: A study of virtual manipulation of elastic objects with destruction. In: Proceedings of the IEEE International Workshop on Robot and Human Communication, pp. 26–31 (1996)
58. Moore, P., Molloy, D.: A survey of computer-based deformable models. In: Machine Vision and Image Processing Conference, 2007. IMVIP 2007. International, pp. 55–66 (2007). doi:10.1109/IMVIP.2007.31
59. Morgenbesser, H.B., Srinivasan, M.A.: Force shading for haptic shape perception. ASME Proc. Dyn. Syst. Control Div. **58**, 407–412 (1996)
60. Morioka, M., Whitehouse, D.J., Griffin, M.J.: Vibrotactile thresholds at the fingertip, volar forearm, large toe, and heel. Somatosens. Motor Res. **25**(2), 101–112 (2008)
61. Moy, G., Wagner, C., Fearing, R.S.: A compliant tactile display for teletaction. In: Robotics and Automation, 2000. Proceedings. ICRA'00. IEEE International Conference on, vol. 4, pp. 3409–3415. IEEE, New York (2000)
62. Nealen, A., Müller, M., Keiser, R., Boxerman, E., Carlson, M.: Physically based deformable models in computer graphics. In: Computer Graphics Forum. Wiley Online Library, vol. 25, pp. 809–836 (2006)
63. Nikitczuk, J., Weinberg, B., Mavroidis, C.: Rehabilitative knee orthosis driven by electrorheological fluid based actuators. In: Robotics and Automation, 2005. ICRA 2005. Proceedings of the 2005 IEEE International Conference on, pp. 2283–2289 (2005). doi:10.1109/ROBOT.2005.1570453
64. Piegl, L.A., Tiller, W.: The NURBS Book. Springer, Berlin (1997)
65. Riener, R., Quintern, J., Schmidt, G.: Biomechanical model of the human knee evaluated by neuromuscular stimulation. J. Biomech. **29**(9), 1157–1167 (1996)
66. Rizzo, R., Sgambelluri, N., Scilingo, E.P., Raugi, M., Bicchi, A.: Electromagnetic modeling and design of haptic interface prototypes based on magnetorheological fluids. IEEE Trans. Magn. **43**(9), 3586–3600 (2007). doi:10.1109/TMAG.2007.901351
67. Ruspini, D.C., Kolarov, K., Khatib, O.: The haptic display of complex graphical environments. In: Proceedings of the 24th Annual Conference on Computer Graphics and Interactive Techniques, SIGGRAPH '97, pp. 345–352. ACM Press/Addison-Wesley Publishing Co., New York (1997). doi:10.1145/258734.258878
68. Salisbury, K., Tarr, C.: Haptic rendering of surfaces defined by implicit functions. In: Proceedings of the ASME 6th Annual Symposium on Haptic Interfaces for Virtual Environment and Teleoperator System, pp. 61–68 (1997)
69. Schmidt, R.F., Thews, G.: Die Physiologie des Menschen. Springer, Berlin (1990)
70. Schostek, S., Schurr, M.O., Buess, G.F.: Review on aspects of artificial tactile feedback in laparoscopic surgery. Med. Eng. Phys. **31**(8), 887–898 (2009)
71. Sgambelluri, N., Scilingo, E.P., Bicchi, A., Rizzo, R., Raugi, M.: Advanced modeling and preliminary psychophysical experiments for a free-hand haptic device. In: Proc. IEEE/RSJ Int. Conf. on Robots and Intelligent Systems—IROS06, pp. 1558–1563 (2006)

72. Shinohara, M., Shimizu, Y., Mochizuki, A.: Three-dimensional tactile display for the blind. IEEE Trans. Rehabil. Eng. **6**(3), 249–256 (1998). doi:10.1109/86.712218
73. Siciliano, O., Khatib, B. (eds.): Handbook of Robotics. Springer, Berlin (2008)
74. Sledd, A.: Performance enhancement of a haptic arm exoskeleton. In: Haptic Interfaces for Virtual Environment and Teleoperator Systems, 2006 14th Symposium on, pp. 375–381 (2006)
75. Stewart, D.: A platform with six degrees of freedom. Proc. Inst. Mech. Eng. **180**, 371–385 (1965–66)
76. Sung, G.T., Gill, I.S.: Robotic laparoscopic surgery: a comparison of the da Vinci and Zeus systems. Urology **58**(6), 893–898 (2001)
77. Sutter, P.H., Iatridis, J.C., Thakor, N.V.: Response to Reflected-Force Feedback to Fingers in Teleoperations. In: Proceedings of the NASA Conference on Space Telerobotics (1989)
78. Tan, H.Z., Pang, X.D., Durlach, N.I.: Manual resolution of length, force, and compliance. Adv. Robot. **42**, 13–18 (1992)
79. Tan, H.Z., Srinivasan, M.A., Eberman, B., Cheng, B.: Human factors for the design of force-reflecting haptic interfaces. Dyn. Syst. Control **55**(1), 353–359 (1994)
80. Thompson, T.V. II, Cohen, E.: Direct haptic rendering of complex trimmed NURBS models. In: Proceeding ACM SIGGRAPH 2005 Courses, pp. 89–96 (2005). doi:10.1145/1198555.1198609
81. Thompson, T.V. II, Johnson, D.E., Cohen, E.: Direct haptic rendering of sculptured models. In: Proceedings of the 1997 Symposium on Interactive 3D Graphics, pp. 167–176 (1997). doi:10.1145/253284.253336
82. Ueberle, M., Mock, N., Buss, M.: Design, control, and evaluation of a hyper-redundant haptic device. In: Ferre, M., Buss, M., Aracil, R., Melchiorri, C., Balaguer, C. (eds.) Advances in Telerobotics. Springer Tracts in Advanced Robotics, vol. 31, pp. 25–44. Springer, Berlin (2007). http://dx.doi.org/10.1007/978-3-540-71364-7_3
83. Van der Linde, R.Q., Lammertse, P., Frederiksen, E., Ruiter, B.: The HapticMaster, a new high-performance haptic interface (2002)
84. van Eijden, T.M., Weijs, W.A., Kouwenhoven, E., Verburg, J.: Forces acting on the patella during maximal voluntary contraction of the quadriceps femoris muscle at different knee flexion/extension angles. Acta Anat. **129**(4), 310–314 (1987)
85. Vischer, P., Clavel, R.: Kinematic calibration of the parallel delta robot. Robotica **16**(02), 207–218 (1998)
86. Wang, Q., Hayward, V.: Tactile synthesis and perceptual inverse problems seen from the viewpoint of contact mechanics. ACM Trans. Appl. Percept. **5**(2), 7 (2008)
87. Wang, Q., Hayward, V.: Biomechanically optimized distributed tactile transducer based on lateral skin deformation. Int. J. Robot. Res. **29**(4), 323–335 (2009)
88. Weinstein, S.: Intensive and extensive aspects of tactile sensitivity as a function of body part, sex, and laterality. In: Kenshalo, D.R. (ed.) The Skin Senses, Springfield, IL, pp. 195–218 (1968)
89. Winter, D.A.: Biomechanics and Motor Control of Human Movement, 3rd edn. Wiley, New York (1990)
90. Zilles, C.B., Salisbury, J.K.: A constraint-based god-object method for haptic display. In: Intelligent Robots and Systems 'Human Robot Interaction and Cooperative Robots', Proceedings. 1995 IEEE/RSJ International Conference on, vol. 3. Chicago, IL, USA, pp. 146–151 (1995)
91. Zimmermann, M.: Mechanoreceptors of the glaborous skin and tactile acuity. In: Studies in Neurophysiology Presented to A.K., p. 267. Cambridge University Press, Cambridge (1978)
92. Zotterman, Y.: Sensory Functions of the Skin in Primates. Pergamon, Oxford (1976)

Chapter 5
Auditory Aspects

5.1 What Are Auditory Displays?

The term *Auditory Display* was introduced around 1992 when the first International Conference on Auditory Display (ICAD) [21] was organized. Before that time, no clear definition on auditory displays existed. In one of the first definitions an auditory display was described as "the use of sound to communicate information about the state of a computing device to a user." [25]. This definition distinguished auditory displays from auditory interfaces. While auditory displays only concern themselves with the use of sound to communicate from the computing device to the user, auditory interfaces may also use sound processing to communicate from the user to the device [25]. A more recent and more general definition of auditory displays includes "all possible transmissions which finally lead to audible perceptions for the user. This could range from loudspeakers over headphones to bone conduction devices." [15]. In addition, this definition also includes aspects concerning the user (user, task, background sound, constraints) and the application (rehabilitation training, movement training in sports), since they are essential for the design and implementation of auditory displays [15].

5.2 Auditory Sense and Perception

Human auditory perception is related to the detection and location of a sound source in space but also to the discrimination of different sound properties such as pitch, volume, timbre, and tempo. Hearing allows humans to detect danger and alerts, communicate, or enjoy music or particular sounds. The loss of hearing ability can lead to social isolation due to limited communicational capabilities. In general, spatial hearing is based on interaural volume, time and spectral composition differences. Remodeling an acoustic scenario without considering all the features that carry the information will most likely sound unnatural to the human and may even impair the extraction of the desired information from the signal. For instance, modeling

R. Riener, M. Harders, *Virtual Reality in Medicine*,
DOI 10.1007/978-1-4471-4011-5_5, © Springer-Verlag London 2012

the distance to a sound source by only setting the signal volume will not work, unless the brain recognizes the sound pattern and, therefore, knows about the typical volume level of the sound source. However, well-designed sound feedback can significantly enhance immersion into virtual environments [2, 35] or may be even required to generate a match between the participant's proprioceptive feedback about body movements and the information generated on the displays [37]. Thus, sound can play a very important role for the effectiveness of virtual training scenarios in medical applications.

5.2.1 Anatomy and Physiology

The human detects auditory stimuli with the ears. The ear consists of three parts, the outer ear, the middle ear, and the inner ear. The outer ear includes the pinna and the auditory canal (Fig. 5.1). Its function is mainly the conduction of sound to the eardrum (tympanic membrane). The sound induced vibration of the eardrum is transferred to the three ear bones (ossicles: malleus, incus, stapes) inside the middle ear, which is filled with a watery liquid. The lever action of the ear bones prevents a loss of the sound signal, which would occur during a sound conduction from air to water. Such a sound signal loss between water and air would occur, because transversal sound waves in air cannot transfer their energy to longitudinal sound waves in water and thus sound waves are fully reflected at water-air transitions. The sound is, thus, transferred by movements of the ear bones and causes vibrations of the oval window. The vibrations of the oval window then induce longitudinal waves in the fluid of the inner ear. The cochlea of the inner ear is traversed by the basilar membrane, which is stiffer at its beginning than at its end. Due to the mechanical properties of the basilar membrane, the traveling longitudinal wave causes a maximum at a frequency-specific location in the cochlea (frequency dispersion). The displacement of the basilar membrane induces action potentials of the hair cells at the frequency-specific location. The signal is conducted through the auditory nerve to the brain [9].

5.2.2 Perception

Humans can perceive frequencies between 16 Hz and 20 kHz (Table 5.1) [33]. The unit of sound pressure level is decibel (dB). This logarithmic scale of sound pressure represents closely the human perception of loudness. The sound pressure level at which humans can hear a sound (hearing threshold) depends on the frequency. At 1 kHz it is approximately 0 dB, which corresponds to a sound pressure of $2 \cdot 10^{-5}$ N/m^2. The hearing threshold is smallest in the range of 2–4 kHz, which is approximately the frequency range of speaking [9] (Fig. 5.2). With age, the sensitivity to higher frequencies decreases.

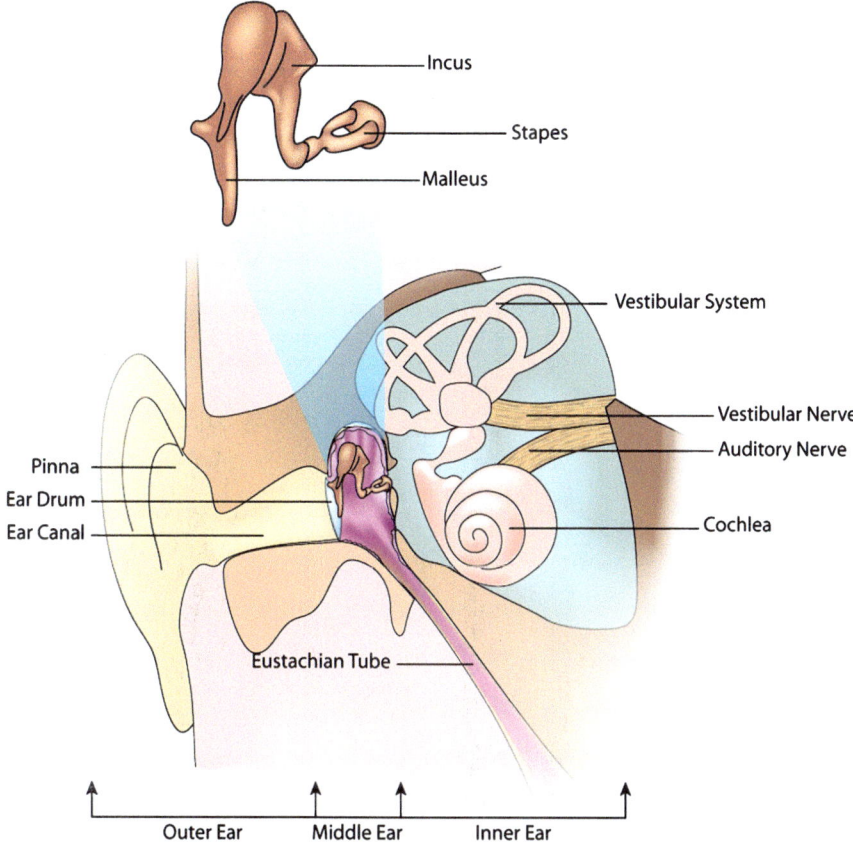

Fig. 5.1 Anatomy of the human ear; © ADInstruments Pty Ltd. Reproduced with permission

Table 5.1 Auditory perception ranges

Frequency range	16–20 Hz to 20 kHz	[13, 33]
Highest frequency sensitivity	2–4 kHz	[13]
Frequency resolution	approx. 3 Hz, at 1 kHz	
Auditory threshold	0 dB SPL[a] ($2 \cdot 10^{-5}$ N/m^2), at 1 kHz	[34]
Just-noticeable difference:		
ITD[b]	10 µs or less	[1]
ILD[c]	0.5–1 dB	[1]
Directional resolution:		
horizontal plane (azimuth)	> 1°	[6, 30]
vertical plane (elevation)	approx. 4°–17°	[1, 6]
Distance resolution	< 20% of distance	[5]

[a]Sound pressure level; [b]Interaural time differences; [c]Interaural level differences

Fig. 5.2 Relation of frequency and sound pressure within the human hearing range. (**a**) Illustration of equal-loudness countours (for details see [6, 40]); (**b**) Approximate human audible range

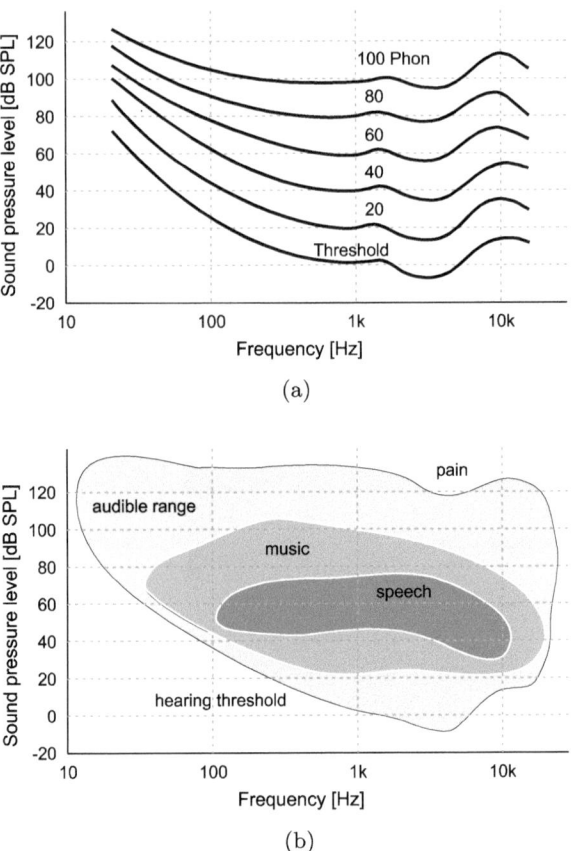

(a)

(b)

Two binaural and one monaural position stimuli are involved in direction detection of a sound source [13]. The term binaural hearing means the auditory processes, which are involved in the comparison of the sounds received by each ear. The three position stimuli are described in the following sections.

First, interaural time differences (ITDs) arise if a sound reaches the two ears at a slightly different instant of time. To be more precise, ITDs are the arrival-time differences between the input signals at the two ears [6]. In real life, ITDs are never very large: sound travels at about 340 m/s, and so it takes, at most, about $6 \cdot 10^{-4}$ s to travel the distance from one ear to the other, which is approximately 20 cm. Nevertheless, the auditory system can easily detect such interaural timing differences and uses them to determine the direction of a sound source. Time differences occur, if the sound source is placed outside the listener's median plane. Time differences increase the more laterally the sound source is placed. Under optimal conditions, listeners can detect interaural timing differences as small as $1 \cdot 10^{-5}$ s. ITDs provide the primary cue for determining sound directions for low-frequency sounds [1]. An ambiguous situation can occur for wavelengths smaller than the diameter of the

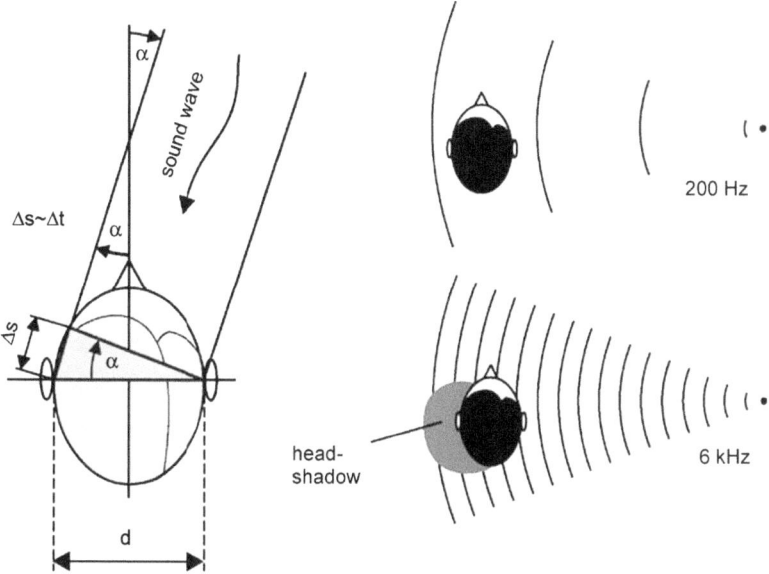

Fig. 5.3 Principles of the appearance of interaural time and interaural level differences (ITD and ILD). *On the left* the principle of time-delay between the two ears dependent on the sound source position angle is shown. *On the right* the principle of frequency and position-dependent damping of the sound signal is illustrated, the so-called head-shadow effect. [46] (© 2006, IEEE)

head (above 1,500 Hz), because then the phase does not necessarily correspond to a unique sound source angle [46].

Second, interaural level differences (ILDs) are used to determine sound source directions. The sound intensity reaching the ear depends on the distance of the sound source and the presence and type of obstacles located between source and ear. Since the two ears are located on opposite sides of the head, the sound will reach the closest ear first. Before the sound is perceived by the other ear, it is shadowed by the head. As a consequence, the sound intensity perceived by the first ear is higher than that of the latter ear. This effect is also used to locate sound sources. ILDs are best evaluated at high frequencies [1]. Low frequency sound is not so much affected by the head shadow effect, because the wavelength of low frequency sounds is longer than the width of the head (Fig. 5.3). This is the reason why subwoofers of Hi-Fi systems, which provide low-frequency sound (bass) can be placed at an arbitrary location, whereas the loudspeakers for high-frequency sound must be placed carefully to get the desired stereo effects.

Third, monaural position stimuli (monaural hearing) are involved in the detection of sound source direction. Dependent on the sound waves' direction of incidence, the sound waves undergo a direction-dependent transformation, or spectral filtering [17]. This filtering depends on the listener's body properties: head, upper torso, and pinnae i.e. the listener's external ears. Mathematically, this anatomical filtering can be described by two digital filters (one per ear) that reflect the personal spectral properties of interaural and monaural cues necessary for sound localization. This mathematical description is called head-related transfer function (HRTF) [13]. While ITD and ILD mainly give information about the sound source direction in the azimuthal plane, they may become ambiguous for elevation angles of incidence. Ambiguities in ITD and ILD occur, when they are equal for both ears. This is the case when a sound source is equidistant to both ears. In contrary to ITD and ILD, spectral cues allow to distinguish the location of sound sources placed in the vertical plane of the head. The distance from a sound source cannot be determined by position stimuli. For sound source distance detection, the overall level of a sound, the amount of reverberation in a room relative to the original sound, and (for very distant sounds, such as thunder) the timbre of the sound are integrated. For known sounds, experience helps to estimate the distance from the sound source.

5.3 Auditory Display Technology

There are many different techniques for generating sound in a virtual environment. The purpose of all of these techniques is to provide the realistic impression to the human listener that the sound is coming from different sources located at different positions in space. Depending on the complexity of each method, the different techniques reach different levels of realism. This section describes the challenges for the technical realization of auditory displays and design principles of the technical approaches.

5.3.1 Challenges for the Design of Auditory Displays

To approximate realistic sound environments, the following challenges should be considered during the technical realization of the auditory display.

- The virtual scenery is spatially distributed, i.e. sound is distributed everywhere in space, resulting in many acoustic sources, especially when sound is reflected on walls and large objects.
- Sound sources can move, i.e. they can change their direction and apparent frequency (Dopplereffect).
- Both ears receive different signals, therefore, different sound signals should be fed into the ears.
- Perception of sound depends on the individual head-ear geometry. The head-related transfer function (HRTF) can be used to adapt the sound to the individual head-ear geometry.
- One must be aware of ergonomic issues, e.g. a portable acoustic display must be lightweight in order to be comfortable and acceptable for the user.

5.3.2 Examples of Auditory Displays

The two basic approaches for displaying auditory signals are headphones and loud-speakers. A more complex system based on stereo hearing is the principle of wave field synthesis. This section presents some details of each system.

5.3.2.1 Headphones

Headphones are the simplest solution for displaying sound to the VR user. They are often used together with head-mounted displays. Headphones can produce stereo sound, and they can suppress noise from the surrounding environment. The characteristics of the sound are independent of the user's position and orientation. Therefore, the user may perceive the sound as unrealistic when moving the head.

HRTF-based spatial audio systems can synthesize 3D sound for VR use for a pair of normal headphones. Sound is placed in space by a finite impulse response filter whose settings are determined by the HRTF measurements of a specific user.

A given sound wave input (parameterized as frequency and source location) is always pre-filtered via the diffraction and reflection properties of the human body dimensions. These include mainly those of the head, pinnae and torso. The sound then reaches the transduction machinery of the eardrum and inner ear (Fig. 5.1). Biologically, the source-location-specific prefiltering effects of these external structures aid in the neural determination of source location, particularly the determination of the source's elevation. The transfer function, derived from linear systems analysis, is the complex ratio between the output signal spectrum and the input signal spectrum as a function of frequency. Lehnert and Blauert [24] initially defined the transfer function as the free-field transfer function (FFTF). Other methods describe the usage of the free-field to eardrum transfer function [45] or the pressure transformation from the free-field to the eardrum [36]. Less specific descriptions include the pinna transfer function, the outer ear transfer function, the pinna response, or directional transfer function (DTF) [8].

The transfer function $H(s)$ of any linear time-invariant system (LTI-system) at the complex frequency s is:

$$H(s) = \frac{Output(s)}{Input(s)}, \tag{5.1}$$

while the HRTF $H(s)$ is the Fourier transform of the head-related impulse response (HRIR) $h(t)$.

The HRIR is derived from the differences in arrival time and intensity of the sound in both ears, which, therefore, deliver valuable information about the sound source and its location. This information leads to the impulse response, which relates the source location to the ear location. Measuring the HRIR, $h(t)$, at the eardrum for the impulse $\Delta(t)$ placed at the given source location, is one method of finding the corresponding HRTF. To minimize various disturbances like the influence of early reflections or reverberations on the measured response, HRTFs are mostly measured in an anechoic chamber and at small angular increments. However, even with small increments, interpolation can lead to front-back confusion, and optimizing the interpolation procedure is an active area of research [3, 46, 47].

The HRTF measurement can be determined by measuring the impulse response at each ear of the user from 144 different sound sources (see [45]) surrounding the subject in order to get a spatial resolution of about 2° between sound sources. When a simulated sound is moved, the new sound response is interpolated from the four nearest measured points, which allows smooth motions of the sound. HRTF-based algorithms can simulate some aspects of room acoustics very accurately such as echoes or room reverberation. It can be combined with the location of the head, which is detected by a head tracker in order to select the appropriate sound feedback. In commercially available hearing aid technology, algorithms such as the Cetera Algorithm [42, 43] are implemented. This algorithm can help the user to locate sound sources and to focus on one sound or voice even when being in a noisy environment due to HRTF-based matching of the pose of the wearer's ears.

5.3.2.2 Mono, Stereo, and Surround Loudspeaker Systems

Sound can also be displayed by loudspeakers. They are often used together with a visual display system. Compared to headphones, loudspeakers can be used by multiple users. Another advantage is that the user does not have to wear equipment covering the ears (i.e. headphones). The following setups are common:

- **Mono loudspeakers** create a center sound field from one audio speaker (Fig. 5.4(a)). Therefore, only a static sound can be simulated. When using the speaker together with a graphical display, sound and image location may be perceived as separate sources.
- **Stereo loudspeaker** systems reproduce the sound using two independent audio speakers. The system can simulate a natural dynamic sound (e.g. a moving sound source) that can be heard from various directions. However, the optimal sound quality can only be found at a particular point in space called *sweet spot*. Therefore, the listener must be located equidistantly from each loudspeaker at about 1.2 times the distance between the loudspeakers (Fig. 5.4(b)).
- **Surround sound** systems may be used to extend the sweet spot region of the stereo sound for a more realistic audio environment. Surround sound can be created using several loudspeakers placed around the subjects to display the sound coming from different directions. A popular surround system is the Dolby Surround sound system (Dolby 5.1 system consists of five full range speakers, placed around the listener and one low frequency channel usually using a subwoofer). This technology is commonly used in public cinemas and is also commercially available for home cinemas. However, technology is still pushed to systems that provide even higher realism of audio environments than provided by Dolby Surround systems. The latest invention in this context are wave field synthesis systems (see next subsection).

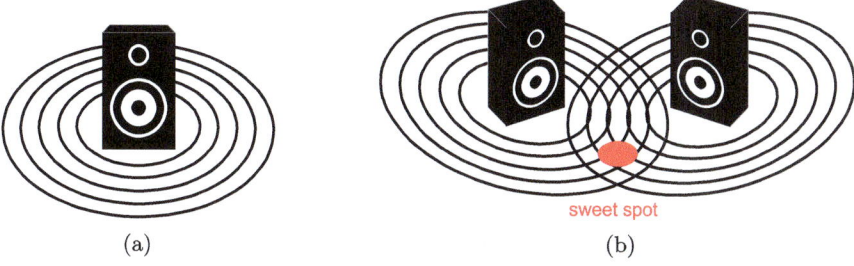

(a) (b)

Fig. 5.4 Propagation of sound waves. (**a**) Sound waves coming from a mono loudspeaker; (**b**) Interacting sound waves coming from stereo loudspeakers. The listener's position should be in the "sweet spot", where the sound system sounds best

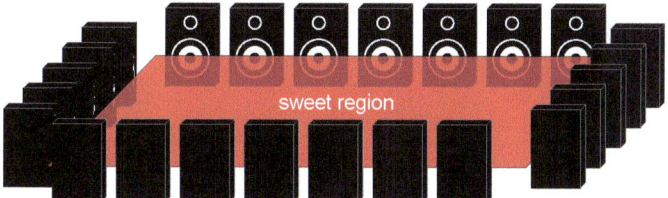

Fig. 5.5 In a wave field synthesis system the "sweet spot" location is extended to a "sweet region". Within this region the listener gets the impression of being within a genuine sound field indistinguishable from a real sound field

5.3.2.3 Wave Field Synthesis

The theory of wave field synthesis (WFS) has been initially invented at the Technical University of Delft and was then developed further within the CARROUSO project at Fraunhofer Gesellschaft (FhG), Germany and the cinema Lindenlichtspiele in Ilmenau, Germany. In contrast to other multi-channel approaches, it is based on fundamental acoustic principles. Wave field synthesis is a technology that reproduces a sound field for a large listening zone from a large number of loudspeakers (Fig. 5.5). The basic principle of WFS is based on the Huygens principle. Huygens stated that any point of a wave front of a propagating wave at any instant conforms to the envelope of spherical waves emanating from every point on the wave front at the prior instant (Fig. 5.6). This principle can be used to synthesize acoustic wave fronts of an arbitrary shape. By placing the loudspeakers on an arbitrary fixed curve and by weighting and delaying the driving signals, an acoustic wave front can be synthesized with a loudspeaker array.

The mathematical formulation of this principle is given by the Kirchhoff-Helmholtz integral (Eq. (5.2)), which can be derived by using the wave equation.

$$P(\mathbf{r}, \omega) = \frac{1}{4\pi} \oint_S \left[P(\mathbf{r}_S, \omega) \frac{\partial}{\partial \mathbf{n}} \left(\frac{e^{jk|\mathbf{r}-\mathbf{r}_S|}}{|\mathbf{r}-\mathbf{r}_S|} \right) - \frac{\partial P(\mathbf{r}_S, \omega)}{\partial \mathbf{n}} \frac{e^{jk|\mathbf{r}-\mathbf{r}_S|}}{|\mathbf{r}-\mathbf{r}_S|} \right] d\mathbf{S} \quad (5.2)$$

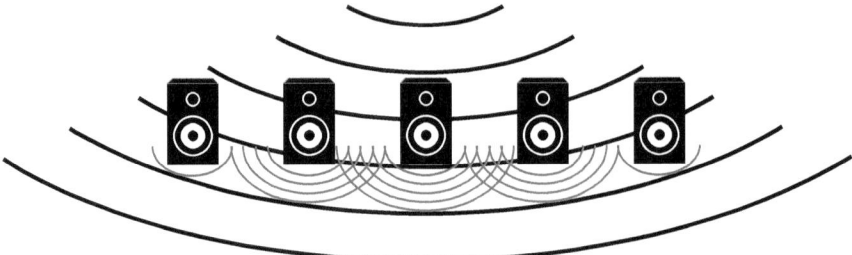

Fig. 5.6 Interaction of several loud speakers in order to form a common wave front. In this way plane waves can also be generated, which create the impression of sound coming from sound sources located far away from the listener or located at any other place

Fig. 5.7 Illustration of the parameters used in Eq. (5.2) of the Kirchhoff-Helmholtz integral (image adapted from [4])

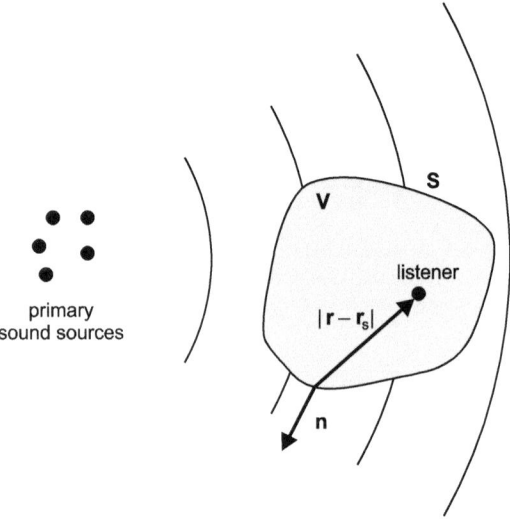

where $\mathbf{S}$ denotes the surface of an enclosed space $\mathbf{V}$, $(\mathbf{r} - \mathbf{r}_S)$ the vector from a surface point $\mathbf{r}_S$ to a listener position $\mathbf{r}$ within the surface $\mathbf{S}$, $P(\mathbf{r}_S, \omega)$ the Fourier transform of the pressure distribution on $\mathbf{S}$, k the wave number and $\mathbf{n}$ the surface normal (Fig. 5.7 illustrates the parameters used in the Kirchhoff-Helmholtz integral). The Kirchhoff-Helmholtz integral states that at any listening point within the source-free volume $\mathbf{V}$ the sound pressure $P(\mathbf{r}_S, \omega)$ can be calculated if both the sound pressure and its gradient are known on the surface enclosing the volume. This can be used to synthesize a wave field within the surface $\mathbf{S}$ by setting the appropriate pressure distribution $P(\mathbf{r}_S, \omega)$. This fact is used for WFS-based sound reproduction. In order to arrive at a realizable system, the volume is constrained under consideration to a plane, and so the surface $\mathbf{S}$ is a line, and since the sound is produced by loudspeakers, a spatial discretization of sound sources is the result (Fig. 5.8). The above approach can also be extended to the case that sources lie inside the volume $\mathbf{V}$. This allows to place acoustic sources between the listener and the loudspeakers within

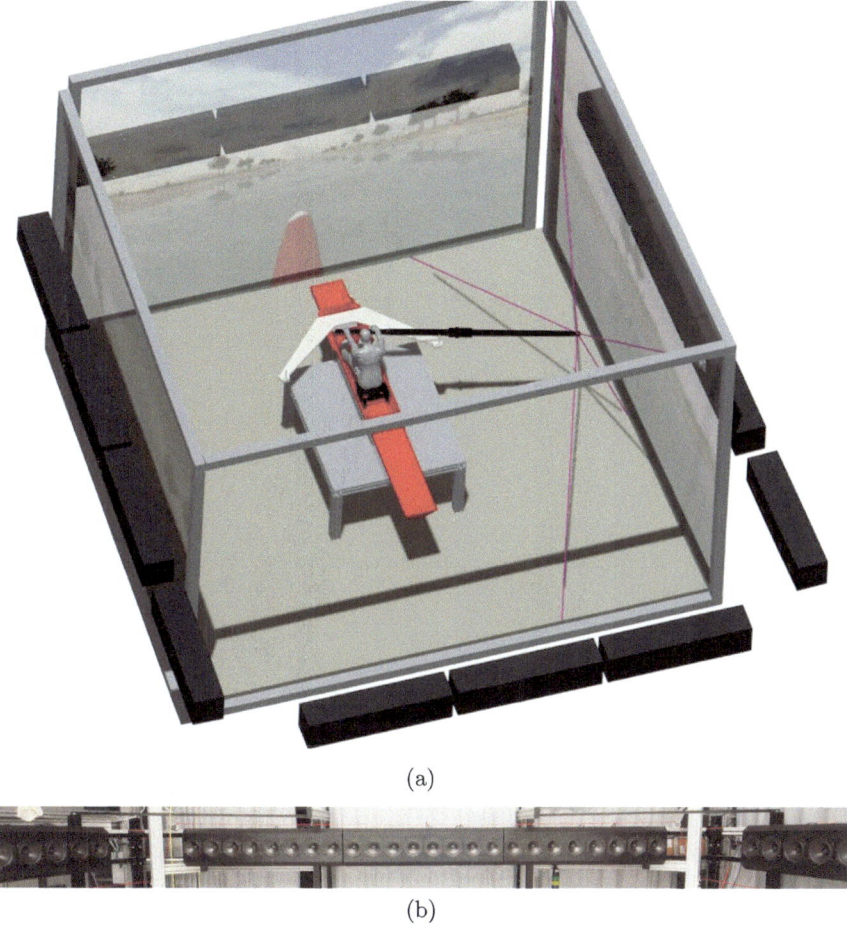

(a)

(b)

Fig. 5.8 Wave field synthesis applied in the M^3 rowing simulator of the Sensory-Motor Systems Lab, ETH Zurich. Virtual sound sources can be generated at arbitrary positions of a horizontal plane. (**a**) Three projection screens and sound panels with speakers; (**b**) The system includes a circular arrangement of 112 speakers, complemented by 4 subwoofers for low-frequency sound

the reproduction area (focused sources). This is not possible with traditional stereo or surround setups [4].

5.3.2.4 Sound Focusing

Sound focusing is a technique which provides high quality sound resolution at a specific point in space, whereas in the surrounding areas sound is hardly noticeable.

To focus sound at super-resolution within a defined volume, techniques like *time-reverse focusing* are used. Time-reverse focusing takes advantage of the Huygens

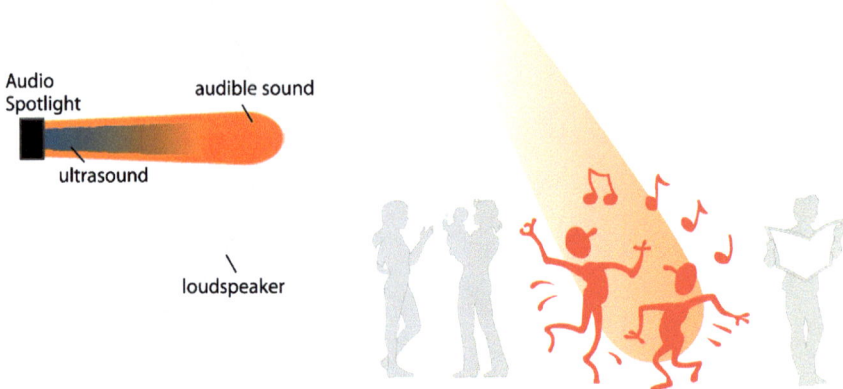

Fig. 5.9 Example for a setup on the sound focusing system "Audio Spotlight" by Holosonics Research Labs, Inc. [29]. The sound is focused on the target listener and nearby people can hardly hear the projected sound

principle, which enables the generation of time-reversal waves in non-dissipative fluids. To generate such time-reversal waves, microphones are placed on a surface around the volume of interest and sound is emitted from this volume. The sound is recorded sufficiently long in order to also record sound reflections during sound propagation. In a further step, the microphones are replaced by loudspeakers and the recorded sound is reversed in time. In this way, spatial and temporal focusing of the sound on the volume of interest i.e. sound focusing volume can be achieved efficiently and easily. From a theoretical point of view, the time-reversing focusing technique can be explained by reversion of a non-dissipatively diverging wave field emitted by one sound source (invariant wave equation). Reversing this diverging wave field yields convergence of the sound waves in the original sound source i.e. the sound focusing volume [47]. Commonly, instead of realizing sound focusing by an array of conventional loudspeakers, sound at super resolution is created by ultra-directional sound systems. Such ultra-directional sound systems "excite" the air itself and, thus, sound can be generated with even more directivity than by conventional loudspeakers. By projecting the sound to a specific location, only the target listeners can hear the sound. Nearby persons can hardly hear it (Fig. 5.9) [29].

5.4 Auditory Rendering

Due to the development of high-capacity computer technology, sound is not any-more restricted to simple replay of prerecorded samples. Sound has made its way towards virtual reality, where rendering of sound is used for creating virtual auditory environments analogous to graphics rendering (see [12]). There are two major principles to render the acoustic information to a virtual environment, which are presented in the following sections.

5.4.1 Display of Pre-recorded Sound Samples

Any acoustic scenario can be rendered using a set of different pre-recorded sound samples. The sound samples are usually static and non-parameterized. To simulate different virtual situations, often a large number of sound samples is required. These different sound samples may be played simultaneously and/or one after the other depending on the user activity and interaction with the virtual scenario. This principle is commonly used to render the background scenario in virtual environments by adding e.g. twittering birds, rushing waters, machine noise, or music. This first principle of pre-recorded sound samples is often combined with the second principle.

5.4.2 Real-Time Synthesizing of Sound

The second principle of sound rendering is either based on real-time synthesizing of sound sources as they are generated by the physical properties of the sound emitting components and materials, or on modulating the sound signals as they appear in the vicinity of the ear of the listener [44].

- **Real-time synthesizing of sound sources**, also called Model-Based Sonification (MBS), are used to mimic the physical properties of sound emitting components and materials. MBS is based on mathematical modeling of the underlying physical principles, which cause the production of sound waves. MBS sonification models describe and configure dynamic processes that behave like real instruments that do not produce any sound without external interactions. In other words: "the data is used to build an instrument or sound-capable object, while the playing is left to the user. The user excites the sonification model and receives acoustic responses that are determined by the temporal evolution of the model" [15]. MBS is especially used for describing the physical phenomena, which occur in string instruments. In many cases, these models are able to synthesize high-quality sounds e.g. the sound of a guitar [19]. Good mathematical models are also capable of taking into account any kind of sound effects that also result from playing an instrument in different ways e.g. a cord is plugged at different locations, or intensities, a cord is plugged by a finger, or excited using a bow. A good overview on the degree of details that may be implemented in mathematical models used for synthesizing sounds is given in [11]. The biggest challenge until now in real-time synthesizing of sound sources using physical models is, to find a good trade-off between the degree of realism a model can reproduce and the needed calculation time in order to obtain sounds in real-time. A detailed introduction to MBS can be found in [14, 16].

- **Synthetic sound rendering**, also called Parameter-Mapping Sonification, is the second principle for real-time synthesizing of sound [26, 28]. In Parameter-Mapping Sonification, data values are mapped to acoustic attributes of a sound (in other words: the data "play" an instrument) [15]. Synthetic sound rendering comprises techniques such as: frequency modulation (FM) synthesis, additive synthesis, subtractive synthesis, wave shaping, frustum tracing [23] and many more. Especially cheap rendering techniques in terms of calculation time, cost of programs/material, and implementation difficulty, are parametric models. These models are controlled only by a few parameters e.g.: pitch, amplitude, and decay time while still providing pleasant sounds [20]. A good trade-off between calculation time and sound quality are the so-called spectral models. These rather realistic models are mostly obtained through modal analysis of elastic body vibrations and imitation of sound production mechanisms [39]. Each model is then associated with the modal characteristics of its original sound source and is spatio-temporally located in the virtual scenario. For sound rendering, the synthetic sound sources emit sound, which is reflected by the virtual environment and recorded by a virtual microphone, which is placed in the same location as the human listener. The virtually recorded sound is finally displayed by the sound system. The complexity of the calculation process in order to finally display the sound depends on the kind of sound system e.g. mono, stereo, dolby-surround, wave field synthesis. A more detailed description of how sound is rendered by realistic spectral models can be found in [32, 41]. A good and more detailed overview of the development of sound rendering through digital synthesis in history and the corresponding methods is given in [12, 38].

5.4.3 Sound Triggering

A further important aspect in rendering sound especially in combination with other modalities in virtual environments is the synchronization of sounds. There are basically three ways to synchronize the sound with the visual scenario in virtual environments: time-based triggering, position-based triggering, and collision-based triggering.

- In **time-based triggering**, the current simulation time is used as a trigger in order to start, stop or change sounds in a virtual environment.
- In **position-based triggering**, the current position of the user is used as a trigger in order to start, stop or change sounds in a virtual environment.
- In **collision-based triggering**, the collision between objects in a virtual scenario is detected. The detected collision can be used as a trigger in order to start, stop or change sounds in a virtual environment. The intensity, duration or any other aspects of the collision can be used to modulate the sound of the collision [41].

5.5 Application of Auditory Displays in Medical VR

Auditory displays applied in VR have become quite important also in the field of medicine [31]. They are used for data analysis (sonification), training of emergency situations, virtual surgery, or medical procedures. In all of these situations sound can play a crucial role through acquisition of enhanced skills and dexterity, increased effectiveness, or facilitated navigation through training in sound-enhanced medical VR scenarios. In a study with skilled sonar operators it has been found that learning on how target sound patterns are produced showed positive implications on classification of auditory patterns [18]. Another example for successful application of auditory displays are assistive technologies for blind users. This study confirmed that attainable skilled performance levels are more important than the level of performance achieved on first exposure [10]. In the future, more complex psychological studies could reveal the positive influence of sound on higher-level cognitive processes, since learning ties together basic perception with higher-level cognitive processes [22]. In addition to research in psychoacoustics that has focused so far on single auditory dimensions (e.g., pitch), further research is needed to investigate how performance with auditory displays changes with practice to improve our understanding of adaptive capabilities [27]. This becomes obvious, since auditory events in the real world change dynamically, and, thus, sound perception has to adapt to simultaneous changes in frequency, intensity, and often location [22]. The unique capabilities of the auditory system to use such covariation to define perceptual events and "scenes" [7] can potentially be exploited to create meaningful and compelling data displays [22]. This is especially important for being able to design new powerful VR environments enhanced by auditory displays for skills training dedicated to medical applications.

References

1. Akeroyd, M.A.: The psychoacoustics of binaural hearing. Int. J. Audiol. **45**(s1), 25–33 (2006)
2. Algazi, V.R., Duda, R.O.: Immersive spatial sound for mobile multimedia. In: Proceedings of the Seventh IEEE International Symposium on Multimedia, pp. 739–746. IEEE Computer Society, Washington (2005)
3. Begault, D.R.: 3D Sound for Virtual Reality and Multimedia. NASA, Washington (1994)
4. Berkhout, A.J., De Vries, D., Vogel, P.: Acoustic control by wave field synthesis. J. Acoust. Soc. Am. **93**(5), 2764–2778 (1993). doi:10.1121/1.405852
5. Blauert, J.: Räumliches Hören, Neue Ergebnisse und Trends seit 1972. Hirzel Verlag, Stuttgart (1985)
6. Blauert, J.: Spatial Hearing: the Psychophysics of Human Sound Localization. MIT Press, Cambridge (1997)
7. Bregman, A.S.: Auditory scene analysis: the perceptual organization of sound (1994)
8. Brown, C.P., Duda, R.O.: A structural model for binaural sound synthesis. IEEE Trans. Speech Audio Process. **6**(5), 476–488 (1998)
9. Deetjen, P., Speckmann, E.J., Hescheler, J.: Physiologie, 4th edn. Elsevier, Urban und Fischer Verlag, München (2005)
10. Earl, C.L., Leventhal, J.D.: A survey of windows screen reader users: recent improvements in accessibility. J. Vis. Impair. Blind. **93**(3), 174–176 (1999)

11. Fletcher, N.H., Rossing, T.D.: The Physics of Musical Instruments, 2nd edn. Springer, Berlin (1998)
12. Funkhouser, T.: Sounds good to me! computational sound for graphics, virtual reality, and interactive systems. In: SIGGRAPH 2002 (2002)
13. Goldstein, E.B.: Wahrnehmungspsychologie: Der Grundkurs, 7th edn. Springer, Berlin (2008)
14. Hermann, T.: Sonification for Exploratory Data Analysis. Bielefeld University, Bielefeld (2002)
15. Hermann, T.: Taxonomy and definitions for sonification and auditory display. In: Proceedings of the 14th ICAD, Paris (2008). www.sonification.de/main-def.shtml
16. Hermann, T., Ritter, H.: Listen to your data: model-based sonification for data analysis. In: Advances in Intelligent Computing and Multimedia Systems, pp. 189–194 (1999)
17. Hofman, P.M., Van Riswick, J.G.A., Van Opstal, A.J.: Relearning sound localization with new ears. Nat. Neurosci. 1(5), 417–421 (1998)
18. Howard, J.H., et al.: Acquisition of acoustic pattern categories by exemplar observation. Org. Behav. Hum. Perform. 30(2), 157–173 (1982)
19. Karjalainen, M., Välimäki, V., Jánosy, Z.: Towards high-quality sound synthesis of the guitar and string instruments. In: International Computer Music Conference, Tokyo, Japan, pp. 56–63 (1993)
20. Karplus, K., Strong, A.: Digital synthesis of plucked-string and drum timbres. Comput. Music J. 7(2), 43–55 (1983)
21. Kramer, G., Santa Fe Institute: Auditory Display: Sonification, Audification, and Auditory Interfaces, p. 672. Addison-Wesley, Reading (1994)
22. Kramer, G., Walker, B., Bonebright, T., Cook, P., Flowers, J.H., Miner, N., Neuhoff, J.: Sonification report: status of the field and research agenda. Faculty publications, Department of Psychology, University of Nebraska–Lincoln (2010)
23. Lauterbach, C., Chandak, A., Manocha, D.: Interactive sound rendering in complex and dynamic scenes using frustum tracing. IEEE Trans. Vis. Comput. Graph. 13(6), 1672–1679 (2007)
24. Lehnert, H.: Principles of binaural room simulation. Appl. Acoust. 36(3–4), 259–291 (1992)
25. McGookin, D.K., Brewster, S.A.: Understanding concurrent earcons: applying auditory scene analysis principles to concurrent earcon recognition. ACM Trans. Appl. Percept. 1(2), 130–155 (2004)
26. Naef, M., Staadt, O., Gross, M.: Spatialized audio rendering for immersive virtual environments. In: Proceedings of the ACM Symposium on Virtual Reality Software and Technology, pp. 65–72 (2002)
27. Neuhoff, J.G.: Perceptual bias for rising tones. Nature 395(6698), 123–124 (1998)
28. Noser, H.: Synthetic vision and audition for digital actors. EUROGRAPHICS 14(3), 325–336 (1995)
29. Pompei, F.: Spotlight of sound. Technical report (2009)
30. Saberi, K., Dostal, L., Sadralodabai, T., Perrott, D.: Minimum audible angles for horizontal, vertical, and oblique orientations: lateral and dorsal planes. Acustica 75(1), 57–61 (1991)
31. Sanderson, P.: Advanced auditory displays and head-mounted displays: advantages and disadvantages for monitoring by the distracted anesthesiologist. Anesth. Analg. 106(6), 1787–1797 (2008)
32. Saviola, L., Huopaniemi, J., Lokki, T., Väänänen, R.: Creating interactive virtual acoustic environments. J. Audio Eng. Soc. 47(9), 675–705 (1999)
33. Schmidt, R.F.: Fundamentals of Sensory Physiology. Springer, Berlin (1986)
34. Schmidt, R.F., Thews, G.: Die Physiologie des Menschen. Springer, Berlin (1990)
35. Serafin, S., Serafin, G.: Sound design to enhance presence in photorealistic virtual reality. In: Proceedings of the 2004 International Conference on Auditory Display, pp. 6–9. Citeseer, Princeton (2004)
36. Shaw, E.: Transformation of sound-pressure level from the free field to the eardrum presented in numerical form. J. Acoust. Soc. Am. 78(3), 1120–1123 (1985)

37. Slater, M., Linakis, V., Usoh, M., Kooper, R.: Immersion, presence, and performance in virtual environments: an experiment with tri-dimensional chess. In: ACM Virtual Reality Software and Technology (VRST), pp. 163–172. Citeseer, Princeton (1996)

38. Smith, J.O.: Viewpoints on the history of digital synthesis. In: Proceedings of the International Computer Music Conference. Citeseer, Princeton (1991)

39. Smith, J.O.: Virtual acoustic musical instruments: review and update. J. New Music Res. **33**(3), 283–304 (2004)

40. Suzuki, Y., Takeshima, H.: Equal-loudness-level contours for pure tones. J. Acoust. Soc. Am. **116**(2), 918 (2004). doi:10.1121/1.1763601

41. Takala, T., Hahn, J.: Sound rendering. In: Proceedings of the 19th Annual Conference on Computer Graphics and Interactive Techniques, p. 220. ACM, New York (1992)

42. Van Tasell, D.J.: New DSP instrument designed to maximize binaural benefits. Hear. J. **51**, 40–51 (1998)

43. Viveros, J.A.T.: Aplicación de técnica de grabación y mezcla binaural para audio comercial y/o pubicitario (2009)

44. Wand, M.: A real-time sound rendering algorithm for complex scenes (2003)

45. Wightman, F.: Headphone simulation of free-field listening. I: Stimulus synthesis. J. Acoust. Soc. Am. **85**(2), 858–867 (1989)

46. Willert, V., Eggert, J., Adamy, J., Stahl, R., Korner, E.: A probabilistic model for binaural sound localization. IEEE Trans. Syst. Man Cybern., Part B, Cybern. **36**(5), 982–994 (2006)

47. Yon, S., Tanter, M., Fink, M.: Sound focusing in rooms: the time-reversal approach. J. Acoust. Soc. Am. **113**(3), 1533–1543 (2002)

Chapter 6
Olfactory and Gustatory Aspects

6.1 What Are Olfactory and Gustatory Displays?

Humans both smell and taste information by chemoreceptors that respond to chemical stimuli. The sense of smell (olfactory sense) and the sense of taste (gustatory sense) are functionally coupled. In general, the sense of smell influences the sense of taste. Without the sense of smell (olfaction), the ability to taste (gustation) may be reduced. In this chapter, simulations of olfactory aspects are discussed first, followed by a description of gustatory aspects. The provision of olfactory feedback in VR environments can enhance the level of realism of different training scenarios. Gustatory simulations are mostly developed for research purposes or entertainment. Olfactory and gustatory displays enable the artificial representation of certain smells and tastes, respectively. They are less popular in VR systems than visual, auditory, and haptic displays, most probably because their contribution to enhance presence and immersion is believed to be limited. The technical design and realization of *realistic*, but also *practical* olfactory and gustatory displays is challenging. The challenges are highlighted in this chapter.

6.2 Olfactory Sense and Perception

Our sense of smell detects chemical molecules that are released by substances in our environment. Odorants in form of chemical molecules are dissolved into the ambient air and inhaled through the nose or the mouth (Fig. 6.1). Humans have about 10 to 30 million olfactory receptor cells located in the regio olfactoria in the nose. An odorant contains different structural elements and can therefore bind to different receptor types. Consequently, an odor (synonym: scent) is determined by the activity of an ensemble of multiple receptor cells. An odor can consist of hundreds of different odorants. It is assumed that the human can distinguish some thousands of odors. The threshold of perception largely differs between odors. It can be e.g. 1×10^7 molecules/ml air for hydrogen sulfide (bad eggs, fecal matter) or 1×10^{14} molecules/ml air for geraniol (rose oil). The perception is highly dependent on

R. Riener, M. Harders, *Virtual Reality in Medicine*, 149
DOI 10.1007/978-1-4471-4011-5_6, © Springer-Verlag London 2012

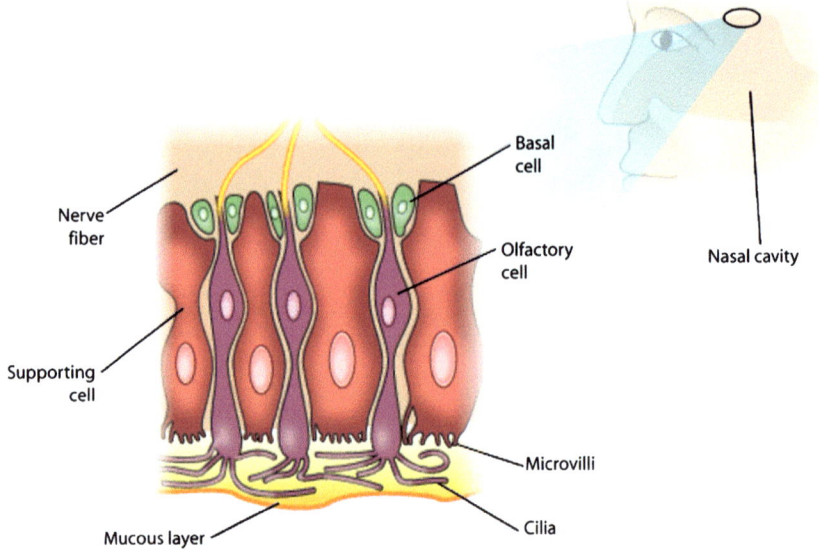

Fig. 6.1   Olfactory epithelium; © ADInstruments Pty Ltd. Reproduced with permission

external circumstances and may vary among ethnic groups. Practically, the olfactory sense works as a warning system for danger, bad food or hygienics. Odors also have an influence on sexual behavior, well-being and social relationships (e.g. mutual mother-child identification). Odors can induce salivation and the secretion of gastric juice [2]. Olfaction has been described to have the following characteristics [8, 12]:

- Olfaction is *nominal*. It has a good absolute sensitivity and an even better quality discrimination, which is more important.
- It is a *near* sense, as the odorants need direct contact with the olfactory receptor cells in the nose.
- It is a *hidden sense*. Olfaction is seldom in the focus of attention, but can subjectively influence the attentional and emotional state of the human.
- Olfaction is very subjective as well as *emotional* and *associative*, as odors are often associated with emotional experiences.
- It is a *special memory*, with a strong relation to emotion. It is rather an episodic than a semantic memory.

6.3 Olfactory Display Technology

6.3.1 Design Principles

The simulation of odors is challenging because odors cannot be described by compressed information as it is the case for colors and sound (i.e. frequency, intensity).

Odors can be produced by releasing small portions of odor samples in the form of vapor into the ambient environment. A number of primary odors may be combined to generate new odors. So far, the major problem with emitting odors has been that the odor diffuses to a wide area, and that it does not dissipate quickly. Various odor parameters such as flow rate, concentration, duration, and direction need to be characterized. Therefore, technological advances in odor storage, mixing, delivery, and removal are required to produce real-time synthesized odor, which can quickly adapt to the change of the situation in the virtual environment. In summary, the main challenges of the design of olfactory displays are

- the generation of a large variety of different odors,
- the mixture of odors, as odors cannot be reduced to a subset of simple parameters such as possible in visual and auditory displays,
- the storage of odors,
- the precise transport of odors to the nose,
- the maintenance of odors in a desired area, and
- the exchange or removal of odors in real-time.

In its most general form, an olfactory display consists of an odor storage, control, and delivery component. Odor components can be stored in a liquid phase, in gel, and solid waxes [1]. An algorithm controls the mixing ratios, concentrations, and timing of the delivery. The odor liquid can be delivered by using inkjet printer technology or heat-induced methods, whereas the odor gels can be released thermally or electro-statically. Once released, odors can be dispersed using a general air ventilation system [12].

Not many olfactory displays have been developed so far, and most often, the devices have stayed in their prototype version. In order to give an insight into different rendering approaches, we refer to the displays introduced exemplarily in Sect. 6.3.2 and Sect. 6.3.3. Olfactory display devices can mainly be separated into stationary or desktop devices and wearable or wireless devices.

6.3.2 Stationary Devices

- **iSmell** A digital scent synthesizer called iSmell has been developed by DigiScents, Inc. The device consists of pots of oils infused with different scents. A combination of pots is heated according to the code received from the computer, thereby evaporating those oils. A fan blows the heated vapors out of the pots. The iSmell was claimed to be able to create thousands of everyday scents with scent cartridges of 128 primary odors. These primary odors are blended to generate other smells that closely replicate common natural and man-made odors, but it is unclear if this claim has ever been scientifically proven. However, DigiScents closed down in April 2001, without having commercialized the iSmell device [16].

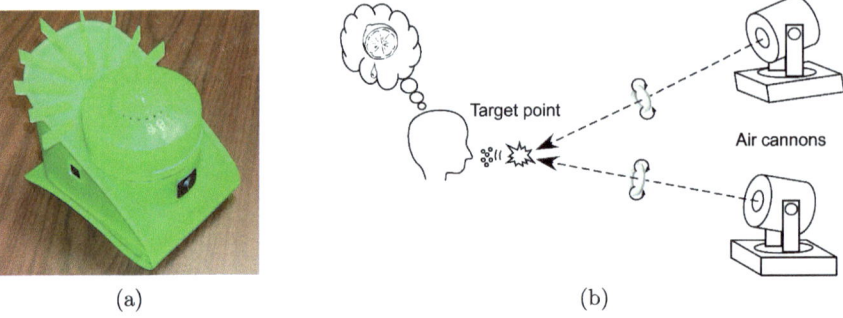

Fig. 6.2 Two examples of stationary olfactory displays. (**a**) TriSenx Scent Dome™ can generate dozens of aromas [16] (© 2004, IEEE); (**b**) Projection-based olfactory display system: SpotScents [10] (© 2006, IEEE)

- **Solenoid Valves-Based Olfactory Display** A research group at Tokyo Institute of Technology has developed an olfactory display system, which can blend up to 31 primary odor components. Thus, theoretically, 2×10^9 combinations of smell are possible [11]. High speed solenoid valves are used as selective switches to control the concentration of each odor component. The time period between on/off states of the high speed solenoid valves is about 1 ms. 32 sample tubes are used in the current system. 31 tubes are filled with different primary odors in liquid form, while one empty tube is used to supply air to the outlet. The vapor of each primary odor is carried out of the tube by a carrier gas. Only one odor component is allowed to flow to the output at a certain time. Time division multiplexing technique is used to mix the odor components. The output odor is produced with a cycle time of 1 s.
- **Scent Palette** The Scent Palette (Envirodine Studios, Canton, GA) allows delivering short and longer burst of scents into a virtual environment. The scents are stored in a gel and enclosed in an airtight chamber with compressed air. Four electric fans inside the Scent Palette generate an air stream in order to release the scent into the room [1, 13].
- **Scent Dome** TriSenx Holdings, Inc. (Savannah, GA) has released a consumer olfactory display product called Scent Dome™. Scent Dome consists of 20 base scents which can generate dozens of aromas by software control (see [14]). The scents are dispersed out of the top of the scent cartridge by a small fan (Fig. 6.2(a)).
- **Projection-Based Olfactory Display** The projection-based olfactory display (scent projector) delivers localized odors to the human nose through free space by incorporating nose-tracking function rather than scattering scented air by simply diffusing it into the atmosphere [18]. The air cannon in the device generates scanted vortex rings that can travel several meters. A limitation is that the user feels an unnatural airflow when the vortex rings reach the face. To reduce this sensation, a later version of the scent projector used two air cannons, each launching

vortex rings [10]. The rings collide at a target point creating a small spot of scents (Fig. 6.2(b)). The user feels the scent as coming with a small breeze. However, the system is not applicable for larger spaces or outdoors, as the firing range is limited and environmental factors such as wind can disturb the delivery of the odor [1, 17].

- **Aroma-Chip based Olfactory Display** An aroma-chip based olfactory display system was developed with the goal that it can easily be used by everyone at home [7]. In this system, a Peltier module controls temperature and, thereby, the gel-sol transition of the temperature sensitive hydrogel of the card type aroma-chip. The hydrogel is mixed with aromatic fragrances, which are released in the sol phase. Interestingly, to drive the release of different odors, dual tone multi-frequency (DTMF) signals were used. These signals, which were on sound tracks of a video tape, triggered the release of different aromatic fragrances.
- **Piezoelectric Perfume Diffusion Technology** Osmooze® introduces a piezoelectric perfume diffusion technology. The perfume passes through a needle towards a bevel edged tip. A piezoelectric ceramic disk induces a vibration (200 Hz) of the needle in order to form droplets of odors. A small ventilator blows the droplets into the room. Another approach, the Osmooze® GEL technology, allows the storage of odorants in a dry state for small volumes. An air stream passes over the gel cartridge, releasing the odorant into the environment.

6.3.3 Wearable Devices

- **ICT Scent Collar** In collaboration with the Institute for Creative Technologies ICT (University of Southern California, USA), AntroTronix, Inc. (Silver Spring, Maryland, USA) has released an olfactory display called Scent Collar or Scent Necklace (Fig. 6.3(a)). In the prototype version, the device can provide four different scents. Each unique scent is contained in an individual cartridge embedded in a lightweight wearable collar that fits around a user's neck [15]. The amount and duration of the scent released are wirelessly controlled via Bluetooth by simulations or games.
- **Sniffman** Another wearable olfactory display "Sniffman" has been developed by Ruetz Technologies (Munich, Germany) and utilized by im.ve, University of Hamburg, to enrich VEs through im.ve's odor-extended VR system. Up to 32 different odors can be released in different concentrations and time intervals [3]. A plug-in controls the synchronization of the smell for example in a VE and sends its commands by radio signal to a device worn around the neck. Different odors are released from an injection nozzle to a heating plate. After evaporation, the odors are released into the air and are then smelled by the user (Fig. 6.3(b)).
- **"Odor Field" Concept** The idea of an "odor field" in a virtual environment is to release odors by a wearable olfactory display depending on the spatial position of the user [17]. The concept of the "odor field" was tested with two prototypes of olfactory displays. The first one transfers odorized air by four DC motor air

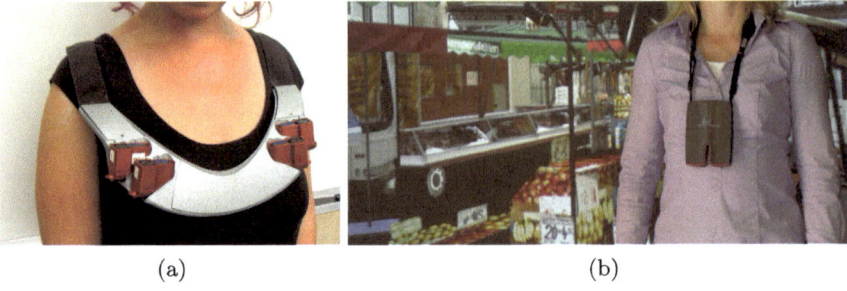

Fig. 6.3   Wearable olfactory displays. (**a**) ICT Scent Collar, by courtesy of J. Morie, University of Southern California; (**b**) Sniffman in combination with virtual marketplace; by courtesy of S. Beckhaus, University of Hamburg

Fig. 6.4   "Odor field" concept using radio-frequency identification (RFID) tag space combined with a wearable olfactory display; [17] (© 2006, IEEE)

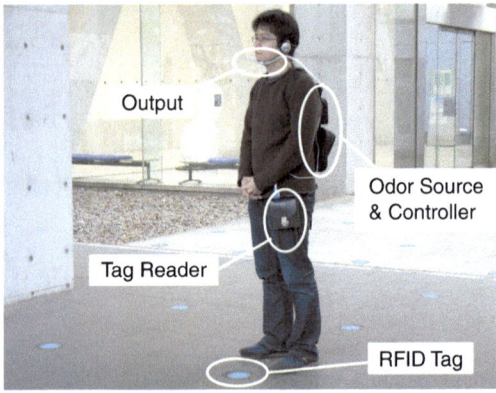

pumps to the user's nose. One air pump was used for non-odor airflow. Three air pumps were connected to three odor filters which contained the perfume materials. The odor strength was adjusted by controlling the proportion of non-odor airflow to odor airflow. Silicon tubes were used for the connections, because silicon is nearly odorless and nontoxic to humans. By placing the odor presenting unit close to the user's nose, odors could be quickly switched and external disturbances such as wind could be minimized. The wearable olfactory display was combined with a radio-frequency identification (RFID) tag space in order to build an odor field. Tests showed that users can perceive the spatial odor information, however, wind made it still difficult to perceive the odor (Fig. 6.4).

The second prototype was constructed in order to allow the display of many odors while still remaining a small, wearable device. The odors were stored in the liquid phase. The inkjet head device of the odor presenting unit released odor droplets directly to the user's nose, where it vaporized (Fig. 6.5). This allowed a subtle control of odor strength. In order to save perfume material and to minimize the amount of odors spread into the environment, the breathing of the user was detected by a respiration sensor. Thus, the perfume material was only released

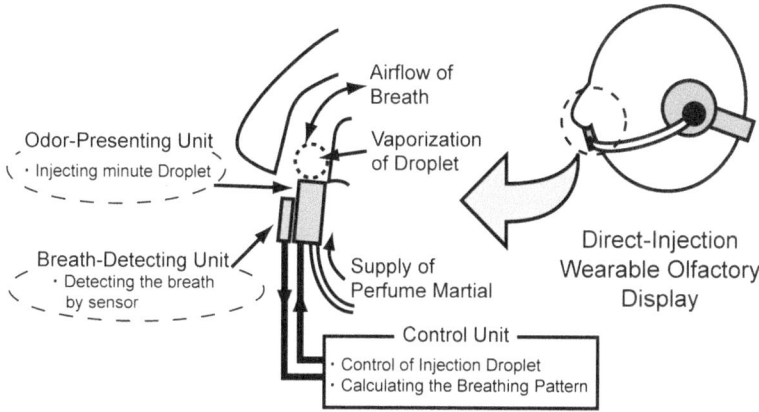

Fig. 6.5 Direct-injection wearable olfactory display system; [17] (© 2006, IEEE)

during inhalation. Indeed, the second prototype was evaluated to be superior to the first one in terms of operating life and stability of odor strength presentation.

- **Further Wearable Devices** The ScentKiosk Scent dispenser can release three odors to the user's nose via a tube (www.scentair.com). Exchangeable single scent cartridges facilitate different scenarios. The system can be applied for data visualization or virtual reality applications. However, as the tube lengths are limited, mobility is constrained [16]. Aromajet has developed a small aroma-dispensing device called Pinoke. The device can be worn but also be placed in front of a monitor (www.aromajet.com). Aromajet provides a kiosk system, which allows a costumer to create different odors [16].

6.4 Gustatory Sense and Perception

The perception of taste (gustation) refers to the ability to detect the flavor of substances such as foods and drinks. Taste is sensed by taste cells contained in bundles called taste buds located on the tongue and in the mucosa of the cheek, palate, pharynx (throat), and larynx (Fig. 6.6). The human can distinguish roughly among five different flavors: sweet, sour, salty, bitter, and umami. Umami is a nutriment with high concentration of the amino acid Glutamate, first described by Japanese scientists sometimes translated as the flavor of broth or meat. The brain integrates information of several different taste cells to identify a taste. The threshold of unspecific sensation is lowest for bitter substances (e.g. nicotine: 1.6×10^{-5} mol/l) and highest for sweet and salty substances (e.g. sucrose or NaCl: 1×10^{-2} mol/l). The main task of the gustatory sense is the detection of spoiled or poisoned food, and the induction of salivation and secretion of gastric juice. In common with odors, tastes may influence our mood and feelings [2].

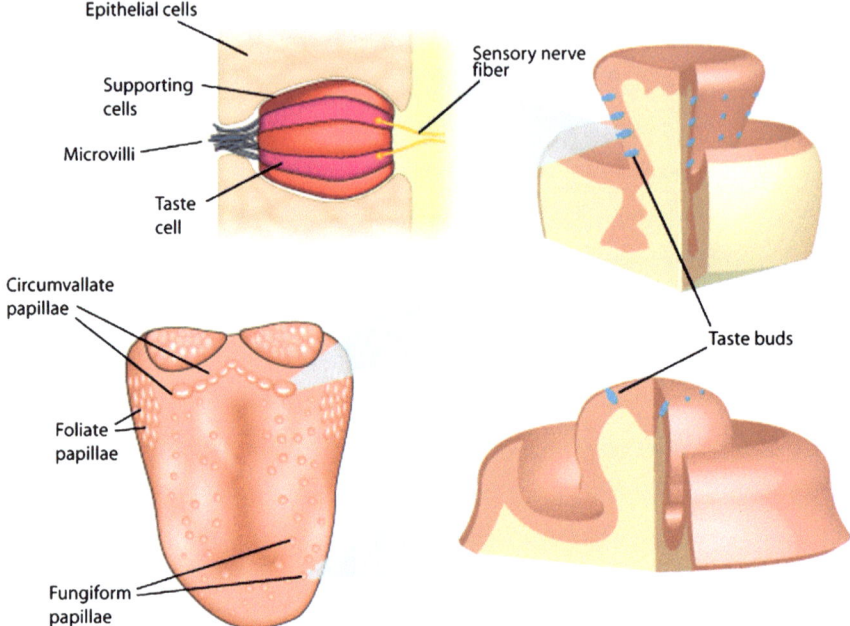

Fig. 6.6 Human tongue and taste buds; © ADInstruments Pty Ltd. Reproduced with permission

6.5 Gustatory Display Technology

6.5.1 Design Principles

Eating or drinking does not only include the sense of taste, but also the haptic sense. The sensation of the consistence of food and drinks influences the perception of food quality. The main challenges in the design of olfactory displays are

- the generation of a huge variety of different tastes,
- the mixture of tastes, as tastes cannot be reduced to a subset of simple parameters,
- the storage of tastes,
- the simulation of the haptic aspects of chewing and drinking,
- the exchange or removal of tastes in real-time, and
- the adherence of hygienics.

In order to illustrate how gustatory impressions can be rendered, exemplary devices are described in the following sections. The sections are separated in taste simulation, food simulation, and drinking simulation.

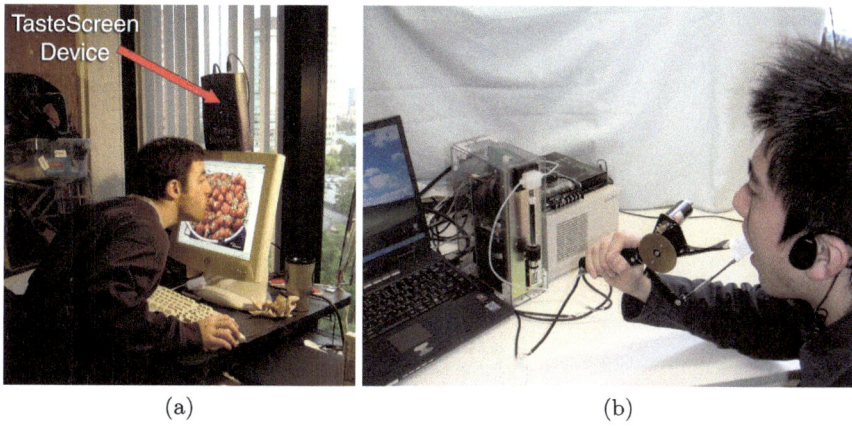

Fig. 6.7 Examples of a taste and a food simulator system. (**a**) TasteScreen from Stanford University [9]; by courtesy of Dan Aminzade; (**b**) The Food Simulator provides taste, smell, and haptic feedback; by courtesy of Hiroo Iwata

6.5.2 Taste Simulation

The TasteScreen consists of an LCD monitor and a USB device placed on its top. The device includes twenty small plastic cartridges each containing a flavoring agent [9]. By combining the flavoring agents, different flavors can be produced. The flavors are mixed in a deployment chamber and then dispensed. The user can lick the thin liquid residue with the tongue from the screen (Fig. 6.7(a)).

6.5.3 Food Simulation

The food simulator, introduced by Iwata et al. (2003) can reproduce taste and smell of food, biting force, but also provides auditory feedback [6]. The taste sensation is generated using a micro injector containing chemical compounds, whereas a vaporizer delivers the smell of the food (Fig. 6.7(b)).

6.5.4 Drinking Simulation

The straw-like User Interface (SUI) simulates drinking by controlling pressure, sound, and vibration of an ordinary straw [4, 5]. A solenoid motor controls the valve to regulate pressure. One loudspeaker is used to generate vibrations in the straw, another one to provide sound feedback. When experiencing the Straw-like User Interface, an integration of pictures of the food, sound, and sensory feedback gives a virtual drinking sensation to the user (Fig. 6.8).

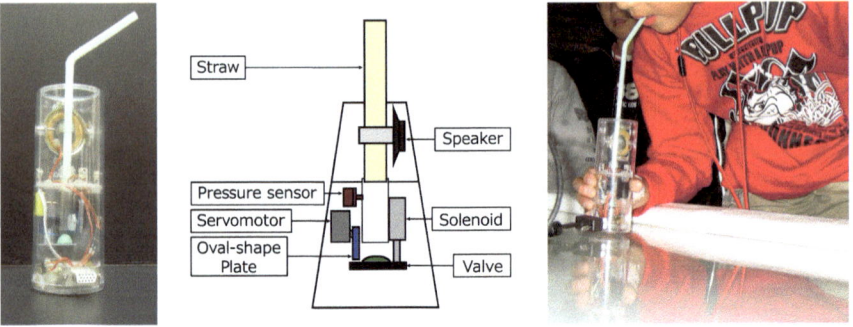

Fig. 6.8 Virtual drinking simulator using a Straw-Like User Interface, by courtesy of Masahiko Inami

6.6 Applications of Olfactory and Gustatory Displays in Medical VR

Olfactory displays are mostly used to increase the level of realism in a virtual environment, e.g. in firefighter training or for entertainment. Odors can not only influence mood and vigilance, but can also decrease stress as well as increase learning performance [12, 16]. Therefore, olfactory displays can also be applied as therapeutic devices to affect mental stress or treating psychological disorders or phobia as well as for aromatherapy on pain and depression. For example, virtual reality scenarios could enhance the treatment of Post Traumatic Stress Disorder (PTSD) of war veterans, victims of kidnapping or terrorist attacks, as special odors experienced in the traumatic event, can be reproduced, released selectively, and combined with a visual and auditory scenario [13].

In addition to psychological treatments, olfactory displays could facilitate the learning of diagnostic decision making for medical students [1]. Some disorders can be identified based on specific odors of the patient. Medical students could be trained in a VE in order to learn to identify odors that accompany these specific disorders. Moreover, in a tele-surgical environment, where doctors perform operations with a robotic device, odors could be displayed to represent human tissue to enhance the experience [14].

Similar to odors, tastes can have significant impacts on the emotional state of a human. Therefore, they could potentially be used to treat psychological disorders. However, gustatory displays, but also olfactory displays, have rarely been applied in the field of medical VR to date.

References

1. Chen, Y.: Olfactory display: development and application in virtual reality therapy. In: Proceedings of the 16th International Conference on Artificial Reality and Telexistence-Workshops, pp. 580–584. IEEE Computer Society, Washington (2006)

2. Deetjen, P., Speckmann, E.J., Hescheler, J.: Physiologie, 4th edn. Elsevier, Urban und Fischer Verlag, München (2005)
3. Haselhoff, S., Beckhaus, S.: Benutzerindividuelle, tragbare Geruchsausgabe in virtuellen Umgebungen. In: Virtuelle und Erweiterte Realität, 3. Workshop der GI-Fachgruppe VR/AR, Koblenz, September, pp. 83–94. Shaker Verlag, Aachen (2006)
4. Hashimoto, Y., Nagaya, N., Kojima, M., Miyajima, S., Ohtaki, J., Yamamoto, A., Mitani, T., Inami, M.: Straw-like user interface: virtual experience of the sensation of drinking using a straw. In: Proceedings of the ACM SIGCHI International Conference on Advances in Computer Entertainment Technology, Hollywood, California, USA, p. 50. ACM, New York (2006)
5. Hashimoto, Y., Inami, M., Kajimoto, H.: Straw-like user interface (II): a new method of presenting auditory sensations for a more natural experience. In: Proceedings of the 6th International Conference EuroHaptics, Haptics: Perception, Devices and Scenarios, Madrid, Spain, p. 484. Springer, Berlin (2008)
6. Iwata, H., Yano, H., Uemura, T., Moriya, T.: Food simulator. In: ICAT International Conference on Artificial Reality and Telexistence, Tokyo, Japan, pp. 173–178 (2003)
7. Kim, D.W., Lee, D.W., Miura, M., Nishimoto, K., Kawakami, Y., Kunifuji, S.: Aroma-chip based olfactory display. In: Proceedings of the Second International Conference on Knowledge, Information and Creativity Support Systems. JAIST Press, Nomi (2007)
8. Köster, E.P.: The specific characteristics of the sense of smell. In: Olfaction, Taste and Cognition, pp. 27–44 (2002)
9. Maynes-Aminzade, D.: Edible bits: seamless interfaces between people, data and food. In: Proceedings of the ACM Conference on Human Factors in Computing Systems, pp. 2207–2210. Citeseer, Princeton (2005)
10. Nakaizumi, F., Yanagida, Y., Noma, H., Hosaka, K.: SpotScents: a novel method of natural scent delivery using multiple scent projectors. In: Virtual Reality Conference, 2006, pp. 207–212. Citeseer, Princeton (2006)
11. Nakamoto, T., Minh, H.P.D.: Improvement of olfactory display using solenoid valves. In: Proceedings of IEEE Virtual Reality, pp. 179–186 (2007)
12. Richard, E., Tijou, A., Richard, P., Ferrier, J.L.: Multi-modal virtual environments for education with haptic and olfactory feedback. Virtual Real. 10(3), 207–225 (2006)
13. Rizzo, A., Pair, J., Graap, K., Manson, B., McNerney, P.J., Wiederhold, B., Wiederhold, M., Spira, J.: A virtual reality exposure therapy application for Iraq War military personnel with post traumatic stress disorder: from training to toy to treatment. In: Roy, M.J. (ed.) Novel Approaches to the Diagnosis and Treatment of Posttraumatic Stress Disorder, pp. 235–250. IOS Press, Amsterdam (2006)·
14. Spencer, B.S.: Using the sense of smell in telemedical environments. In: Medical and Care Compunetics, vol. 1, pp. 135–142 (2004)
15. Tortell, R., Luigi, D.P., Dozois, A., Bouchard, S., Morie, J.F., Ilan, D.: The effects of scent and game play experience on memory of a virtual environment. Virtual Real. 11(1), 61–68 (2007)
16. Washburn, D.A., Jones, L.M.: Could olfactory displays improve data visualization? Comput. Sci. Eng. 6(6), 80–83 (2004)
17. Yamada, T., Yokoyama, S., Tanikawa, T., Hirota, K., Hirose, M.: Wearable olfactory display: using odor in outdoor environment. In: Virtual Reality Conference, pp. 199–206 (2006)
18. Yanagida, Y., Kawato, S., Noma, H., Tomono, A., Tetsutani, N.: Projection-based olfactory display with nose tracking. In: IEEE Virtual Reality Conference, pp. 43–50 (2004). http://vrlab.meijo-u.ac.jp/~yanagida/scent/index.html

Chapter 7
Virtual Reality for Rehabilitation

7.1 Rationale for the Use of Virtual Reality in Rehabilitation

Rehabilitation has the goal to restore previously lost movement capabilities, to learn compensatory movements or to treat cognitive and psychological deficits that enable subjects to cope with daily life. Virtual reality technologies in rehabilitation are thereby mostly employed in physiotherapy, occupational therapy, and psychotherapy. Applications in physiotherapy and occupational therapy consist, for instance recovery of limb functionality after disease or accident. In psychotherapy, VR is mostly used to treat phobias or stress trauma.

The three key concepts of physiological rehabilitation are repetition of the movement that needs to be rehabilitated, active participation of the patient and performance feedback. Movement repetition is important both for motor learning and the corresponding cortical changes [33, 34]. Active participation in gait training was shown to increase therapy outcome [35]. Same is true for the rehabilitation of the upper extremities when stroke patients are forced to use their paretic arm due to constraint induced movement therapy (CIMT) [5]. The repeated practice must also be linked to incremental success at some task or goal. In the intact nervous system, this is achieved by trial and error practice, with feedback about the performance success provided by the senses (e.g., vision, proprioception).

VR is a powerful tool to motivate the patients to active participation, while providing augmented performance feedback. VR in rehabilitation provides motivating training that can be superior to training in a real situation [18, 50]. It was shown that increased motivation [36] and active participation [26] can lead to increased efficiency and advancements of motor learning in neuro-rehabilitation. Enriched environments, highly functional and task-oriented practice environments were shown to be necessary for motor re-learning and recovery after stroke [26]. Additionally, VR can be utilized to test different methods of motor training, types of feedback provided, and practice schedules with regard to their effectiveness in improving motor function in patients. VR technology provides a convenient mechanism for manipulating these factors, setting up automatic training schedules and for training, testing, and recording participants' motor responses.

R. Riener, M. Harders, *Virtual Reality in Medicine*,
DOI 10.1007/978-1-4471-4011-5_7, © Springer-Verlag London 2012

Fig. 7.1 VR application in
ankle rehabilitation using the
Rutgers Ankle; Copyright
Rutgers Tele-Rehabilitation
Institute. Reprinted by
permission

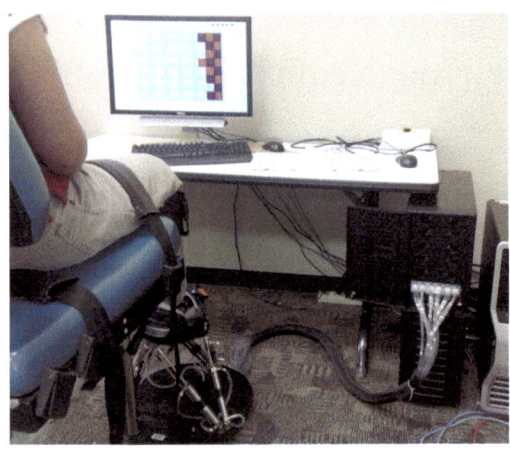

7.2   Virtual Reality Supported Physiotherapy

7.2.1   Ankle Rehabilitation

At Rutgers University, Burdea and colleagues developed the VR supported haptic
device Rutgers Ankle [14]. The system consists of a Stewart platform-type haptic
interface that provides 6 degrees of freedom resistive forces to the patient's foot,
in response to his or her performance in a game-like VR exercise (Fig. 7.1). The
patient is treated in a sitting posture, with the foot attached via a footplate to the
device. Two exercise games have been developed. In the first one, the patient uses
the foot to steer a virtual airplane through a virtual sky. As the plane moves forward,
a series of open square hoops are presented on the screen. The goal is for the patient
to maneuver the plane through the hoops without hitting the sides. This is done
by mapping the ankle movement to the flight path, where for instance ankle dorsi-
extension can cause the nose of the plane to point upward, elevation can cause the
plane to go toward the left, etc. The difficulty level can be adjusted by changing
the number and placement of hoops, airplane speed, and the amount of resistance
provided by the haptic interface.

A second game calls for the patient to pilot a virtual speedboat over the ocean
while avoiding buoys, again by moving the ankle up and down or in and out. A recent addition to these games is the ability to apply task-related haptic effects such
as a jolt when a buoy or hoop is hit, or to change the environmental conditions by
adding turbulence to the air or water implemented by generating a low-frequency
side-to-side vibration of the platform. Another group of researchers has used VR
technology to train obstacle avoidance during walking in chronic post-stroke patients [24]. They compared real world and virtual world obstacle avoidance training. Patients who received VR training showed significantly greater improvements
in fast paced velocity than patients who trained with real objects. Improvements in
obstacle clearance and step length of the non-paretic side were also higher in the

VR group, but not significantly. The Rutgers Ankle system has been tested on patients with orthopedic disorders. A pilot study was conducted on three patients with ankle injuries. Case 1 was a 14-year-old patient, 2 weeks after grade 1 ankle sprain. Case 2 was a 15-year-old patient, 5 months after grade 2 ankle sprain. Case 3 was a 56-year-old patient, 2 months after bimalleolar fracture. Patients received five treatment sessions over a 2-week period, sessions were 30 min, delivered two to three times per week. A sixth session was used for the post test. The treatment consisted of piloting a virtual airplane through hoops, at progressive levels of difficulty, as described earlier for the stroke patients. Cases 1 and 3 were also receiving concomitant physical therapy for their ankle problem. Case 2 received only the VR therapy. Each case is discussed separately, and different measures are presented for each participant. The authors report that all three participants improved. However, only for participant 2 could these changes be attributed to the VR treatment, as the other participants were receiving additional therapy at the same time. The most consistent improvement across the three participants was in task accuracy, defined as the number of hoops entered versus the missed ones. All were able to reach 100% accuracy, from a starting point of 40%, 65%, and 25%, for cases 1, 2, and 3, respectively. Improvements of varying amounts in ankle range of motion and torque production, one leg stance time, stair descent time, and speed of target hoop acquisition were also noted in one or more participants.

A recent study by Mirelman et al. [39] compared robotic intervention using the Rutgers Ankle system for patients exercising with and without an attached VR system. The researchers did not only compare standard neurological tests for both groups, but also investigated the distance walked and the steps taken in every day life using an accelerometer based system. The group that received VR augmented training showed greater changes in walking velocity, distance and number of steps taken.

7.2.2 Gait Rehabilitation

7.2.2.1 Treadmill Training

Treadmill training is part of a rehabilitation program administered to patients with neurological gait disorders in order to improve existing but limited walking capabilities [11]. Some clinical research groups are using VR systems that are coupled to treadmills, which are commonly used in rehabilitation. Baram and Miller studied the effects of VR on the walking abilities of multiple sclerosis patients. In 16 patients, they found an average short-term improvement of 24% increase in walking speed compared to baseline after exercising with VR [3]. Using a treadmill mounted on a 6 degree of freedom motion platform with a coupled VR system, Fung et al. could not only investigate walking, but also turning movements. This system provided auditory and visual feedback on gait performance and resulted in increased gait speed [13].

7.2.2.2 Treatment of Parkinson's Disease

One of the primary symptoms of Parkinson's disease (PD) is hypokinesia, or difficulty in the initiation and continuation of motions, in particular during ambulation. These symptoms tend to worsen as the disease progresses. Although the symptoms can be mitigated by drugs such as L-dopa, these drugs can become less effective over time and may produce unwanted side effects, such as correaform and athetotic movements. Thus, a complimentary method to treat hypokinetic gait in PD could offer patients a way to delay or reduce drug use while still maintaining or improving gait function. Such an alternative method is based on an interesting phenomenon associated with patients with PD termed *kinesia paradoxa*. Patients with PD, who are unable to ambulate, or even unable to initiate a step on open ground are, paradoxically, able to step over objects placed in their path with little difficulty. Weghorst and colleagues have conducted a number of studies to ascertain, whether VR technology provides a way to take advantage of this phenomenon and facilitate walking in PD patients by presenting virtual objects overlaid on the natural world [54].

7.2.2.3 Robot-Assisted Gait Training

Several devices for robot-assisted gait training have been developed over the last decades and were shown to cause significant improvement of gait function in patients suffering from stroke or spinal cord injury [22, 37]. Robots for treadmill walking typically consist of a body weight support system, a treadmill and an exoskeletal or end-effector based actuated mechanism driving the limbs of the patient. Examples are the Lokomat [12, 44], which uses actuators in hips and knees to automate treadmill walking, the WalkTrainer, which combines robot-assisted walking with functional electrical stimulation [49], the Bowden cable driven LOPES robot [52] and the Autoambulator (www.autoambulator.com) by HealthSouth Inc.

In the following section, the principles of VR in gait rehabilitation will be explained on the example of the Lokomat gait orthosis (Fig. 7.2). The Lokomat gait orthosis was developed in the Spinal Cord Injury Center at the University Hospital Balgrist for improvement and automation of neurorehabilitative treadmill training [12, 44]. It consists of two actuated leg orthoses, which are strapped to the patient's legs. On each orthosis, two motors, one at the hip joint and one at the knee joint, guide the patient's legs along a physiological walking pattern. The orthosis is synchronized with the belt speed of a treadmill. Together with the body weight support system, the orthosis allows even non-ambulatory patients to perform walking movements.

- **Visual rendering** Initially, in order to address patient-specific motor deficits, therapists and physicians can define the requirements for a VR based rehabilitation training. In a project with cerebral palsy children, the motor function training aims to increase the maximal force output of hip and knee flexors/extensors, to exercise and improve maximum joint range of motion, speed adaptation during walking, translation of visual input into motor output (eye/head coordination)

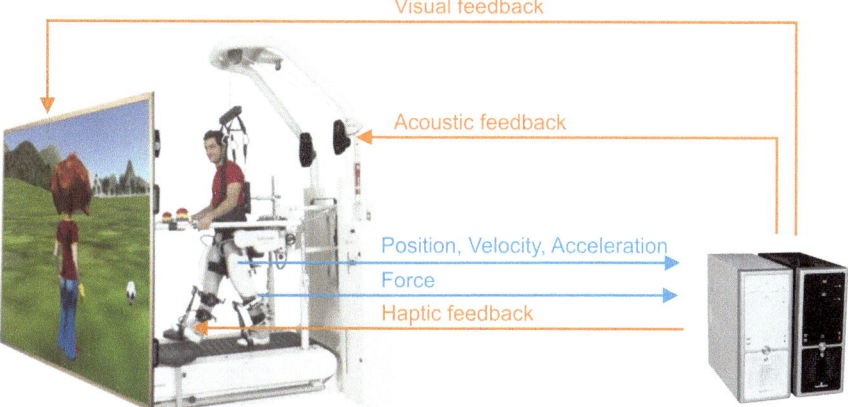

Fig. 7.2 The Lokomat VR setup

Table 7.1 Therapy goals of a virtual scenario used with cerebral palsy patients

	Soccer	Obstacle	Traffic	Snow
Muscle strength		+		+
Range of motion	+	+		
Walking speed	+		+	
Limb coordination	+	+		
Cognition	+		+	

and initiation/termination of gait. Four training scenarios of daily living were implemented as virtual tasks that address the above-mentioned training goals (Fig. 7.3) [28]. For muscle strengthening and to increase the range of motion, the patients wade through snow in a virtual world or kick a virtual soccer ball. In order to exercise the starting and stopping of gait and the increase and decrease of walking speed, the patients have to walk within a street traffic scenario, where they have to cross a street at a traffic light. Patients exercise gait-eye coordination (translation of visual input into motor output) and leg motion coordination in the street traffic scenario and in an obstacle course (Table 7.1).

Studies in healthy subjects showed that VR enabled healthy subjects to perform more accurate movements during obstacle stepping performed with the

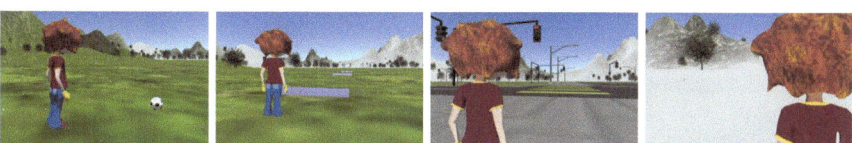

Fig. 7.3 Virtual gait parcours for children with cerebral palsy. *From left to right*: soccer scenario, obstacle overstepping, traffic scenario and walking through snow

Lokomat [55]. Subjects were given auditory, visual and haptic feedback on their foot clearance and the distance to obstacles they had to overstep. Performance was measured as foot clearance over the obstacle and the number of obstacles hit. This study showed that subjects had higher performance with auditory feedback than with visual feedback. Additionally, the authors showed that 3D vision did not improve performance compared to 2D vision. In patients, a Lokomat study by Bruetsch et al. showed that VR had the potential to increase active participation of children with cerebral palsy [10] compared to gait therapy alone. Participation was thereby quantified by EMG measurements.

- **Acoustic rendering** Sound should be properly timed with a visual or haptic event. In order to create a realistic impression, the sound should not be delayed more than 20 ms after the occurrence of the visual and haptic event. An example is the collision of the foot with a virtual obstacle. When the foot impacts the virtual wall, the graphical and haptic displays show the foot contact with the wall with a minimal time shift to the acoustics.

- **Haptic rendering** The Lokomat system is an input device used to translate the patient's movements into avatar movement within the virtual environment. The Lokomat system also serves as a haptic display, performing at a sampling frequency of 1,000 Hz. This renders force feedback as resulting from the interactions of the patient with virtual objects. The Lokomat was not built to be a haptic display. It only has motors in hip and knee joints, whereas the ankle joint cannot be actuated. Therefore, contact forces on the toes cannot be displayed directly. Nevertheless, it is possible to produce a quasi-realistic haptic perception by tricking the tactile system with synchronized visual and acoustic cues into believing the interaction would happen at the toes.

  Impedance control is normally used to display haptic objects in the virtual environment. Typical sampling times for haptic rendering lie in the area of 500–1,000 Hz. Below 500 Hz, the rendering of stiff objects will become unstable yielding vibrations. To guarantee the required update rate, the haptic rendering is, therefore, directly included within the Lokomat control architecture. An impedance controller computes a corrective force from the difference between desired and real position. It implements a spring-damper system as an internal impedance model. The reaction force is computed from the stiffness of the spring-damper system. Stability problems can occur, when the controller has to display an infinitely stiff wall, i.e. an infinitely high spring constant. Then, an infinitesimally small penetration of the object would result in infinitely high forces. Computation of the contact forces can be done by impulse based methods or by penalty based methods. An impulsive force is applied on contact of the foot with the object and pushes the foot out of the virtual object. Thereby, the position of the foot in Cartesian space must be computed as a function of hip and knee angles and length of shank and thigh. When shank length is known, estimation of the length of thigh and foot can be done with the method of Winter [57]. Then, during contact with the object, the desired haptic interaction forces, $\mathbf{F}$, can be computed. In penalty based methods, the interaction force will be computed depending upon the penetration depth $\delta\mathbf{x}$ and/or velocity $\dot{\mathbf{x}}$. Additional friction terms can help creating a realistic feeling. Thereby, it is possible to use the following linear viscoelastic relationship

$$\mathbf{F} = k\Delta\mathbf{x} + b\dot{\mathbf{x}}, \quad \text{if } \Delta\mathbf{x} > 0 \tag{7.1}$$

or a weighted spring-damper system

$$\mathbf{F} = k\Delta\mathbf{x} + b\Delta\mathbf{x}\dot{\mathbf{x}}, \quad \text{if } \Delta\mathbf{x} > 0 \tag{7.2}$$

otherwise

$$\mathbf{F} = \mathbf{0}, \quad \text{if } \Delta\mathbf{x} \leq 0 \tag{7.3}$$

where k is the spring coefficient and b the damping coefficient.

7.2.3 Arm Rehabilitation

7.2.3.1 Motivation for Robot Aided Arm Therapy

Arm rehabilitation is applied in neurorehabilitation for patients with paralyzed upper extremities due to lesions of the central or peripheral nervous system, e.g. after stroke or spinal cord injury. The goals of the therapy are to recover motor function, to improve movement coordination, to learn new motion strategies ("trick movements"), and/or to prevent secondary complications such as muscle atrophy, osteoporosis, and spasticity.

The advantages of robotic training are that the therapist can get assisted, e.g. relieved from the weight of the patient's arm, the training can get longer and more intensive (up to 20 times more movement repetitions per training session), and the movements can be measured and used for therapy assessment. Furthermore, special VR technologies can make the training much more entertaining and motivating as well as task-oriented and functional and, thus, more relevant for daily living activities.

Examples of arm robots are the MIT-Manus [31], which allows planar movements (Fig. 7.4(a)), the T-WREX (commercialized as Armeo®Spring, Hocoma AG, Switzerland) [19, 20], a passive, gravity-balancing orthosis with 5 degrees of freedom (Fig. 7.4(b)), the Bi-Manu-Track [16] for the training of distal functions (Fig. 7.4(c)) and ARMin [40], an active device with 7 degrees of freedom (Fig. 7.6).

One of the key elements for a successful rehabilitation is the motivation of the patient. It is also known that task-orientated training improves motor recovery in patients [4]. Audiovisual displays can ideally be used to present tasks and instructions to the patient [1, 2, 9, 25, 38, 42, 58]. Therefore, most systems are connected to a visual display or even virtual environment, where the robot acts as an input device for playing games and performing tasks (Fig. 7.5). The movement can be represented by a virtual avatar, by projecting a real camera image to the virtual world or by mapping the subjects movement to any other object (e.g. virtual ball or virtual car). During motor training also cognitive tasks can be exercised.

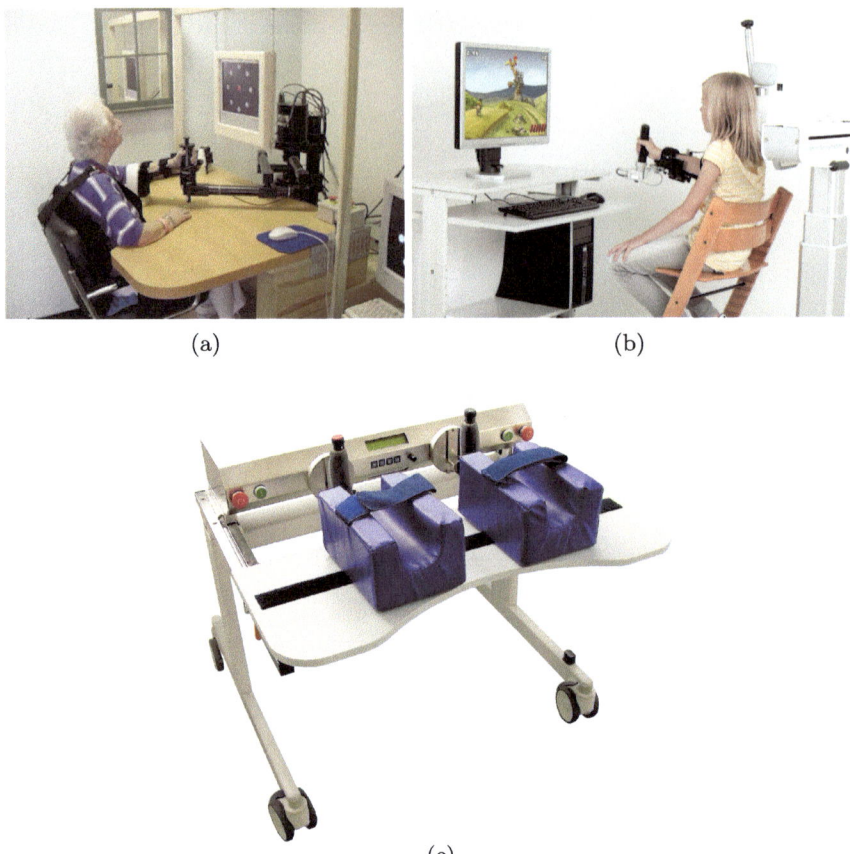

Fig. 7.4 Examples of arm rehabilitation robots. (**a**) MIT-Manus used for therapy at Burke Rehabilitation Hospital (White Plains, NY), originally published in [31]; with kind permission from
Springer Science+Business Media B.V.; (**b**) Armeo®Spring Pediatric, Hocoma AG, Switzerland;
(**c**) Bi-Manu-Track, by courtesy of B. Brandl-Hesse

7.2.3.2 Virtual Reality Applications with ARMin

ARMin was developed at ETH Zurich in collaboration with Balgrist University Hospital. The newest version of the device consists of seven active degrees of freedom
(Table 7.2) and allows the training of functional movements (Fig. 7.6). The exoskeleton is attached to the patients arm with two cuffs, one on the upper and one
on the lower arm [40].

ARMin is connected to a virtual environment to provide visual and auditory feedback. The system has two computers, a control system with the real-time operating
system Matlab xPC-Target and a host computer with the graphical user interface.
The API of xPC is used to poll the needed data from the control system. For

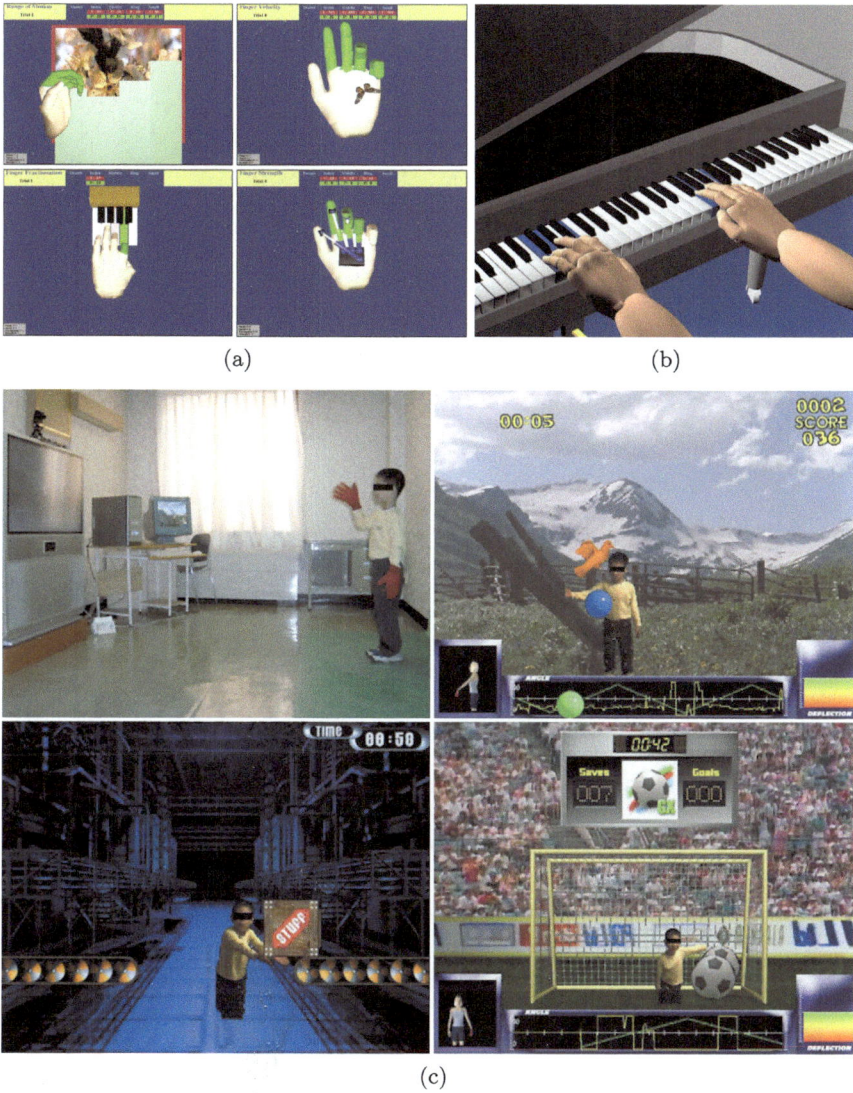

(a)   (b)

(c)

Fig. 7.5 Examples of VR applications with different motor tasks of the upper extremities. (**a**) Finger movements; by courtesy of S.A. Adamovich; (**b**) Piano task; by courtesy of S.A. Adamovich; (**c**) Projection of a camera image to the virtual world; figure by [58], with kind permission of John Wiley & Sons Ltd

graphical rendering the GIANTS game engine (http://www.giants-software.com) and Coin3D (http://www.coin3d.org/) was used.

There are currently three different modes used for training, i.e. mobilization mode, simple games, and activities of daily living (ADL).

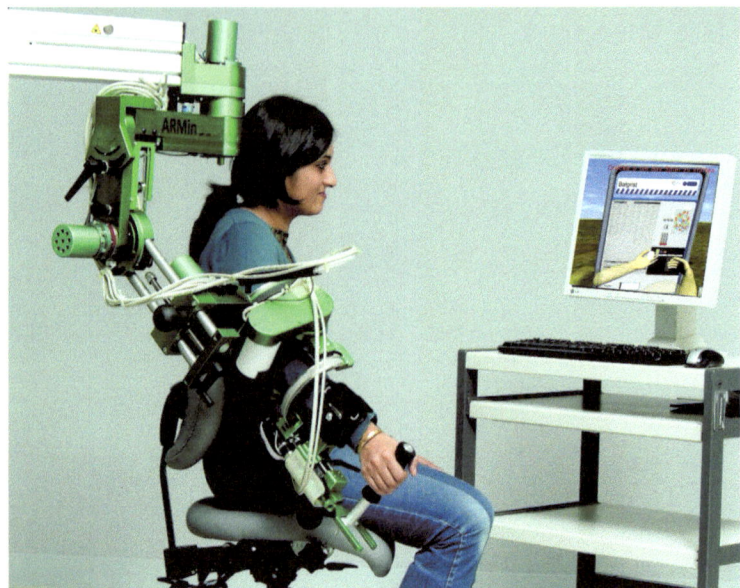

Fig. 7.6 ARMin III with 7 degrees of freedom

Table 7.2 Range of motion of ARMin III

Axis	Range of Motion
Arm elevation q_1	$40°\ldots125°$
Plane of elevation q_2	$-40°\ldots140°$
Int./ext. shoulder rotation q_3	$-90°\ldots90°$
Elbow flexion/extension q_4	$0°\ldots120°$
Forearm pro./supination q_5	$-90°\ldots90°$
Wrist flexion/extension q_6	$-40°\ldots40°$
Hand open and close q_7	$0°\ldots64°$

- **Mobilization mode** In the mobilization mode the therapist is able to teach and repeat movements. The therapist determines the choice of joints to be moved as well as the range of motion and speed of the movement. The movement taught by the therapist is smoothened and then stored by the robot. A position controller repeats the stored trajectory, while the patient can remain completely passive. The joint angles of the robot are mapped to a virtual avatar on the screen (Fig. 7.7). The goal of this mode is to foster blood circulation, reduce spasticity in the hemiparetic arm, prevent joint contractures, train muscle strength, etc.
- **Game mode** To train joint movements simple games have been implemented. In the ball game the patient controls a virtual bar to catch a ball (Fig. 7.8(a)). The joint to be involved and the range of motion are selected by the therapist. The handle position x_{handle} is calculated by mapping the range of motion of the joint

Fig. 7.7 Avatar used in the mobilization mode

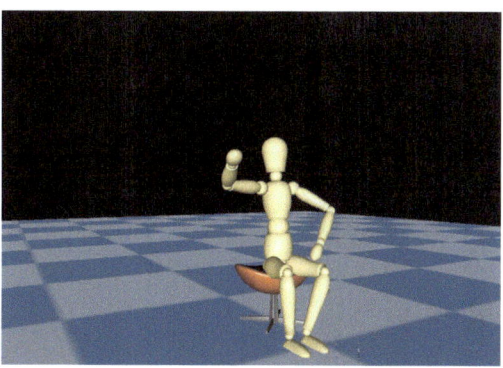

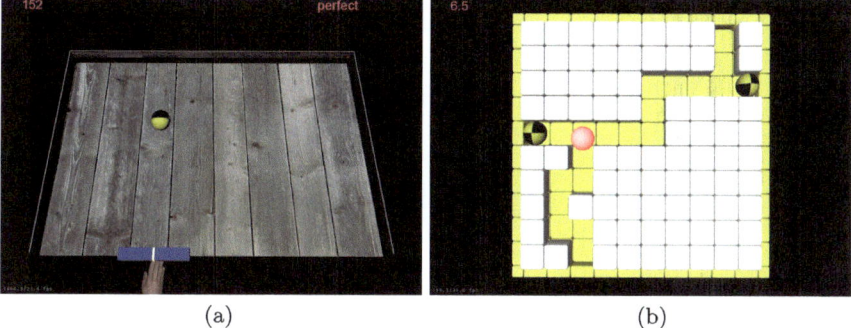

(a)   (b)

Fig. 7.8 Game mode. (**a**) Ball game; (**b**) Labyrinth game

to the interval $[0,1]$ of the x-axis of the virtual world with,

$$x_{handle} = \frac{q_i - q_{i_{min}}}{q_{i_{max}} - q_{i_{min}}}, \tag{7.4}$$

where q_i is the actual angle of the selected joint, $q_{i_{min}}$ the minimal desired angle of joint i and $q_{i_{max}}$ the maximal desired angle of joint i.

Furthermore, difficulty level, amount of support and ball behavior are adjustable to the patients needs. The robot supports the patient with an as-much-as-needed control strategy by applying a force F_x to the handle.

$$F_x = \begin{cases} 0 & \text{if } y_{ball} > 0.5, \\ K(x_{ball} - x_{hand}) \cdot (1 - y_{ball}) - B\frac{dx_{hand}}{dt} & \text{if } y_{ball} \leq 0.5, \end{cases} \tag{7.5}$$

where y_{ball} is the height of the ball, K is a constant value that can be adjusted by the therapist and B is a damping factor. Typical values are $K = 10$ N/m and $B = 0.01$ Ns/m.

In another game, coordination can be trained by moving a ball through a randomly generated labyrinth (Fig. 7.8(b)). Again, the workspace is adjustable by

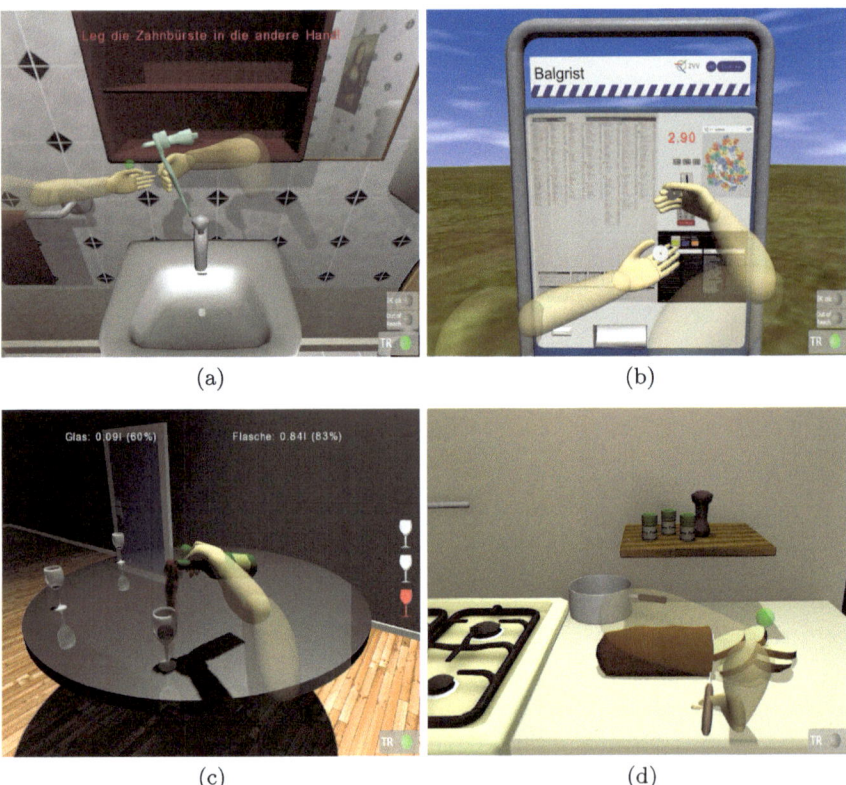

Fig. 7.9 Activities of Daily Living that can be trained with ARMin III. (**a**) Bathroom; (**b**) Ticket machine; (**c**) Dining room; (**d**) Cutting bread

the therapist and then mapped to the plane representing the labyrinth. The walls are haptically rendered with a penalty based approach.

To train coordination, the force applied against the walls must not exceed a given threshold. Otherwise, the patient has to restart from the beginning of the labyrinth. Additionally, appealing sound is given as a reward, when the end of the labyrinth is reached.

- **Activities of daily living mode** A third mode enables the training of ADL (Fig. 7.9(a)–7.9(d)). The patient has to perform functional movements with the whole arm to achieve the tasks and train activities he can use in daily life. Realistic tasks have been implemented according to a list defined by several criteria (e.g. importance in daily life, feasiblility with ARMin). Besides the visual feedback, auditory feedback is applied to maximally involve the patient in the virtual world. Furthermore, perception when interacting with objects is mimicked by sound feedback. As third modality haptic feedback has been implemented to support the patient (e.g. haptic table) or to enhance the level of realism by adding friction and weight to objects. To simplify collision detection only the end-effector

Fig. 7.10 Representation of
patient-cooperative control
strategy in the virtual world

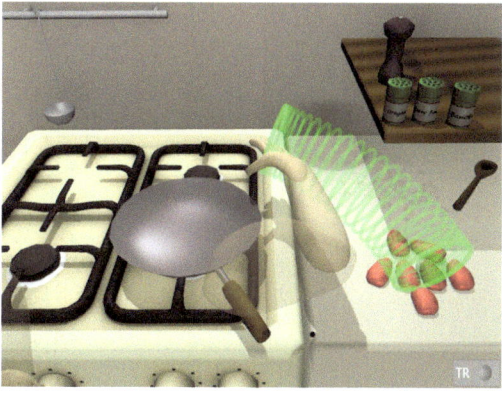

position (representing the hand), is considered for haptic interaction. Virtual objects are rendered as cylinders or cuboids. To calculate the haptic feedback each object is modeled by a spring-damper system. When a collision occurs the calculated force is applied at the end-effector by the controller. While the visual and auditory feedback have a sampling rate of 60 Hz, the haptic feedback is rendered with 1 kHz.

During the rehabilitation of patients it is important that the training is linked to the real world in order to maximize the transfer to daily life. Realistic behavior of objects is provided by the physics and collision detection engine of GIANTS. Instead of 3D-vision, lighting and shadow effects help to perceive visual depth in the virtual world.

Important in rehabilitation therapy is the adaptability of the virtual world to the skills of the patient. Therefore, the avatar can be moved by the therapist to a position, where the patient can reach all objects needed within the range of movement available to him.

The ADL training system has been evaluated with healthy subjects and stroke patients [15]. Besides using the visual feedback to present the task and arm movement it was also used to display the virtual tunnel of the patient-cooperative control strategy (Fig. 7.10).

7.2.4 Future Directions

Most rehabilitation efforts using VR have involved cognitive rehabilitation, a topic reviewed in [48]. There have been few attempts to work with motor retraining in the acquired brain injury population using virtual environments. Researchers from the University of Texas have begun to evaluate the use of VR as a diagnostic tool for ADL skills. They have developed a virtual kitchen environment and a test task while making soup and a sandwich.

The psychological or mental state of subjects, in particular motivation, was shown to have major influence on the outcome of the rehabilitation [35, 36, 47].

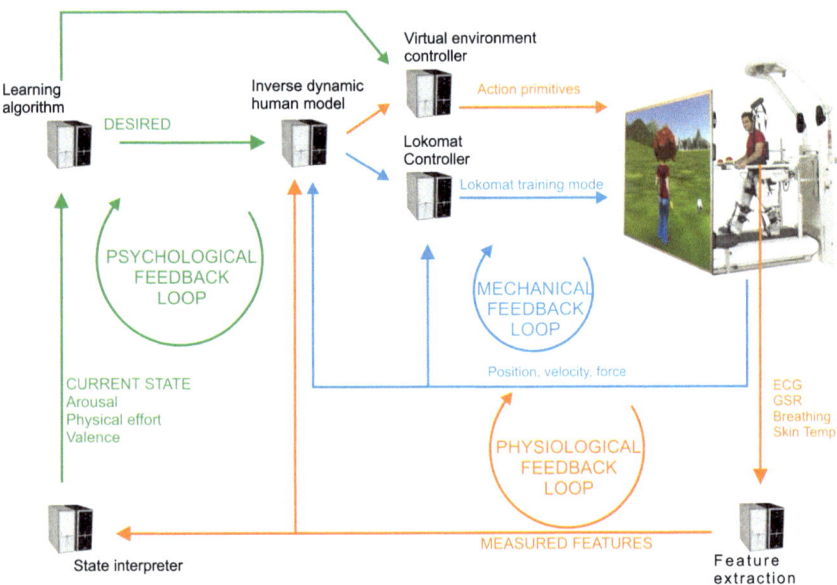

Fig. 7.11 Closed loop control of the psycho-physiological state of patients during gait rehabilitation

While motivation itself can only be quantified via questionnaires, recent research efforts are directed towards improving rehabilitation outcome by automatically controlling cognitive loading of the subject during gait and upper extremity training [29, 30, 41, 45]. Cognitive load is thereby defined as the amount of attention and focus the patient has to dedicate towards a rehabilitation task in order to successfully fulfill this task [29]. It is desirable to control cognitive load, as research in healthy subjects suggests that motor learning decreases in the presence of a distracting cognitive task, which presents a cognitively over-challenging situation [43, 51]. A task which is too easy for the subject will be perceived as boring, a task which is too difficult will over-stress the subject, while an optimally challenging task should induce maximal motivation and cognitive participation.

Quantifying cognitive load during the training can be achieved by evaluation of physiological quantities such as ECG, GSR, breathing frequency and skin temperature [30]. This is possible, as all psychological quantities as behavioral, social and emotional aspects are reflected in physiological signals of the body [21]. Using auto-adaptive linear classification methods [29], these physiological signals can be used to determine the cognitive load in real-time. By adapting the training environment and task difficulty of the virtual environment, it is possible to control the physiological and psychological state of subjects during gait and arm rehabilitation in a closed loop fashion (Fig. 7.11).

7.3 Wheelchair Mobility and Functional ADL Training

The treatment of unilateral neglect has been developed by Webster et al. [53]. They examined whether the use of a computer assisted therapy (CAT) system in combination with a wheelchair simulator device would be effective in improving real world performance on a wheelchair obstacle course in a group of patients with stroke and unilateral neglect syndrome. In addition, they examined, whether this training influenced the number of falls experienced by participants during their inpatient hospital stay. Forty patients (38 men, two women) with right hemisphere stroke participated. All patients were right handed and showed evidence of unilateral neglect, defined as specific scores on two standard tests of neglect, the Random Letter Cancellation Test and the Rey-Osterrieth Complex Figure test. The patients who had received the VR-CAT training made fewer errors, and hit significantly fewer ($p \leq 0.0001$) obstacles with the left side of their wheelchair during the real world wheelchair obstacle course test than did participants in the control group, who had not received this training (1.3 vs. 5.1 collisions). In addition, participants in the VR-trained group sustained significantly fewer falls ($p \leq 0.02$) than those in the control group (two of 19 patients in CAT group; eight of 19 in the control group). The virtual performance tests, conducted on participants in the CAT group, showed improved performance after the training for both the video tracking and VR wheelchair obstacle test, indicating that learning in the virtual world had occurred.

7.4 Balance Training

A preliminary report on the use of VR in balance training has been provided by Jacobson et al. [23]. The authors describe a VR system they have developed for balance training of subjects with vestibular disorders, which they call the *Balance Near Automatic Virtual Environment (BNAVE)*. Subjects with peripheral vestibular disorders frequently suffer from disequilibrium during standing and walking, and visual blurring during head movements. They are often treated in vestibular rehabilitation programs by exposure to situations that stimulate their symptoms in order to promote habituation. Typically, patients are taken through a graded type exposure that progressively adds situations and positions that provoke and increase their symptoms (e.g., dizziness, motion sickness, loss of balance). VR technologies can support such a training, as large immersive visual fields can be created and changed rapidly to suit patient needs. The BNAVE system developed by Jacobson et al. [23] is a spatially immersive, stereoscopic, projection-based VR system that encompasses a subject's entire horizontal field of view, and most of the vertical field of view, when looking forward (view angle, 200° horizontal, 95° vertical). The validity of the system's immersion was tested in a pilot study. Both normal and vestibular-impaired subjects responded to the visual stimuli provided by the BNAVE system with substantial greater head movements (range, 100–300% increase) and body sway movements (3.3 vs. 9.2 cm) in synchrony with the visual motion. The results confirmed the robust effect of the visual stimuli provided by the system on postural responses.

Fig. 7.12 VR simulation in psychotherapy. (**a**) Simulator for the treatment of aviatophobia (fear of flying); by courtesy of Prof. A. Mühlberger, University of Würzburg, Germany; (**b**) Driving simulators are used to reduce driving anxiety but also for clinical assessments for driving fitness in patients suffering from Parkinson, Alzheimer, and visual neglect; by courtesy of ST Software Simulator systems, Groningen, Netherlands

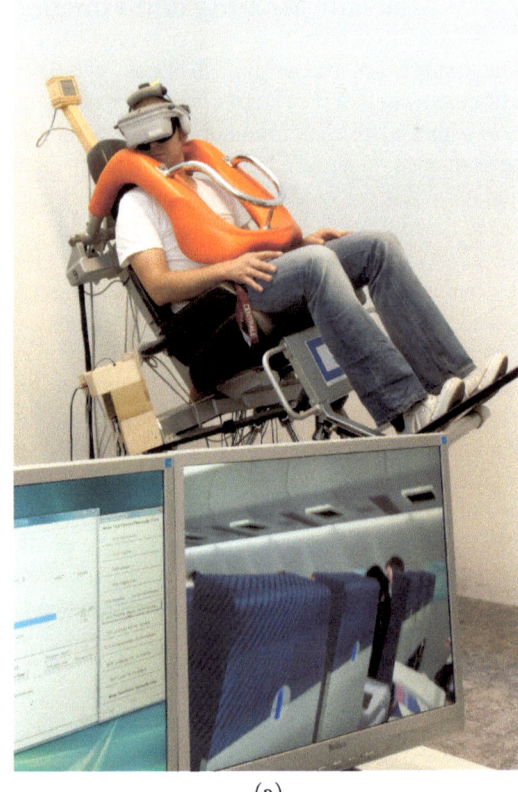

(a)

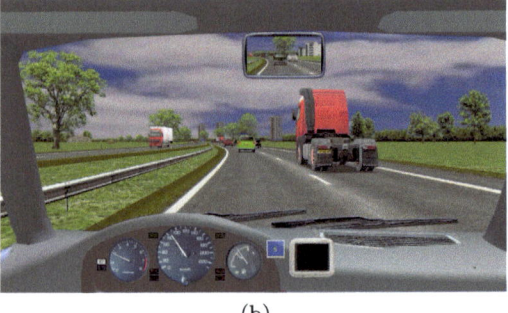

(b)

7.5 VR Supported Psychotherapy

Wiederhold and Wiederhold [56] were one of the first who recognized the potential of VR as a tool in psychotherapy, in order to treat patients suffering from different phobias. Examples are acrophobia (fear of height), aviatophobia (fear of flying), fear of driving, social phobias, claustrophobia (fear of small spaces) or agoraphobia (fear of large spaces) (Fig. 7.12). Comprehensive reviews were presented by Krijn et al., 2004 [32] and Brahnam and Jain, 2011 [8].

Virtual environments mimic scary situations under controllable and save conditions. Arachnophobia, for example, can be treated with a virtual spider simulation, in which the patient can explore his boundaries in a safe environment. By letting the patient relive traumatic situations in simulation, the patient can learn to process the memory. The study of Hoffman et al. [17] demonstrated that the congruence of visual, auditory and haptic sense is crucial for VR supported treatment of phobias. In the treatment of arachnophobia (fear of spiders), Hoffman et al. [17] demonstrated a clinically significant decrease in behavioral avoidance and subjective fear after only one hour of treatment with a VR scenario. A third treatment group that received a plastic spider as haptic input additionally to the visual input had the strongest decrease of fear. Botella and colleagues successfully treated aviatophobia [7] and claustrophobia [6] using a VR system. They could show that the effects of this VR supported psychotherapy persisted even months after the therapy session. In the treatment of social phobias, the comparison of VR supported psychotherapy against standard behavioral therapy was investigated by Klinger et al. [27]. Data was evaluated from 36 patients that were either assigned to a VR intervention group or to a standard behavioral therapy group. The authors found no evidence of superiority of one treatment over the other.

While VR might not be superior in situations that can easily be mimicked such as social situations [27], VR supported psychotherapy might in the future be particularly successful in traumatic situations, which the patient cannot relive easily or alone such as plane crashes or war situations [46].

References

1. Adamovich, S.V., Merians, A.S., Boian, R., Lewis, J.A., Tremaine, M., Burdea, G.S., Recce, M., Poizner, H.: A virtual reality-based exercise system for hand rehabilitation post-stroke. Presence **14**(2), 161–174 (2005)
2. Adamovich, S.V., Fluet, G.G., Mathai, A., Qiu, Q., Lewis, J., Merians, A.S.: Design of a complex virtual reality simulation to train finger motion for persons with hemiparesis: a proof of concept study. J. NeuroEng. Rehabil. **28**(6), 28–38 (2009)
3. Baram, Y., Miller, A.: Virtual reality cues for improvement of gait in patients with multiple sclerosis. Neurology **66**(2), 178–181 (2006)
4. Bayona, N.A., Bitensky, J., Salter, K., Teasell, R.: The role of task-specific training in rehabilitation therapies. Top. Stroke Rehabil. **12**(3), 58–65 (2005)
5. Bonaiuti, D., Rebasti, L., Sioli, P.: The constraint induced movement therapy: a systematic review of randomised controlled trials on the adult stroke patients. Eur. J. Phys. Rehabil. Med. **43**(2), 139–146 (2007)
6. Botella, C., Banos, R., Perpina, C., Villa, H., Alcaniz, M., Rey, A.: Virtual reality treatment of claustrophobia: a case report. Behav. Res. Ther. **36**(2), 239–246 (1998)
7. Botella, C., Osma, J., Garcia-Palacios, A., Quero, S., Banos, R.M.: Treatment of flying phobia using virtual reality: data from a 1-year follow-up using a multiple baseline design. Clin. Psychol. Psychother. **11**(5), 311–323 (2004)
8. Brahnam, S., Jain, L.C.: Advanced Computational Intelligence Paradigms in Healthcare 6: Virtual Reality in Psychotherapy, Rehabilitation, and Assessment. Studies in Computational Intelligence, vol. 337. Springer, Berlin (2011)

 9. Broeren, J., Claesson, L., Goude, D., Rydmark, M., Sunnerhagen, K.S.: Virtual rehabilitation
    in an activity centre for community-dwelling persons with stroke. Cerebrovasc. Dis. **26**(3),
    289–296 (2008)
10. Brütsch, K., Schuler, T., Koenig, A., Zimmerli, L., Merillat-Koeneke, S., Lunenburger, L.,
    Riener, R., Jancke, L., Meyer-Heim, A.: Influence of virtual reality soccer game on walk-
    ing performance in robotic assisted gait training for children. J. NeuroEng. Rehabil. **7**(1), 15
    (2010)
11. Cherng, R.J., Liu, C.F., Lau, T.W., Hong, R.B.: Effect of treadmill training with body weight
    support on gait and gross motor function in children with spastic cerebral palsy. Am. J. Phys.
    Med. Rehabil. **86**(7), 548–555 (2007)
12. Colombo, G., Joerg, M., Schreier, R., Dietz, V.: Treadmill training of paraplegic patients using
    a robotic orthosis. J. Rehabil. Res. Dev. **37**(6), 693–700 (2000)
13. Fung, J., Richards, C.L., Malouin, F., McFadyen, B.J., Lamontagne, A.: A treadmill and mo-
    tion coupled virtual reality system for gait training post-stroke. Cyperpsychol. Behav. **9**(2),
    157–162 (2006)
14. Girone, M., Burdea, G., Bouzit, M., Popescu, V., Deutsch, J.E.: Orthopedic rehabilitation us-
    ing the "Rutgers ankle" interface. Med. Meets Virtual Real. **70**, 89–95 (2000)
15. Guidali, M., Duschau-Wicke, A., Broggi, S., Klamroth-Marganska, V., Nef, T., Riener, R.:
    A robotic system to train activities of daily living in a virtual environment. Med. Biol. Eng.
    Comput. (2011). doi:10.1007/s11517-011-0809-0
16. Hesse, S., Werner, C., Pohl, M., Rueckriem, S., Mehrholz, J., Lingnau, M.L.: Computerized
    arm training improves the motor control of the severely affected arm after stroke. Stroke **36**,
    1960–1966 (2005)
17. Hoffman, H., Garcia-Palacios, A., Carlin, A., Furness, A. III, Botella-Arbona, C.: Interfaces
    that heal: coupling real and virtual objects to treat spider phobia. Int. J. Hum.-Comput. Interact.
    16(2), 283–300 (2003)
18. Holden, M.K.: Virtual environments for motor rehabilitation: review. Cyberpsychol. Behav.
    8(3), 187–211 (2005)
19. Housman, S.J., Le, V., Rahman, T., Sanchez, R.J., Reinkensmeyer, D.J.: Arm-training with
    t-wrex after chronic stroke: preliminary results of a randomized controlled trial. In: Rehabil-
    itation Robotics, 2007. ICORR 2007. IEEE 10th International Conference on, pp. 562–568
    (2007). doi:10.1109/ICORR.2007.4428481
20. Housman, S.J., Scott, K.M., Reinkensmeyer, D.J.: A randomized controlled trial of
    gravity-supported, computer-enhanced arm exercise for individuals with severe hemipare-
    sis. Neurorehabil. Neural Repair **23**(5), 505–514 (2009). doi:10.1177/1545968308331148.
    http://nnr.sagepub.com/content/23/5/505.full.pdf+html
21. Hugdahl, K.: Psychophysiology: The Mind-Body Perspective. Harvard University Press, Cam-
    bridge (1995)
22. Husemann, B., Muller, F., Krewer, C., Heller, S., Koenig, E.: Effects of locomotion training
    with assistance of a robot-driven gait orthosis in hemiparetic patients after stroke: a random-
    ized controlled pilot study. Stroke **38**(2), 349–354 (2007)
23. Jacobson, J., Redfern, M., Furman, J., Whitney, S., Sparto, P., Wilson, J., Hodges, L.: Balance
    NAVE: a virtual reality facility for research and rehabilitation of balance disorders. In: Pro-
    ceedings of the ACM Symposium on Virtual Reality Software and Technology, pp. 103–109
    (2001)
24. Jaffe, D.L., Brown, D.A., Pierson-Carey, C.D., Buckley, E.L., Lew, H.L.: Stepping over ob-
    stacles to improve walking in individuals with poststroke hemiplegia. J. Rehabil. Res. Dev.
    41(3), 283–292 (2004)
25. Jang, S.H., You, S.H., Hallett, M., Cho, Y.W., Park, C., Cho, S., Lee, H., Kim, T.: Cortical
    reorganization and associated functional motor recovery after virtual reality in patients with
    chronic stroke: an experimenter-blind preliminary study. Arch. Phys. Med. Rehabil. **86**(11),
    2218–2223 (2005)
26. Johnson, M.J.: Recent trends in robot-assisted therapy environments to improve real-life func-
    tional performance after stroke. J. NeuroEng. Rehabil. **3**, 29 (2006)

27. Klinger, E., Bouchard, S., Légeron, P., Roy, S., Lauer, F., Chemin, I., Nugues, P.: Virtual reality therapy versus cognitive behavior therapy for social phobia: a preliminary controlled study. Cyberpsychol. Behav. **8**(1), 76–88 (2005)

28. Koenig, A., Wellner, M., Koneke, S., Meyer-Heim, A., Lunenburger, L., Riener, R.: Virtual gait training for children with cerebral palsy using the Lokomat gait orthosis. Stud. Health Technol. Inform. **132**, 204–209 (2008)

29. Koenig, A., Novak, D., Pulfer, M., Omlin, X., Perreault, E., Zimmerli, L., Mihelj, M., Riener, R.: Real-time closed-loop control of cognitive load in neurological patients during robot-assisted gait training. IEEE Trans. Neural Syst. Rehabil. Eng. **19**(4), 453–464 (2011). doi:10.1109/TNSRE.2011.2160460

30. Koenig, A., Omlin, X., Zimmerli, L., Sapa, M., Krewer, C., Bolliger, M., Mueller, F., Riener, R.: Psychological state estimation from physiological recordings during robot assisted gait rehabilitation. J. Rehabil. Res. Dev. **48**(4), 367–386 (2011)

31. Krebs, H.I., Hogan, N., Volpe, B.T., Aisen, M.L., Edelstein, L., Diels, C.: Overview of clinical trials with MIT-MANUS: a robot-aided neuro-rehabilitation facility. Technol. Health Care **7**(6), 419–423 (1999)

32. Krijn, M., Emmelkamp, P., Olafsson, R., Biemond, R.: Virtual reality exposure therapy of anxiety disorders: a review. Clin. Psychol. Rev. **24**(3), 259–281 (2004)

33. Kwakkel, G., Wagenaar, R.C., Koelman, T.W., Lankhorst, G.J., Koetsier, J.C.: Effects of intensity of rehabilitation after stroke. A research synthesis. Stroke **28**(8), 1550–1556 (1997)

34. Kwakkel, G., Kollen, B.J., Wagenaar, R.C.: Long term effects of intensity of upper and lower limb training after stroke: a randomised trial. J. Neurol. Neurosurg. Psychiatry **72**(4), 473–479 (2002)

35. Liebermann, D.G., Buchman, A.S., Franks, I.M.: Enhancement of motor rehabilitation through the use of information technologies. Clin. Biomech. **21**(1), 8–20 (2006)

36. Loureiro, R., Amirabdollahian, F., Cootes, S., Stokes, E., Harwin, W.: Using haptics technology to deliver motivational therapies in stroke patients: concepts and initial pilot studies. In: Proceedings of EuroHaptics 2001, p. 6 (2001)

37. Mayr, A., Kofler, M., Quirbach, E., Matzak, H., Frohlich, K., Saltuari, L.: Prospective, blinded, randomized crossover study of gait rehabilitation in stroke patients using the Lokomat gait orthosis. Neurorehabil. Neural Repair **21**(4), 307–314 (2007)

38. Merians, A.S., Fluet, G.G., Qiu, Q., Saleh, S., Lafond, I., Davidow, A., Adamovich, S.V.: Robotically facilitated virtual rehabilitation of arm transport integrated with finger movement in persons with hemiparesis. J. NeuroEng. Rehabil. **8**(1), 1–10 (2011). doi:10.1186/1743-0003-8-27

39. Mirelman, A., Bonato, P., Deutsch, J.: Comparative study randomized controlled trial research support. Stroke **40**(1), 169–174 (2009)

40. Nef, T., Guidali, M., Riener, R.: ARMin III—arm therapy exoskeleton with an ergonomic shoulder actuation. Appl. Bionics Biomech. **6**(2), 127–142 (2009)

41. Novak, D., Ziherl, J., Olensek, A., Milavec, M., Podobnik, J., Mihelj, M., Munih, M.: Psychophysiological responses to robotic rehabilitation tasks in stroke. IEEE Trans. Neural Syst. Rehabil. Eng. **18**(4), 351–361 (2010)

42. Podobnik, J., Munih, M., Cinkelj, J.: HARMiS—hand and arm rehabilitation system. In: Proceedings of 7th International Conference Series on Disability, Virtual Reality and Associated Technologies, pp. 237–244 (2008)

43. Redding, G.M., Rader, S.D., Lucas, D.R.: Cognitive load and prism adaptation. J. Mot. Behav. **24**(3), 238–246 (1992)

44. Riener, R., Lünenburger, L., Maier, I.C., Colombo, G., Dietz, V.: Locomotor training in subjects with sensori-motor deficits: an overview of the robotic gait orthosis lokomat. J. Healthc. Eng. **1**(2), 197–216 (2010)

45. Riener, R., Munih, M.: Guest editorial: special section on rehabilitation via bio-cooperative control. IEEE Trans. Neural Syst. Rehabil. Eng. **18**(4), 2 (2010)

46. Rizzo, A., Pair, J., Graap, K., Manson, B., McNerney, P.J., Wiederhold, B., Wiederhold, M., Spira, J.: A virtual reality exposure therapy application for Iraq War military personnel with

post traumatic stress disorder: from training to toy to treatment. In: Roy, M.J. (ed.) Novel Approaches to the Diagnosis and Treatment of Posttraumatic Stress Disorder, pp. 235–250. IOS Press, Amsterdam (2006)

47. Robertson, I.H., Murre, J.M.J.: Rehabilitation of brain damage: brain plasticity and principles of guided recovery. Psychol. Bull. **125**(32), 544 (1999)

48. Rose, F.D., Brooks, B.M., Rizzo, A.A.: Virtual reality in brain damage rehabilitation: review. Cyberpsychol. Behav. **8**(3), 241–271 (2005)

49. Stauffer, Y., Allemand, Y., Bouri, M., Fournier, J., Clavel, R., Metrailler, P., Brodard, R., Reynard, F.: The WalkTrainer—a new generation of walking reeducation device combining orthoses and muscle stimulation. IEEE Trans. Neural Syst. Rehabil. Eng. **17**(1), 38–45 (2009)

50. Sveistrup, H.: Motor rehabilitation using virtual reality. J. NeuroEng. Rehabil. **1**(1), 10 (2004)

51. Taylor, J.A., Thoroughman, K.A.: Motor adaptation scaled by the difficulty of a secondary cognitive task. PLoS ONE **3**(6), e2485 (2008)

52. Veneman, J.F., Kruidhof, R., Hekman, E.E., Ekkelenkamp, R., Van Asseldonk, E.H., van der Kooij, H.: Design and evaluation of the LOPES exoskeleton robot for interactive gait rehabilitation. IEEE Trans. Neural Syst. Rehabil. Eng. **15**(3), 379–386 (2007)

53. Webster, J., McFarland, P., Rapport, L., Morrill, B., Roades, L., Abadee, P.: Computer-assisted training for improving wheelchair mobility in unilateral neglect patients. Arch. Phys. Med. Rehabil. **82**(6), 769–775 (2001)

54. Weghorst, S.: Augmented reality and Parkinson's disease. Commun. ACM **40**(8), 47–48 (1997)

55. Wellner, M., Schaufelberger, A., von Zitzewitz, J., Riener, R.: Evaluation of visual and auditory feedback in virtual obstacle walking. Presence **17**(5), 512–524 (2008)

56. Wiederhold, B.K., Wiederhold, M.D.: A review of virtual reality as a psychotherapeutic tool. Cyberpsychol. Behav. **1**(1), 45–52 (1998)

57. Winter, D.A.: Biomechanics and Motor Control of Human Movement, 3rd edn. Wiley, New York (1990)

58. You, S.H., Jang, S.H., Kim, Y.H., Kwon, Y.H., Barrow, I., Hallett, M.: Cortical reorganization induced by virtual reality therapy in a child with hemiparetic cerebral palsy. Dev. Med. Child Neurol. **47**(9), 628–635 (2005). doi:10.1111/j.1469-8749.2005.tb01216.x

Chapter 8
VR for Medical Training

8.1 Introduction

The major advantage of VR-based training is that an interactive and engaging setting enables an operator to learn through a first-person experience. Tasks are represented, which would be dangerous, expensive, or even infeasible to undertake in a real setting.

Immersive training environments using VR technology have been a topic of research in diverse application areas, including fire-fighting, vehicle driving, space missions, triage, emergency handling, maintenance, hazardous material handling, or military activities (see [6, 36] for examples).

In this chapter, we will discuss the use of VR for medical training. First, we will focus on applications in surgical education. A brief review of traditional training options will be provided, followed by a general overview of surgical training in VR. The latter includes a discussion of advantages and disadvantages, as well as a presentation of the key components. Following this, a large number of example systems will be presented. These are categorized into *tool-based* and *phantom-based* applications.

Tool-based training systems belong to a group of medical VR simulators that provide the haptic interface in the form of surgical instruments. These tool-based setups allow medical students and surgeons to perceive kinesthetic and tactile feedback of the real surgical instruments while practicing surgical operations within the artificial scene generated by the computers. Tool-based trainers can be distinguished by the mechanical structure and type of application. Numerous examples of these systems will be provided in Sect. 8.2.

The second group of medical training simulators are regarded as phantom-based training simulators. In contrast to tool-based training simulators, in these the user is in direct contact with an anatomical mock-up—i.e. the *phantom*—rather than a tool. Note that hereby the term phantom should not be confused with the PHANTOM haptic interface (see Fig. 4.1(a)). The notion of phantom-based systems will be outlined in more detail in Sect. 8.3.

R. Riener, M. Harders, *Virtual Reality in Medicine*,
DOI 10.1007/978-1-4471-4011-5_8, © Springer-Verlag London 2012

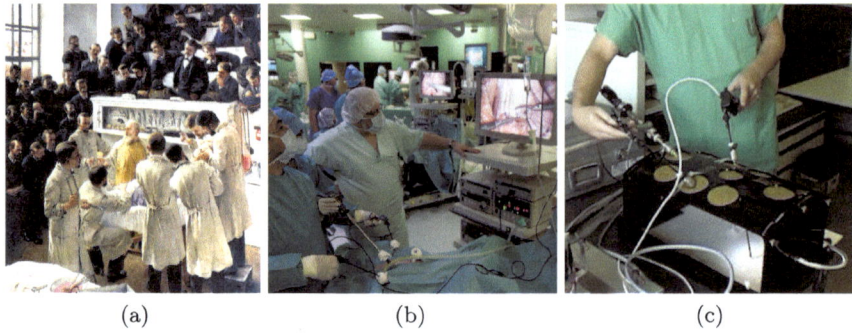

(a)   (b)   (c)

Fig. 8.1 Traditional options for training in surgical education. (**a**) Traditional apprenticeship model of surgical education; (**b**) Training on animal cadavers at IRCAD (courtesy of Luc Soler); (**c**) Training on plastic mock-ups (courtesy of Benoit Herman)

8.1.1 Traditional Training Options

A number of educational options currently exist. Figure 8.1 provides an overview of different approaches. Next to the usually practiced "learning by doing", which involves supervised interventions on real patients, training can also be performed using cadavers, animals, life-like mock-ups, actors, multi-media tools, or simulations. All of these have positive and negative aspects, which are summarized below in Table 8.1.

The different training options should usually be combined in a complementary fashion leveraging the individual advantages. The selection of the means of training needs to be governed by the specific skills that are to be trained. In this sense one has to discriminate between basic manipulative vs. procedural skills. The former include, for instance, hand-eye coordination needed for handling of endoscopic cameras, while the latter relate to more cognitive processes, such as problem identification during intervention and selection of appropriate reaction. As an example, rehearsal of knot tying does probably not require a highly sophisticated simulation environment. Instead, a simple box setup might be sufficient.

8.1.2 Advantages and Disadvantages of Surgical Simulation

The great potential of training approaches using VR techniques in surgical education has already been recognized at the beginning of the 1990s (see [19, 30]). A wide range of systems has been proposed and implemented in recent years, including academic projects as well as commercial products. Overviews can be found in recent review papers [3, 23].

Figure 8.2 depicts two example training systems developed at ETH Zurich, Switzerland. In addition to common single user rehearsal, training environments

Table 8.1 Advantages and disadvantages of non-VR training options

Paradigm	Pros	Cons
Training in operation room	Real behavior of patient, actual environment and tools	Risk to patient, subjective skill evaluation, additional operation-room time/cost, limited exposure to rare cases
Cadavers	Reduced time constraints, exact anatomy	Availability of cadavers, changed tissue behavior, no physiology, one-time use, special preparation required, inappropriate for MIS training
Animals	In-vivo physiology and anatomy	Prohibited in some countries, limited availability of animals, ethical concerns, limited similarity to human anatomy, specialized facilities required, high cost, one-time use
Mock-ups	Relatively inexpensive, usually allows repeated training, effective rehearsal of basic manipulative skills	Needs replacement of components after training, tactile and biomechanical properties of tissue incorrect, limited physiology, low immersion
Non-interactive, PC-based tools	Detailed 3D visualizations, intra-operative movies, self-paced learning, low hardware requirements, limited cost	No tactile information, very limited interactivity, no evaluation, no immersion

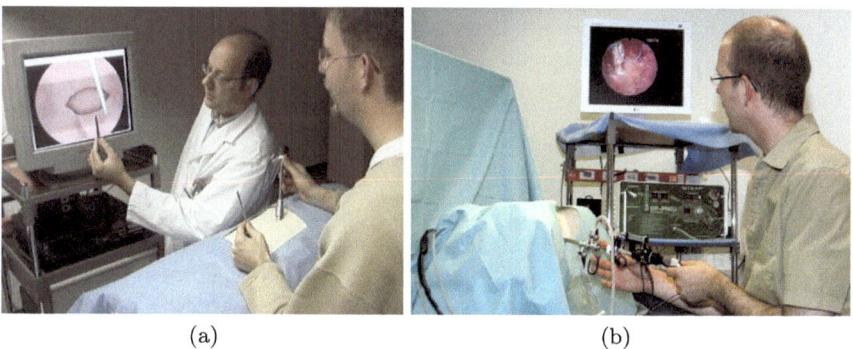

(a)   (b)

Fig. 8.2 Examples of surgical simulator systems. (**a**) Laparoscopic simulator; (**b**) Hysteroscopic simulator

may also be extended to include additional team members, for instance anaesthetists, to carry out team training. It should be noted, that a number of further application areas of surgical simulation techniques have been envisioned in the past, including patient-specific preparation, testing of new interventions, patient education, practitioner certification, student admission, or surgical planning. However, several of these ideas would denote a significant paradigm change. Moreover, the current technology is still immature and needs further development to provide satisfactory solutions for these advanced scenarios.

VR based training offers several benefits over alternative training methods, but can also be associated with certain risks. The following advantages can be identified.

- **No patient involvement** VR training does not directly involve any patients or animals, thus, providing a risk-free environment for surgical education. Patients understandably show resistance to being operated on at the beginning of a resident's learning curve.
- **Objective assessment** VR trainers allow tracking of all user actions in a fully-known simulated environment. The acquired data can be used as a basis for objective assessment without further effort. So far, performance measurement is usually limited to the overall surgical outcome and the subjective judgment of the trainee's skills by the supervising expert. Unfortunately, this occurs through in-training evaluation, which only allows poor reliability. This could be improved through bench-station examination and objective structured assessment of technical skills (OSATS) forms. Nevertheless, a large effort is required compared to assessment on a virtual reality trainer.
- **Availability** Currently, training is dependent on the actual demand of interventions and the availability of appropriate cases. With VR simulators, students can practice, independent of busy operating room schedules or availability of patient cases or cadavers.
- **Training case variability** Nowadays, any surgeon-to-be will experience different cases during the training period. These may be limited to the more common findings. In contrast, a VR-based simulator can offer a large number of different anatomies and pathologies in a compressed period of time.
- **Complication training** High-fidelity surgical simulators have the potential to allow training of rare, but dangerous complications which a trainee might not otherwise experience during the residency program. This may improve surgeons to better anticipate, manage, and even avoid possible complications.
- **Reduced costs** VR simulators have the potential to save costs in education and training. Recent return on investment studies estimated the pay-back period when buying a simulator system. This period was estimated for the case of a teaching hospital to about half a year. Potential savings stem from reduced operation room time for training as well as faster time to competence for the trainees. However, traditional reimbursement models currently do not account for these savings.

VR-based simulation is an appealing option to supplement traditional clinical education. While the great potential of this approach has consistently been recognized, the formal integration of training simulators into the medical curriculum is still lacking. Several factors are likely contributing to this unsatisfactory situation.

- **Unclear training target** There is often a lack of identification of the skill categories to be trained. A clear separation between motor and cognitive skills, as well as other skill factors is sometimes not taken into account.

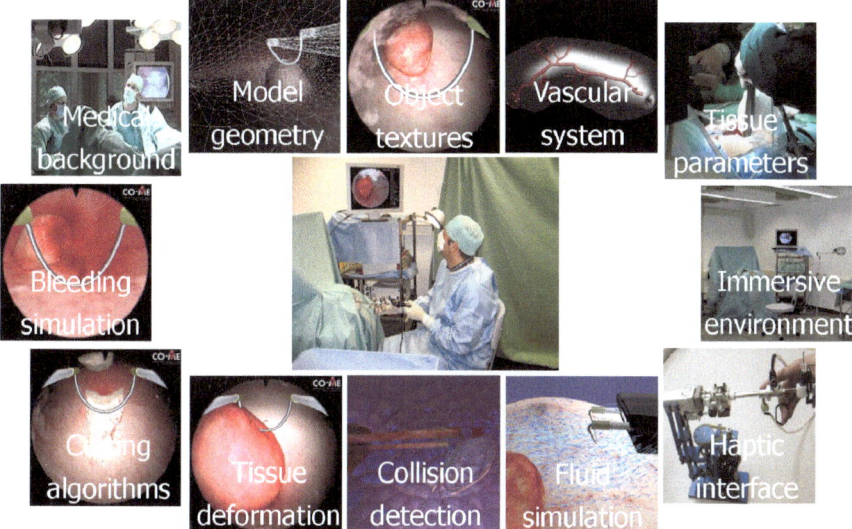

Fig. 8.3 Key modules of a surgical simulator

- **Unknown real-world transfer** The evaluation and validation of existing systems is lacking. Often only the performance improvement on the simulator itself is taken as an indication for successful training, while inside the OR only semi-quantitative measures are available.
- **Curriculum integration** The relation to and advantage over conventional methods is not shown. This is especially disturbing, if only basic motor skills are trained, e.g. placing clips on a tube.
- **Negative training** Effects, such as a possibly reduced performance in a real situation due to an incorrect representation in the simulated environment, are not examined. In the extreme case, incorrectly trained behavior could lead to errors with potentially severe consequences for a patient.
- **Required level of realism** The correlation between level of realism and training effect concerning the specific skills to be trained is not fully known. This is an important factor, since realism usually strongly correlates with complexity (and, thus, with overall cost).

8.1.3 Surgical Simulator Components

In order to build a surgical simulator, several components have to be integrated. In Fig. 8.3 the required key modules are compiled. These elements belong to four major categories. First and foremost is the medical background of the simulated procedure. The next category focuses on the generation of surgical scenes. This includes models of healthy and pathological anatomy, organ textures, vessel structures, as well as tissue deformation parameters. These scenarios are used in the interactive simulation, which is composed of elements of the last two categories. The former denotes the interface elements controlling the simulation, for instance the haptic device or the immersive training environment, while the latter comprises the software modules, which are combined into the virtual representation of the surgery.

- **Medical background** The medical knowledge defines the problem area, identifies the training needs, and influences the system development at all stages. Input data required for the scene generation usually stem from actual patient cases. The system also needs to be evaluated in collaboration with clinical experts to determine the training effect.
- **Model geometry** The first step in a surgical scenario definition process is the generation of the geometrical representation of the scene objects. The latter mainly denote the human organs and possibly their pathological changes. A key component within this respect is the ability to provide different scenes for every training session reflecting the natural variability in cases and patients.
- **Object textures** The next component in the scenario definition is the object surface appearance. Providing correct visual information is indispensable in surgical simulation if a realistic training environment is required. A central point is the appropriate texture generation for healthy and pathologically altered organs.
- **Vascular system** A further key element in a scene definition scheme is the generation and integration of vascular structures. Blood vessels affect surgical simulation on several levels. Firstly, they are the carrier of blood circulation and thus an integral part of a patient physiology model. Moreover, they affect the visual appearance of organ surfaces and thus have to be included into the texturing process. In addition, they have to be part of the geometrical model since they deform with the tissue and are the source of bleeding after cutting
- **Tissue parameters** In order to model the dynamic biomechanical behavior of soft tissue in a surgical scene, appropriate parameters have to be determined for the deformation algorithms. Optimally, these parameters are obtained directly from living human tissue, since the behavior of ex-vivo samples can change considerably.
- **Immersive environment** The sense of presence plays an important role to achieve a training effect. To enable user immersion into the environment, the surrounding and interaction metaphors should be the same as during a real intervention. Optimally, a complete OR is replicated for the simulation, also comprising auditory feedback. For instance, by including an anesthesia simulator, a complete team training setting could be generated.
- **Haptic interface** The haptic device is the human-machine interface between the trainee and the simulator. It renders haptic feedback to the user based on the interaction with the virtual world. Moreover, it provides a natural means for controlling the simulation. In the optimal case, real surgical tools are adapted and equipped with sensors to serve as input devices, while interaction via mouse or keyboard should be avoided.
- **Fluid simulation** Several surgical procedures require the modeling of fluids. For instance, in hysteroscopy the uterus is distended with liquid media to access and

visualize the uterine cavity. Therefore, the real-time modeling of fluid motion is required. Any changing boundary conditions for a fluid solver at the operation site also have to be taken into account.

- **Collision detection** In order to process the interaction between soft and rigid objects in a simulator, efficient collision detection algorithms are required. In addition, an appropriate response to the collisions needs to be determined. A geometrical representation of all scene objects has to be provided to this end, which is usually done during the scene generation step.
- **Tissue deformation** Deformable tissue modeling is a key component in any surgical simulator. Efficient and robust methods are required to deliver dynamic behavior of soft tissue at interactive speed. This usually necessitates the generation of meshes for all deformable objects.
- **Tissue cutting** Interactive simulation of soft tissue cutting is an integral part of surgery simulation. Smooth cuts into the organ models have to be created, while preserving the numerical stability of the underlying deformation computation. The process usually requires a real-time remeshing of the organ models, as well as an update of scene textures.
- **Bleeding simulation** During cutting or strong collisions with organs, vessels can be damaged, which causes bleeding depending on the size of the vessel. Thus, a bleeding model is required to simulate different effects, e.g. oozing or fast spurts. The type of bleeding depends on the information coming from the vascular structure of the scene.

This list of simulator components is still not exhaustive. For instance, a missing key element is the real-time visualization of the surgical intervention. This includes modeling of the endoscopic camera (lighting, distortion), special visual effects (e.g. for smoke or bleeding), object deformation, etc. Another critical simulator module is a system for automatic, objective performance evaluation. A number of other possible advanced modules exist, e.g. patient physiology, biochemical processes, models of neurology or genetics. However, such simulation components are less common and currently only receive little attention in surgical simulator development. In the following, examples of tool-based and phantom-based training systems in medicine will be introduced.

8.2   Tool-Based Applications

8.2.1   Laparoscopy Training

Among all minimally invasive procedures, laparoscopic training devices are the most common surgical simulators available today [9]. Laparoscopic surgery is performed through small incisions using long and thin tools for manipulation and viewing to perform a procedure within the abdomen. During laparoscopy, as during any other minimally invasive procedure, the surgeon's view is occluded by the skin.

Only indirect sight is given through a camera that is inserted into the patient together with the manipulation tools. The use and movement of the tools and camera is not at all intuitive as the surgeon has to perform the movement around the fixed trocars through which the tools enter the body. Orientation within the body and identification of anatomical structures is difficult, because of the unnatural camera image and restricted viewing angle. Furthermore, the surgeon cannot use traditional open surgery devices, and direct palpation with the fingers is also not possible due to the restricted access into the abdominal regions. Therefore, a trainee needs a lot of exercise to learn the complex minimally invasive steps and skills before performing an operation on a living subject. Several simulators have been developed by different research groups for this purpose. Many of those are commercially available (see also [9] for a review).

8.2.2 Basic and Advanced Skill Training

One of the first commercially available laparoscopic training simulators was the Procedicus MIST [32], first sold by Virtual Presence, London, United Kingdom, and then by Mentice AB, Gothenburg, Sweden. The hardware allows for tracking of the tools and provides 4 DOF force feedback (axial force as well as pitch, yaw, and roll torque). The graphical animation is rather abstract: the system enables basic skill training such as knot tying using a series of simple geometric shape manipulation tasks.

LapVR is another laparascopic simulator that is offered by Immersion Medical Inc. It can be used for basic skill training including handling of abstract geometric objects with minimally invasive tools. Other tasks with more realistic virtual environments include camera navigation, cutting and procedural tasks of laparoscopic cholecystectomy (gall bladder removal). The training progress can be recorded and later evaluated together with the training expert. Many other devices have been developed without providing adaquate force feedback, such as the SurgicalSim Education Platform (SEP) produced in partnership between SimSurgery (Oslo, Norway) and Medical Education Technologies (Sarasota, FL, USA) or the Simendo (SIMulator for ENDOscopy) offered by DeltaTech (Rotterdam, Netherlands).

Later, more advanced laparoscopic training with improved haptic feedback and high-fidelity graphics features have been developed and offered by different companies. Simbionix Ltd. sells the LAP Mentor, which comprises Xitact LS500 hardware [20], two laparoscopic tool interfaces and one endoscopic camera. This system allows training of knot tying, suturing, and particular teamwork and decision making tasks.

Other well advanced simulators are the LapSim from Surgical Science AB (Gothenburg, Sweden), the SkillSetPro from Verifi Technologies Inc. [27] or the VSOne system from VEST System One, Select IT VEST Systems (Bremen, Germany), all allowing different advanced laparoscopic training modes such as suturing, camera navigation, and teamwork training. The KISMET software of VSOne supports real-time interactions with deformable objects.

8.2.3 Gynecological Procedures

Several laparoscopic simulators have been developed to support training of particular minimally invasive procedures in the area of gynecology. The SurgicalSim Education Platform (SEP) enables training of embryo removal and general teamwork and decision making. LapSim from Surgical Science AB (Gothenburg, Sweden) can be purchased with a special add on gynecological module. The HystSim simulator by VirtaMed (Zurich, Switzerland) is a multimodal training environment including advanced haptic feedback capabilities that can be used to learn and train hysteroscopy procedures [2]. It is also distributed by Symbionix (Cleveland, Ohio, USA). Diagnostic or surgical tasks can be performed in the uterine cavity on a rather high performance level with respect to physical behavior and visual appearance.

8.2.4 Arthroscopy and Sinuscopy Training

Arthroscopy is a minimally invasive, endoscopic procedure at a joint (mostly knee or shoulder) performed for diagnostic or therapeutic reasons. It requires a small camera and specialized instruments to be inserted into the joint. In this procedure, the operator's tools interact with soft tissue and hard bone of the joint. Nasalendoscopy (sinuscopy or rhinoscopy) refers to similar endoscopic procedures at the endonasal sinus.

8.2.4.1 Arthroscopy Training

The insightArthroVR is an arthroscopy (knee, shoulder) simulator for the training of orthopedic surgeons and can also be used as a tool to plan real surgery (Fig. 8.4). The system consists of a phantom leg or shoulder and a set of arthroscopic instruments. The virtual scene of the arthroscopic camera view is displayed on a screen while the trainee uses the instruments. The system includes graphical and statistical data to evaluate the navigation skills of the trainee during training sessions. Force feedback is provided by the PHANTOM haptic device.

The Virtual Reality Arthroscopy Training Simulator (VRATS) is an interactive medical training system for arthroscopy education [25]. The system provides the virtual environment, including surgical instruments and a phantom knee joint, which allows the user to navigate with a virtual arthroscope. It provides interactive visual feedback while the user interacts with the virtual anatomy of the knee joint. Tissue deformations can be simulated that are caused by collisions between the instruments and soft tissues.

The Virtual Environments Knee Arthroscopy Training System (VE–KATS) has also been developed for training of arthroscopic knee surgery [31]. The simulator consists of a mock surgical probe and an artificial arthroscopic camera used in conjunction with a phantom of the knee. The system provides a real-time interactive

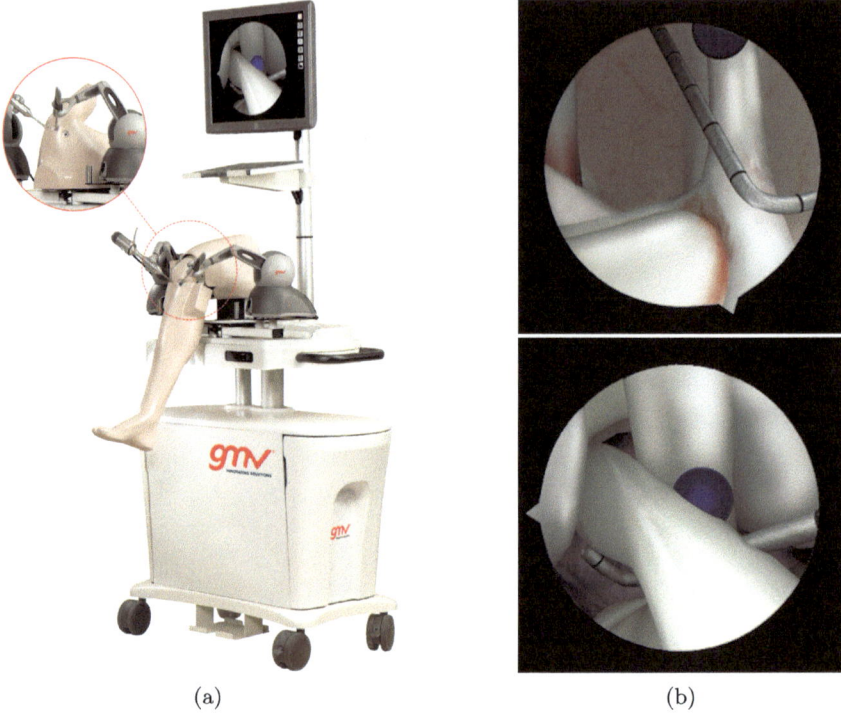

(a)   (b)

Fig. 8.4 Virtual reality arthroscopy trainer, GMV/insightArthroVR; by courtesy of GMV, Madrid, Spain. (**a**) Setup; (**b**) Visualization

view from the arthroscope, showing the position of the instruments and the deformations of soft tissue structures such as ligaments and menisci. Furthermore, the simulator can render the reaction force while the instruments interact with the knee model.

8.2.4.2 Nasal Endoscopy Training

Nasal Endoscopy Simulator (NES) is a VR simulator providing different training levels for endoscopic procedures of the endonasal sinus. The underlying virtual scene is based on simple abstract models as well as on complex 3D geometries. The system provides the opportunity to train the handling of a sinuscope (rhinoscope), to diagnose pathologic cases as well as to perform therapeutic interventions on a virtual situs. The trainee can navigate through the virtual situs using a mock endoscope and perform the therapeutic procedure with mock surgical instruments. The training can be recorded and the recorded data can be used to evaluate the performance of the trainee.

8.2.5 Flexible Endoscopy Training

Flexible endoscopes are cameras combined with long bendable tubes, which allows them to be inserted into natural orifices of the body such as the mouth or anus. The operator guiding the endoscope into the body will feel resistance between the tool and the anatomical structures such as the oesophagus, stomach, bronchi or the colon.

8.2.5.1 Bronchoscopy Training

Several research groups developed VR simulators with the required haptic feedback modality to provide realistic physiological response and appropriate tool behavior and applied those to training of bronchoscopy [37, 38].

8.2.5.2 Gastrointestinal Endoscopy Training

The AccuTouch simulator provides a VR training environment for lower gastrointestinal endoscopy. It enables novices and also experienced physicians to practice motor skills to perform colonoscopy training with a multimodal environment. The system consists of a PC, a physical anatomy model of the body orifice, proxy endoscopes, and several software modules. The system generates and transmits force feedback through the flexible endoscope to provide tactile sensations of the actual procedure.

The GI Mentor simulator (Simbionix, Ltd.) accompanies training of endoscopic procedures for gastrointestinal diagnostic and therapeutic procedures with a large physical mannequin (Fig. 8.5). The system enables the navigation through the lower gastrointestinal tract with a virtual view from the endoscope. As with the AccuTouch, users can simultaneously perceive visual feedback and tactile sensation while performing the procedure.

A comprehensive overview of gastrointestinal endoscopy simulators has been provided by Trifan and Stanciu [34].

8.2.6 Needle Insertion Training

There are several medical procedures, where the physician has to insert a needle into the human body, in order to inject any matter, to extract tissue, or to perform a local intervention. Needle insertions can be challenging, especially when a well defined target area such as a small tumor or a blood vessel must be hit by the practitioner. Typical examples are epidural injections, taking of blood samples, trocar insertions, catheter insertions, biopsies, percutaneous vertebroplasty, lumbar puncture, suturing for wound closure or acupuncture. There exist a variety of different needle insertion simulators that can be used to train such procedures (for review see also Coles et al.

Fig. 8.5 GI Mentor II, by
courtesy of Arjun D. Koch

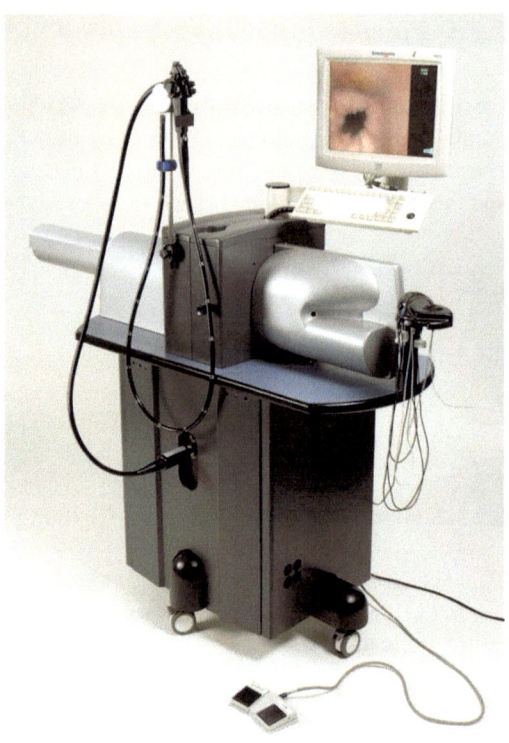

2011 [9]). A needle insertion is commonly realized using commercial haptic display devices with modified end-effectors. One DOF can be sufficient to simulate the penetration force during the insertion process. However, 5 DOF are recommended to accurately simulate needle puncture into an arbitrary location on the human body. Fixing the insertion point on the body reduces this to only 3 DOF.

8.2.6.1 Epidural Injections Training

There are several epidural injection simulators that are attaching a standard syringe to a Sensable PHANTOM display device in order to combine a real interface (syringe) with realistic force feedback when inserting the syringe into the body. One example is the Mediseus Epidural Simulator from Medic Vision [24]. An auditory display provides vocal responses in order to instruct the user and inform about mistakes. The syringe end-effector is connected to a fixed insertion point so that the three translational DOF of the PHANTOM are transformed into one translational and two rotational DOFs.

Another epidural injection simulator using the PHANTOM technology is the EpiSim from Yantric Inc., which was developed at the MIT [11]. The device simulates the resistance (impedance) changes during the injection through the different layers of soft tissue. During the procedure, the simulator displays coronal and sagital views of X-ray images showing the current position of the needle in real-time.

8.2.6.2 Catheter Insertion Training

Immersion Medical produced an intravenous access device called the CathSim Accu-Touch system [10]. The needle can be moved in three DOF (pitch, yaw and depth insertion), while one degree of force feedback is provided in insertion direction. This single force DOF enabled the trainee to feel how the needle passes through different layers of tissue. Later, the CathSim system has been replaced by the Virtual IV intravenous access training simulator, were sold by Immersion and Laerdal.

Another simulator that is used to train catheter insertions was developed by the Center of Advanced Studies, Italy [39]. This system used a head-mounted display system for visual feedback and a PHANTOM display for haptic feedback. Soft tissue deformations were simulated by an incremental viscoelastic model [5].

8.2.6.3 Needle Biopsy Training

Ra et al., 2002 [28] developed a spine needle biopsy simulator incorporating visual and force feedback for training and task planning. Also this system integrates a 3 DOF PHANTOM device, where the endeffector is attached to a needle. Additionally a mannequin is used to provide a realistic scenario. The insertion point is fixed on the lumbar region of the mannequin, thus, transforming the DOF into two rotational and one translational DOF, as it has been realized in other systems such as the mentioned Mediseus Epidural Simulator.

8.2.6.4 Lumbar Puncture Training

As has been pointed out in the review by Coles et al., 2011 [9], lumbar puncture simulators have been developed over the last 18 years. First versions used custom-made haptic feedback that suffered from graphics delay and instability, especially when simulating interactions with high impedances. In 2000, Gorman et al. developed a more successful lumbar puncture simulator that was based on a PHANTOM display device, a mannequin, and a powerful graphics computer [18].

More recently, a lumbar puncture simulator using a 6 DOF force feedback device has been developed [14]. The simulator displays all relevant forces and torques in space while inserting the needle (Fig. 8.6). If the trainee releases the needle, it stays in the correct position and orientation. Needle resistance is calculated on the basis of CT density data. Tissue and needle propagation can be visually displayed in 2D or 3D stereo in real-time.

Fig. 8.6 Lumbar puncture
simulator [14]; by courtesy of
SPRINGER

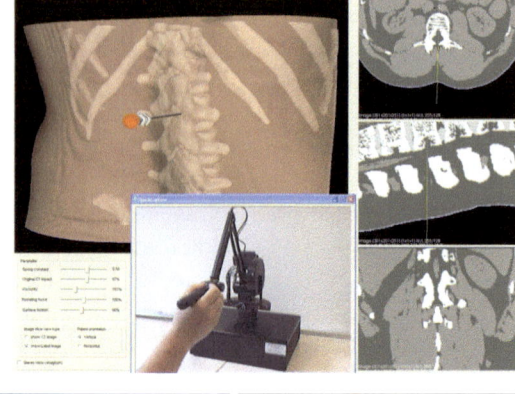

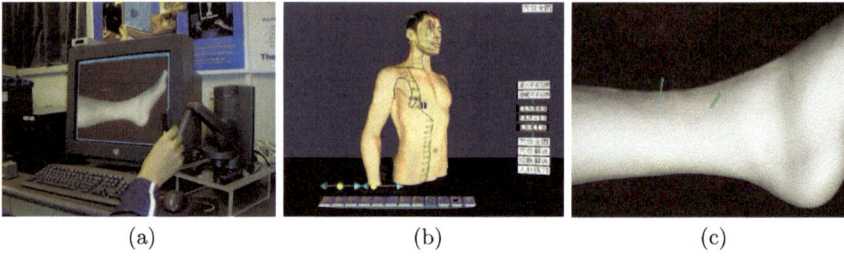

(a)   (b)   (c)

Fig. 8.7 Virtual Acupuncture, Chinese University of Hong Kong. (**a**) Acupuncture Simulator;
(**b**) Graphical user interface; (**c**) Close-up screen shot

8.2.6.5 Virtual Acupuncture Training

A virtual acupuncture simulator has been developed by a research group of The
Chinese University of Hong Kong (Fig. 8.7) [21]. The system aims to use VR technology for teaching and training of Chinese acupuncture. The users can learn and
practice with 3D virtual patients and receive force feedback from a PHANTOM
display device.

8.2.7 Open Surgery Training

Also open surgery requires special skills that can be trained with VR training simulators. These skills can be related to the time management and decision making or
to haptic skills required during certain microsurgical and other open surgical tasks
(see Sect. 8.2.7.1).

8.2.7.1 Skin Surgery Training

A surgery simulator has been developed at the University of Washington [4], aiming
to provide training of suturing of a virtual patient's skin (Fig. 8.8). Based on fast

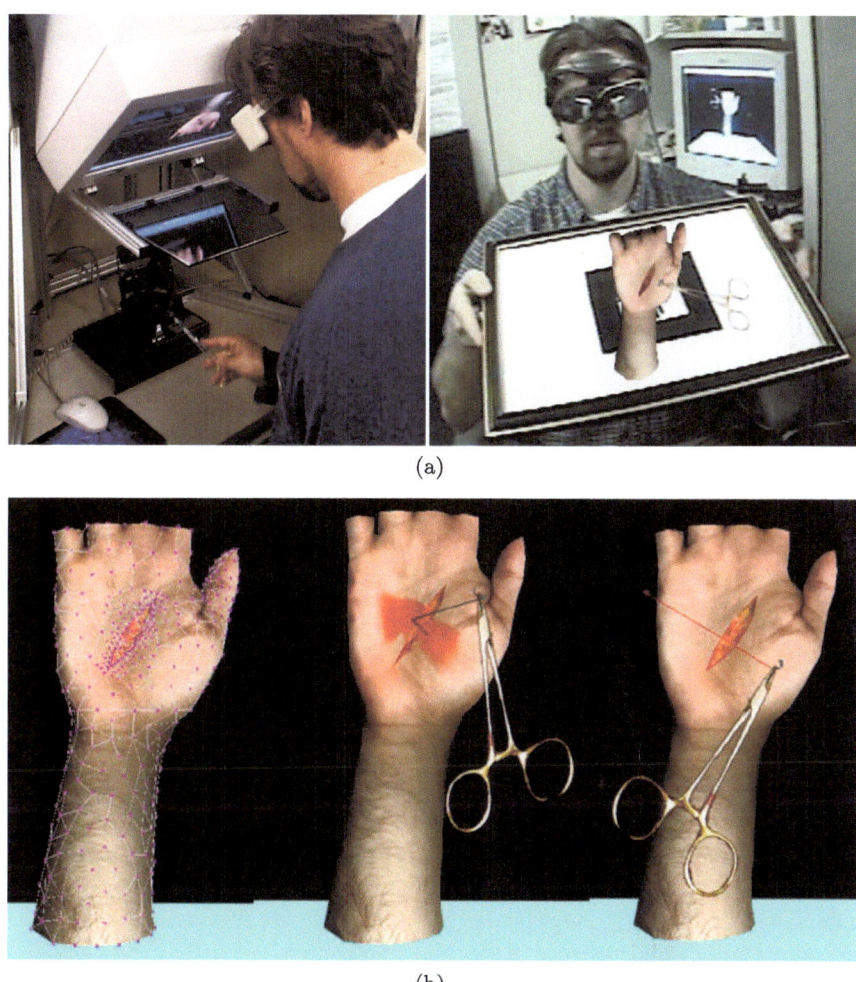

(a)

(b)

Fig. 8.8 Skin Surgery Simulator, University of Washington; © 2004 IEEE. Reprinted, with permission, from [4]. (**a**) Suturing simulator with AR technology; (**b**) Graphical representation

finite element modeling methods the system can display three-dimensional human skin deformations with real-time haptic feedback.

8.2.8 Palpation Training

Physicians palpate human skin or organs with their fingers to locate anatomical landmarks or to feel the presence or absence of anatomical or physiological features (e.g. pulse, respiration function) or abnormalities (e.g. tumor, calcified vessels). This is

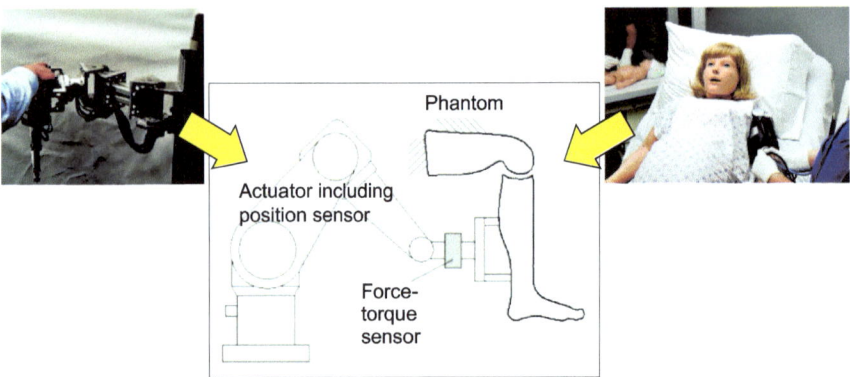

Fig. 8.9 Phantom-based haptic display; by courtesy of Lehrstuhl für Steuerungs- und Regelung-stechnik, TU München (left) and © Gaumard® Scientific 2011 (right)

usually performed for diagnostic purpose or for decision making during an inter-vention. In general, haptic response of palpation requires multi-finger, multi-contact tactile display devices, which would be very challenging for a medical simulator [9]. Therefore, simulation of palpation is mostly ignored, or greatly simplified. Some ap-plications are realized with the Sensable PHANTOM display device, where one or several fingers are attached to the gimbal to produce a certain sensation of touch to the finger tips. Typical applications are palpation of the femoral pulse during in-terventional radiology [8], the brachial pulse [35], the prostate for the diagnosis of cancer [7], the heart during ventricular plastic surgery [33], or the female breast [1]. In another project, the Rutgers Master force feedback glove was used to simulate the palpation of subsurface tumors [22]. One solution to produce rather realistic tactile impressions during particular palpative or manual tasks are *phantom-based training simulators* as they are presented in the following section.

8.3 Phantom-Based Applications

8.3.1 Principle of Phantom-Based Training Simulators

A *phantom*, in the context of training setups, means a passive imitation of an anatomical component. Phantoms are usually made of special polymer materials so that their geometrical appearances, tactile properties and even biomechanical func-tions can be close to the real and physiology. Examples of phantoms are anatomical models of organs, joints, spines, skulls, bones, etc. Such phantoms support basic ed-ucation for medical staff as well as for persons active in the health and sport sector.

Fig. 8.10 Multi-layer
structure of a phantom leg

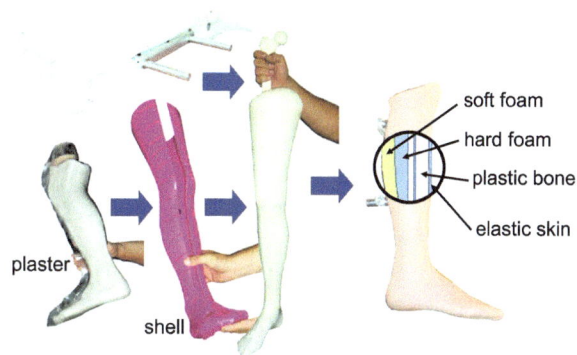

8.3.1.1 Phantom-Based Haptic Displays

The phantom-based haptic display is a new approach that utilizes the integration of
mechatronic actuators and passive anatomical phantoms to provide tactile and kinesthetic feedback to the VR user (Fig. 8.9). The anatomical phantoms can display tactile feedback from their material properties while the mechatronic actuators provide
additional biomechanical force feedback or kinesthetic properties of the simulated
anatomy. The user is not only able to touch the anatomical tissue directly with bare
hands but he can use any medical instruments to interact with the phantom.

The human body consists of internal organs, bone, muscles, fat, and skin. To provide realistic biomechanical properties of the body, the phantoms can be produced
with special multi-layer procedures. Figure 8.10 illustrates an example of how a leg
phantom can be fabricated.

Main advantages of the phantom-based approach are the easiness of the design
and implementation, and the rather high quality of tactile sensations. However, the
use of such haptic display devices can sometimes be inconvenient, especially when
anatomical variations should be simulated, which would require that the phantom
be replaced.

8.3.1.2 Operating Modes

There are two operating modes, which are possible in a phantom-based training
simulator, the teaching and the interactive mode.

- **In the teaching mode** the phantom is automatically driven by the actuator to
  control its positions and movements. The actuator forces the phantom to move
  along pre-defined paths to generate the normal and pathological movements of
  the simulated human organs or limbs. This mode is used to guide or teach the
  medical trainees how to move the organ in a correct manner in order to perform
  clinical examinations of the organ. For example, the simulator can show the users
  how to move a knee joint in order to perform the diagnoses of a ligament rupture.

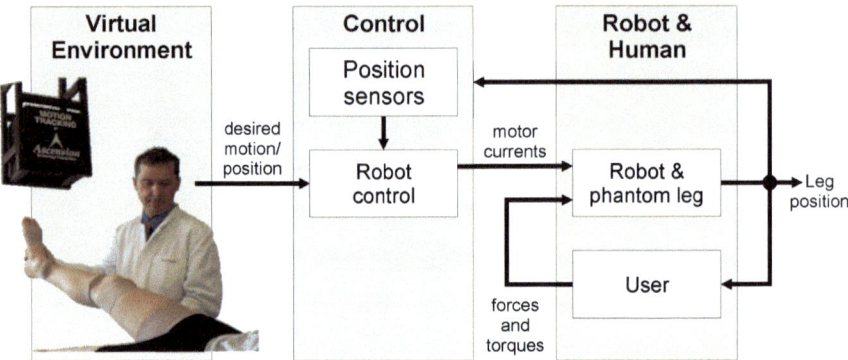

Fig. 8.11 Desired positions are obtained from a pre-recording with a magnetic system

- **In the interactive mode** the simulator works in the same way as typical haptic displays which render forces and movements to react to the actions applied by the trainees. This interaction occurs in real-time so that the trainee has the feeling as if he would interact with a real patient.

8.3.1.3 Control Architectures

There are two conventional control architectures that can be implemented in the phantom-based training simulator, i.e. impedance control and admittance control architectures (see Sect. 4.3.3).

The two approaches are typically used to provide position and force feedback in the interactive mode. In the teaching mode, the controller can be simpler, applying a standard position controller (Fig. 8.11).

8.3.2 The Munich Knee Joint Simulator

The goal of the Munich Knee Joint Simulator is to provide an educational training environment for examinations of knee joint problems [16, 29]. The main components of the simulator consist of an industrial robot and a leg phantom connected to the end of the robot's arm (Fig. 8.12). A force-torque sensor is embedded at the connector between the robot's end-effector and the leg phantom providing the force and moment information of the user's actions. The simulator renders biomechanical force feedback of a healthy and of different pathological knee joints realized by the robot. Tactile feedback is provided by the special materials of the leg phantom. In addition to those main components, a mannequin of the patient body, visual displays and auditory displays are also integrated to the system to make the user environment more realistic.

Fig. 8.12 The Munich Knee
Joint Simulator: A
multimodal platform for
orthopaedic training

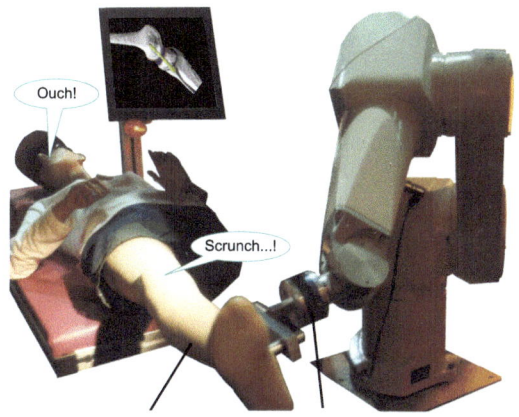

While practicing knee joint diagnoses, the user can see the videos of a medical professional performing the tests with a real patient as well as the virtual animation of the internal structures of the knee joint from the visual display. Loudspeakers in the phantom knee and the head of the mannequin display the sound of the knee joint while being moved and pain reactions of the patients, respectively.

This simulator allows the training of different knee joint evaluation tests to detect rapture of different ligaments (e.g. anterior/posterior cruciate ligament, collateral ligaments) and lesions of the patella tendon and the menisci.

8.3.2.1 Data Acquisition for the Teaching Mode

In the teaching mode, the knee joint movement data is obtained from several knee joint tests performed by a medical expert. The positions and movements of the knee joint are acquired by position and motion tracking systems. Three standard camcorders are used to record the maneuvers of the expert. A magnetic tracking system (Ascension Technology Corp.) with four electromagnetic position sensors is applied to measure the kinematics of the leg while being moved by the expert.

8.3.2.2 Image Data Acquisition

The internal structure of the knee joint consists of bones, ligaments, tendons and muscles. The graphical animation provides a possibility for medical trainees to learn and to understand how the internal structure of the knee joint moves and deforms during the joint movements. The graphical animation is synchronized with the movements of the leg phantom determined by the users.

The information about the internal structures of the knee joint was obtained from CT scan images taken from a cadaver knee joint at different postures (with varying flexion-extension, anterior-posterior, and varus-valgus angles). Figure 8.13 shows

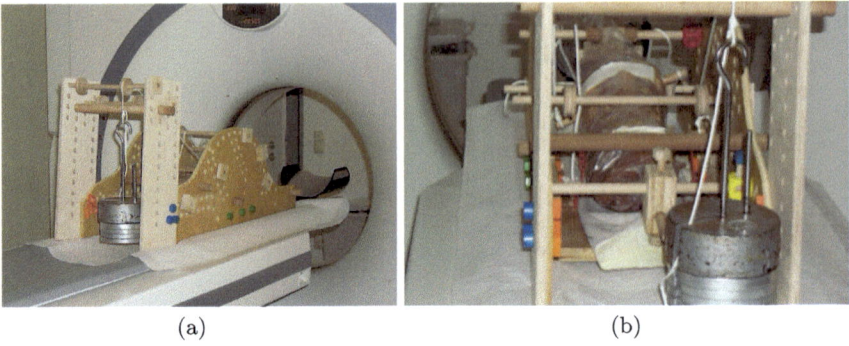

(a)   (b)

Fig. 8.13 Image data acquisition; by courtesy of Rainer Burgkart, TU München. (**a**) Setup for CT recordings; (**b**) The wooden construction enables the adjustment of different knee postures

Fig. 8.14 Knee joint and menisci at different postures

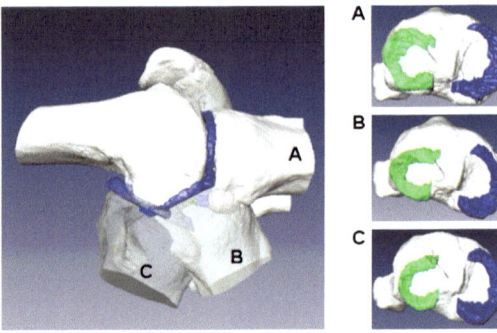

the setup for the image data acquisition including the apparatus for adjusting the posture of the cadaver.

At each posture the 3D geometries of the internal structures (bones, cartilage, ligaments, menisci) were reconstructed and the movements of the internal structures were interpolated from the 3D models (Fig. 8.14). A real-time interpolation method was applied to predict the missing postures.

8.3.2.3 Biomechanical Data Acquisition

The biomechanical data of the knee joint for both healthy and pathologic conditions are required for the haptic display [17]. Elastic joint forces (stiffness characteristics) can be obtained by connecting a cadaver knee joint to a robot and recording the joint forces and torques produced by the robot as a function of the position and orientation of the knee joint. In the experiments, the cadaver shank was rigidly fixed on a table and the thigh was connected to the robot's end-effector via a force-torque sensor. While the robot moves, the positions and orientations of the thigh and the load reactions are recorded. Thus, the elastic properties of the knee joint can be determined [15].

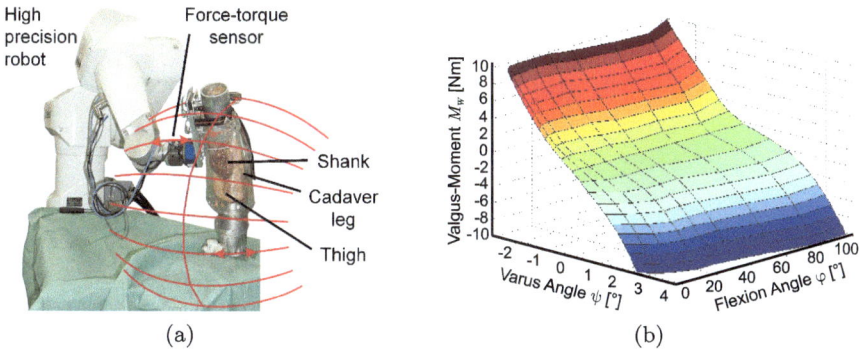

Fig. 8.15 Biomechanical data acquisition. (**a**) Experimental set-up; (**b**) Varus-valgus-load characteristic over varying joint flexion angles

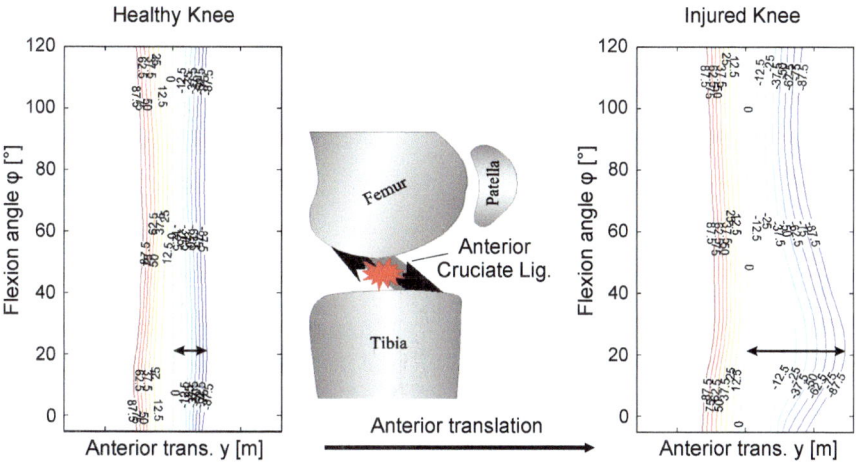

Fig. 8.16 Elastic properties of knee joint in a healthy condition and in a case of anterior cruciate ligament rupture. Level curves in the left and right graphs indicate the regions with equal force levels. The two arrows represent force vectors with magnitudes of 87.5 N each

The setup of the biomechanical data acquisition experiment is illustrated in Fig. 8.15(a). Figure 8.15(b) shows the stiffness characteristic of the healthy knee joint in varus-valgus directions at different knee flexion angles.

To simulate a pathological knee joint, different lesions were modeled (e.g. the anterior cruciate ligament rupture) by dissecting parts of the bones, where the respective ligament is attached instead of directly cutting the ligament. The dissected bone can be re-attached back to the bone by screws, in order to restore the function of the ligament for further measurements. This allows one to replicate a large variety of different ligament ruptures without destroying ligamentous structure.

The experimental results, as shown in Fig. 8.16, present a comparison of the elastic properties of a knee joint under healthy and pathologic conditions (anterior

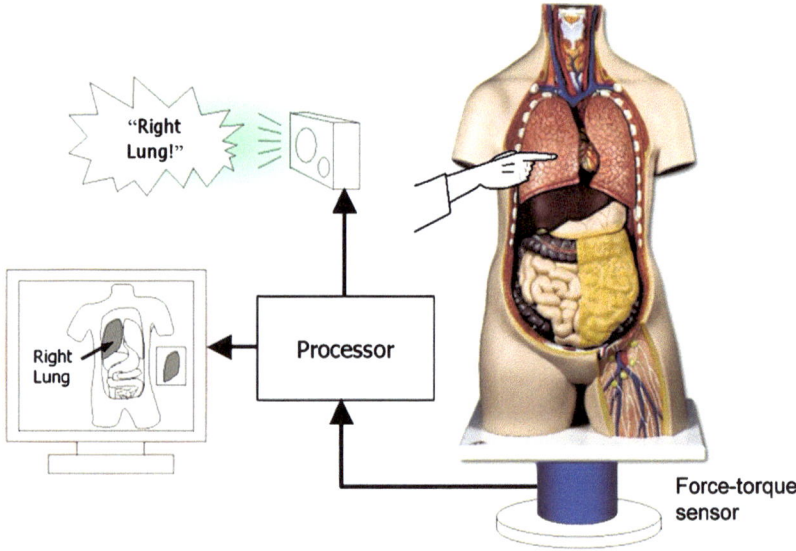

Fig. 8.17   Touch simulator setup exemplified by a torso simulator

cruciate ligament rupture). The data is used to provide training possibilities for the so-called Anterior Drawer Test and Lachmann Test.

8.3.3 Touch Simulators

A touch simulator can be considered as a special case of the phantom-based haptic display. In the touch simulator setup, a phantom is mounted on a force-torque sensor alone and is simply placed on a desk without any additional actuators. When a user touches the phantom, the applied force and moment are measured. The measured force-torque information can be used to determine the user's touch point. With this technique, it is possible to turn a completely passive phantom into an interactive input device, which reacts like a three-dimensional touch display.

The setup of the touch simulator is simple and easy to be applied for any solid object. The users can touch the phantom with a finger or a medical device that can apply a single-point-contact such as a needle. The interactive effects can be produced when the user touches the phantom, including interactive display of the name and function of the touched anatomical region (Fig. 8.17) and the associated cross section images of the anatomy at the touched location.

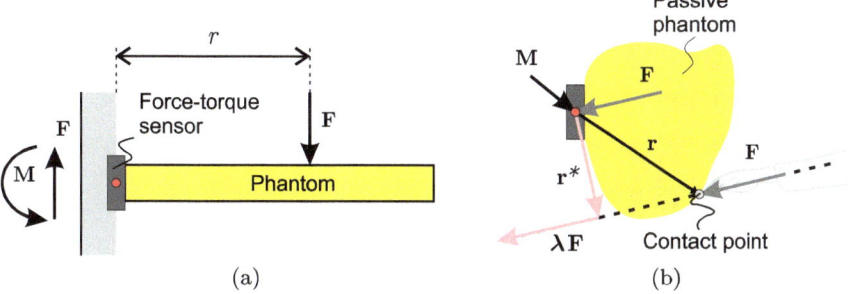

Fig. 8.18 Technical principle. (**a**) One-dimensional case; (**b**) Three-dimensional case

8.3.3.1 Technical Principle

This section shows the technique how the contact locations can be computed by the force-torque information.

Consider a simplified situation in 1D as shown in Fig. 8.18(a). An object representing a phantom is connected to a force-torque sensor and fixed to the ground at one end while the other end is free. When a user applies a force F to the object, the location of the applied force measured from the origin of the sensor (distance r) can be computed from the relationship:

$$M = r \cdot F \quad \Rightarrow \quad r = M/F. \tag{8.1}$$

When the same principle is applied in 3D space, the force, moment and distance relationship can be written in a vector form as:

$$\mathbf{M} = \mathbf{r} \times \mathbf{F}. \tag{8.2}$$

This relationship forms a system of linear equations. Although the vectors $\mathbf{F}$ and $\mathbf{M}$ are known, the system of equations cannot be solved by the Gaussian elimination method. This is because the coefficient matrix of the system is singular, i.e. the determinant of the coefficient matrix is equal to zero. So the solution of the system of equations is not unique (underdetermined system).

From a physical point of view, the solutions of the system lie on the line of action of the contact force intersecting the contact point (Fig. 8.18(b)). Therefore, the contact point solutions can be determined if the line of action and the geometry of the phantom are known.

The mathematical description of the line of action is given in a parametric form as:

$$\mathbf{d}(\lambda) = \mathbf{r}^* + \lambda \cdot \mathbf{F}, \tag{8.3}$$

where

$$\mathbf{r}^* = \frac{\mathbf{F} \times \mathbf{M}}{|\mathbf{F}|^2}. \tag{8.4}$$

Vector $\mathbf{r}^*$ is orthogonal to $\mathbf{F}$ and $\mathbf{M}$; it points from the origin of the sensor to the line of action. The geometry of the phantom used in the touch simulator is described by a polyhedral surface containing a set of connected triangles. This information can be extracted from CT or MR images and 3D surface reconstruction techniques such as the marching cubes algorithm (see Sect. 10.4.2).

The intersection between the line of action and the phantom geometry can be determined from the parameter λ, which is obtained by performing ray-triangle intersection tests between the line of action and each face of the phantom geometry.

The computational procedure to find the intersection point can be summarized as following:

- Calculate the normal vectors of all triangular faces
- Reject the "shadow-sided" triangles whose normal vectors point to the same half space as the direction of the applied force vector ($\mathbf{F} \cdot \mathbf{n} < 0$)
- Perform ray-triangle intersection tests between the line of action and the remaining triangles
- If the computed contact point is found inside the area of the respective triangle, the contact point is the intersection point.

Note that there is no guarantee for a unique solution, because the line of action may intersect the phantom surface more than once. To guarantee the uniqueness of the contact point solution, the applied force must be torque-free and unidirectional (pushing force). Additionally, only a single contact point must be applied and the shape of the object or, at least the interacting region, must be convex [26]. Furthermore, deformations of the object (when the base fixation is too weak or when soft objects are being used) result in limited accuracy of the contact point determination.

On the other hand, advantages are that only a simple sensor technology is required that can be centrally integrated in the object's base. Thus, no adaptations of the object (e.g. electrical contacts) or the environment (e.g. optical navigation system) is required.

8.3.3.2 Applications

Touch simulators can be used for different applications. For example, the interesting regions being touched can be classified (e.g. organs, bones, vessels, etc.); furthermore, object changes (removal or addition of parts) can be detected considering weight changes; and last but not least different commands can be activated when producing a specific temporal contact pattern or when touching particular contact regions.

Touch simulators can be used to support the training of acupuncture, dental procedures, oral implantation, brain anatomy, neurosurgical tasks, etc. (Fig. 8.19) [26].

Fig. 8.19 Examples of touch simulators. (**a**) Simulator for oral implantology; (**b**) BrainTrain system

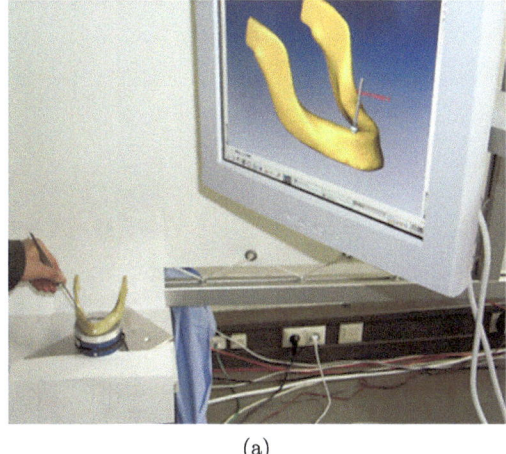

(a)

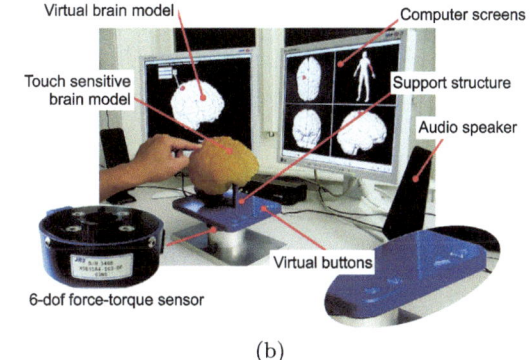

Virtual brain model

Computer screens

Touch sensitive brain model

Support structure

Audio speaker

6-dof force-torque sensor

Virtual buttons

(b)

8.3.4 Delivery Simulators

A delivery simulator aims to provide a training environment for childbirth (Fig. 8.20). A typical setup consists of a baby phantom attached to an actuator system and a phantom of the abdomen and the pelvis of a female body. The simulator displays multi-modal information to the user including graphics, sound, and tactile and kinesthetic impressions presented by the baby phantom. The simulation flow and simulated complications are controlled by the trainer.

The simulator SIMone™ 3B Scientific GmbH includes a biomechanical model of the birth process in order to provide a haptic feeling to the user. The simulator is also equipped with a graphical display in order to give instructions, present signals of the monitoring devices (e.g. cardiotaco graph) or show a real-time animation of the anatomical relationships during delivery, such as the position and orientation of the fetus, fetal head, umbilical cord, and also the forces acting during the process (Fig. 8.21).

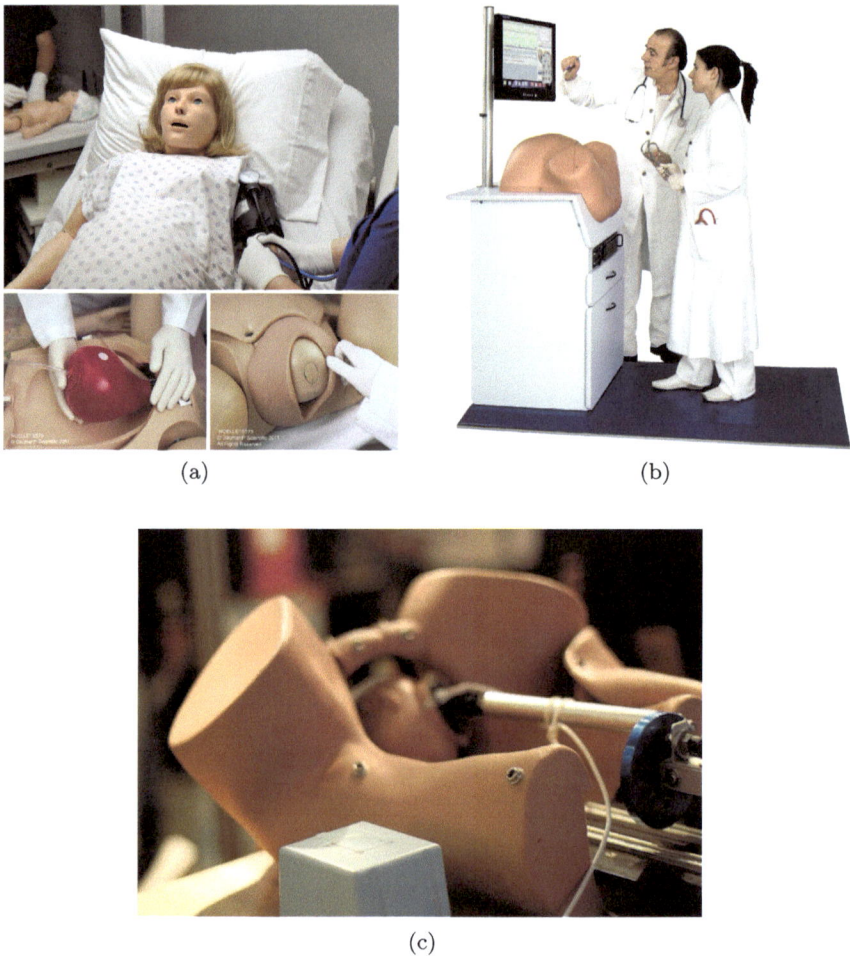

(a)   (b)

(c)

Fig. 8.20 Examples of delivery simulators. (**a**) NOELLE®, © Gaumard®Scientific 2011; (**b**) SI-Mone™, © 3B Scientific GmbH, Hamburg, 2011; (**c**) BirthSim, Ampère Lab, Lyon, France [12, 13]; by courtesy of Richard Moreau

To provide a complete feedback to the user, the simulator would require a model of physiological processes of mother and child. This would provide the user with information such as the fetal heart rate, uterus contractions intensity, blood pressure, or the mother's groaning and breathing.

With such technologies the obstetricians and midwives can learn the techniques of forceps or vacuum extraction and different pulling techniques, while the graphical display provides visual insights into the anatomical and biomechanical structures of mother and child. They can also train the decision making that is important in certain emergency cases, when complications occur like fetal oxygen deficiency, fetal fatigue, or shoulder dystocia.

Fig. 8.21 Graphical display of SIMone™; by courtesy of Rainer Burgkart, TU München

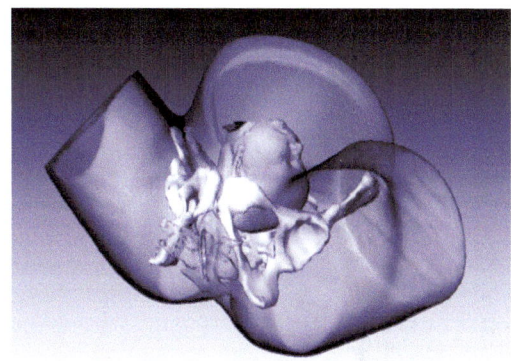

Fig. 8.22 METI anesthesia simulator, photo courtesy of METI® © 2011 METI

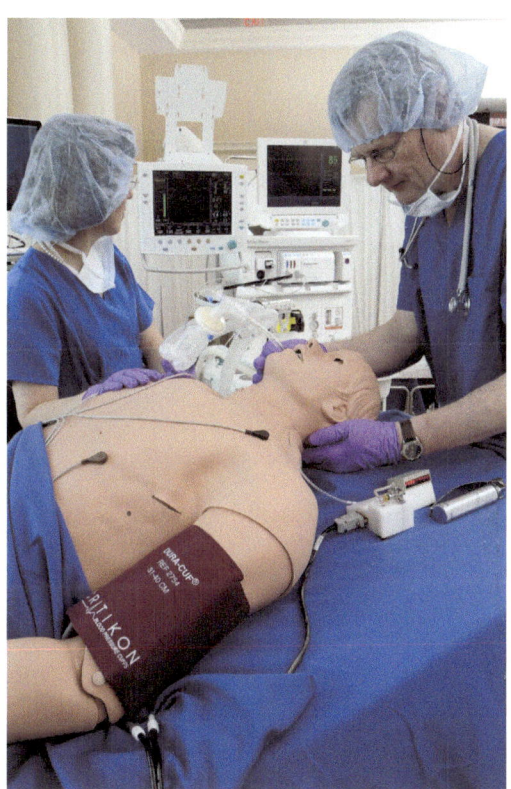

8.3.5 Anesthesia Simulators

Anesthesia simulators serve for training anesthetists in managing patients in the operating room. Such kind of simulator basically consists of a mannequin, actuators and displays, sensors and a processing unit with a computer model of the physiological processes involved during anesthesia (Fig. 8.23). The system is capable

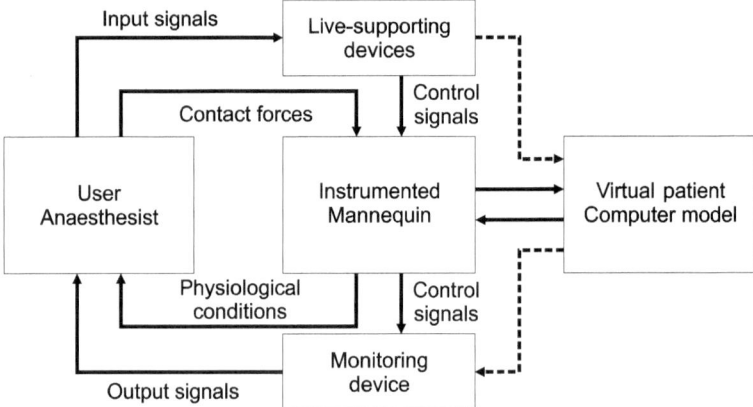

Fig. 8.23   Anesthesia simulator: information flowchart

of simulating palpable pulses, heart and respiration sounds, respiration movements, artificial respiration, intubation, urine production, simulation of kidney function, infusions, injections of different medications, body temperature, pupil reflex, eye movements, indirect blood pressure measurement according to Riva-Rocci, ECG and EEG recordings, neuromuscular transmission, and certain trauma-module cases to simulate fractures, arm movements, thorax drainages. The most famous commercial system is the METI anesthesia simulator (Fig. 8.22).

References

1. Alhalabi, M.O., Daniulaitis, V., Kawasaki, H., Hori, T.: Medical training simulation for palpation of subsurface tumor using hiro. In: Proceedings of the First Joint Eurohaptics Conference and Symposium on Haptic Interfaces for Virtual Environment and Teleoperator Systems, pp. 623–624. IEEE Computer Society, Washington (2005)
2. Bachofen, D., Zatonyi, J., Harders, M., Szekely, G., Fruh, P., Thaler, M.: Enhancing the visual realism of hysteroscopy simulation. Stud. Health Technol. Inform. **119**, 31–36 (2006)
3. Basdogan, C., Sedef, M., Harders, M., Wesarg, S.: VR-Based simulators for training in minimally invasive surgery. IEEE Comput. Graph. Appl. **27**(2), 54–66 (2007). ISI Impact Factor 1.429
4. Berkley, J., Turkiyyah, G., Berg, D., Ganter, M., Weghorst, S.: Real-time finite element modeling for surgery simulation: an application to virtual suturing. IEEE Trans. Vis. Comput. Graph. **10**(3), 314–325 (2004). doi:10.1109/TVCG.2004.1272730
5. Brett, P.N., Parker, T.J., Harrison, A.J., Thomas, T.A., Carr, A.: Simulation of resistance forces acting on surgical needles. Proc. Inst. Mech. Eng. Part H, J. Eng. Med. **211**(4), 335–347 (1997)
6. Burdea, G., Coiffet, P.: Virtual Reality Technology. Wiley, New York (1993)
7. Burdea, G., Patounakis, G., Popescu, V., Weiss, R.E.: Virtual reality-based training for the diagnosis of prostate cancer. IEEE Trans. Biomed. Eng. **46**(10), 1253–1260 (1999). doi:10.1109/10.790503

8. Coles, T., John, N.W., Gould, D.A., Caldwell, D.G.: Haptic palpation for the femoral pulse in virtual interventional radiology. In: Advances in Computer-Human Interactions, 2009. ACHI '09. Second International Conferences on, pp. 193–198 (2009). doi:10.1109/ACHI.2009.61

9. Coles, T.R., Meglan, D., John, N.W.: The role of haptics in medical training simulators: a survey of the state of the art. IEEE Trans. Haptics **4**(1), 51–66 (2011). doi:10.1109/TOH.2010.19

10. Cunningham, R.L., Feldman, P., Feldman, B., Merril, G.L.: Interface device and method for interfacing instruments to vascular access simulation systems (2002). Google Patents. US Patent 6,470,302

11. Dang, T., Annaswamy, T.M., Srinivasan, M.A.: Development and evaluation of an epidural injection simulator with force feedback for medical training. Med. Meets Virtual Real. **81**, 97 (2001)

12. Dupuis, O., Moreau, R., Silveira, R., Pham, M.T., Zentner, A., Cucherat, M., Rudigoz, R.C., Redarce, T.: A new obstetric forceps for the training of junior doctors: a comparison of the spatial dispersion of forceps blade trajectories between junior and senior obstetricians. Am. J. Obstet. Gynecol. **194**(6), 1524–1531 (2006). doi:10.1016/j.ajog.2006.01.013

13. Dupuis, O., Moreau, R., Pham, M.T., Redarce, T.: Assessment of forceps blade orientations during their placement using an instrumented childbirth simulator. Int. J. Obstet. Gynaecol. **116**(2), 327–333 (2009). doi:10.1111/j.1471-0528.2008.02004.x

14. Färber, M., Heller, J., Hummel, F., Gerloff, C., Handels, H.: Virtual reality based training of lumbar punctures using a 6dof haptic device. In: Buzug, T.M., Holz, D., Bongartz, J., Kohl-Bareis, M., Hartmann, U., Weber, S. (eds.) Advances in Medical Engineering. Springer Proceedings in Physics, vol. 114, pp. 236–240. Springer, Berlin (2007). http://dx.doi.org/10.1007/978-3-540-68764-1_39

15. Frey, M., Burgkart, R., Regenfelder, F., Riener, R.: Optimised robot-based system for the exploration of elastic joint properties. Med. Biol. Eng. Comput. **42**(5), 674–678 (2004)

16. Frey, M., Hoogen, J., Burgkart, R., Riener, R.: Physical interaction with a virtual knee joint-the 9 dof haptic display of the Munich knee joint simulator. Presence: Teleoperators and Virtual Environments **15**(5), 570–587 (2006)

17. Frey, M., Riener, R., Michas, C., Regenfelder, F., Burgkart, R.: Elastic properties of an intact and acl-ruptured knee joint: measurement, mathematical modelling, and haptic rendering. J. Biomech. **39**(8), 1371–1382 (2006)

18. Gorman, P., Krummel, T., Webster, R., Smith, M., Hutchens, D.: A prototype haptic lumbar puncture simulator. Med. Meets Virtual Real. **70**, 106 (2000)

19. Green, P.E., Piantanida, T.A., Hill, J.W., Simon, I.B., Satava, R.M.: Telepresence: dexterous procedures in a virtual operating field. Am. Surg. **57**, 192 (1991)

20. Halvorsen, F.H., Elle, O.J., Fosse, E.: Simulators in surgery. Minim. Invasive Ther. Allied Technol. **14**(4–5), 214–223 (2005). doi:10.1080/13645700500243869. http://informahealthcare.com/doi/pdf/10.1080/13645700500243869

21. Heng, P.A., Wong, T.T., Yang, R., Chui, Y.P., Xie, Y.M., Leung, K.S., Leung, P.C.: Intelligent inferencing and haptic simulation for Chinese acupuncture learning and training. IEEE Trans. Inf. Technol. Biomed. **10**(1), 28–41 (2006)

22. Langrana, N., Burdea, G., Ladeji, J., Dinsmore, M.: Human performance using virtual reality tumor palpation simulation. Comput. Graph. **21**(4), 451–458 (1997)

23. Liu, A., Tendick, F., Cleary, K., Kaufmann, C.: A survey of surgical simulation: applications, technology, and education. Presence: Teleoperators and Virtual Environments **12**(6), 599–614 (2003)

24. Mayooran, Z., Watterson, L., Withers, P., Line, J., Arnett, W., Horley, R.: Mediseus epidural: full-procedure training simulator for epidural analgesia in labour. In: SimTecT Healthcare Simulation Conference 2006 (2006)

25. Müller, W., Bockholt, U., Lahmer, A., Voss, G., Börner, M.: VRATS—virtual-reality-arthroskopie-trainingssimulator. Radiologe **40**(3), 290–294 (2000). doi:10.1007/s001170050671

26. Panchaphongsaphak, B., Burgkart, R., Riener, R.: Three-dimensional touch interface for medical education. IEEE Trans. Inf. Technol. Biomed. **11**(3), 251–263 (2007)

27. Pham, T., Roland, L., Benson, K.A., Webster, R.W., Gallagher, A.G., Haluck, R.S.: Smart tutor: a pilot study of a novel adaptive simulation environment. Stud. Health Technol. Inform. **111**, 385–389 (2005)
28. Ra, J.B., Kwon, S.M., Kim, J.K., Yi, J., Kim, K.H., Park, H.W., Kyung, K.U., Kwon, D.S., Kang, H.S., Kwon, S.T., et al.: Spine needle biopsy simulator using visual and force feedback. Comput. Aided Surg. **7**(6), 353–363 (2002)
29. Riener, R., Frey, M., Proll, T., Regenfelder, F., Burgkart, R.: Phantom-based multimodal interactions for medical education and training: the Munich knee joint simulator. IEEE Trans. Inf. Technol. Biomed. **8**(2), 208–216 (2004)
30. Satava, R.M.: Virtual reality surgical simulator: the first steps. Surg. Endosc. **7**(3), 203–205 (1993)
31. Sherman, K.P., Ward, J.W., Wills, D.P., Mohsen, A.M.: A portable virtual environment knee arthroscopy training system with objective scoring. Stud. Health Technol. Inform. **62**, 335 (1999)
32. Taffinder, N., Sutton, C., Fishwick, R.J., McManus, I.C., Darzi, A.: Validation of virtual reality to teach and assess psychomotor skills in laparoscopic surgery: results from randomised controlled studies using the mist VR laparoscopic simulator. Stud. Health Technol. Inform. **50**, 124–130 (1998)
33. Tokuyasu, T., Kitamura, T., Sakaguchi, G., Komeda, M.: Development of training system for left ventricular plastic surgery. In: Biomedical Engineering, IEEE EMBS Asian-Pacific Conference on, pp. 60–61 (2003). doi:10.1109/APBME.2003.1302583
34. Trifan, A., Stanciu, C.: Computer-based simulator for training in gastrointestinal endoscopy. Rev. Med.-Chir. Soc. Med. Nat. Iasi **111**(3), 567–574 (2007)
35. Ullrich, S., Mendoza, J., Ntouba, A., Rossaint, R., Kuhlen, T.: Haptic pulse simulation for virtual palpation. Bildverarb. Med. **10**, 187–191 (2008)
36. Vince, J.: Introduction to Virtual Reality. Springer, Berlin (2004)
37. Vining, D.J., Liu, K., Choplin, R.H., Haponik, E.F.: Virtual bronchoscopy: relationships of virtual reality endobronchial simulations to actual bronchoscopy findings. Chest **109**(2), 549 (1996)
38. Wang, Q., Ou, Y., Xu, Y.: A prototype virtual haptic bronchoscope. In: Intelligent Robots and Systems, IEEE/RSJ International Conference on, vol. 2, pp. 1361–1366 (2002). doi:10.1109/IRDS.2002.1043944
39. Zorcolo, A., Gobbetti, E., Pili, P., Tuveri, M., et al.: Catheter insertion simulation with combined visual and haptic feedback. In: Proceedings of the First Phantom Users Research Symposium. Citeseer, Princeton (1999)

Chapter 9
VR for Planning and Intraoperative Support

9.1 Introduction

The medical training systems we have discussed so far are based on generic data processing and depiction, mostly without the need to refer to individual patient data and individual situations. However, there are numerous medical tasks and applications that require patient-specific data, for instance, to support patient individual diagnosis and therapy. This chapter presents examples of medical VR applications dealing with individual patient-specific data. Most of these examples deal with surgical applications. In the first subsection we present different systems, where concrete patient imaging data are applied for the planning of individual surgical treatments prior to the intervention. In the remaining two subsections we overview applications, where patient imaging data are used to support a surgical treatment during the intervention. In those latter subsections the term *Augmented Reality* (AR) plays a relevant role and will be explained in detail.

9.2 VR for Surgical Planning

Planning of surgical procedures can be supported by visualization of virtual 3D depictions of patient-specific anatomy. In many situations it is helpful to also interact with the displayed anatomical structures in order to plan the different surgical steps required for the individual treatment. However, since it is very complicated to produce patient-individual haptic information most pre-operative (as well as operative) VR applications focus only on the visual modality.

9.2.1 Radiosurgery Planning

Stereotactic radiosurgery (SRS) is applied to treat abnormal lesions, such as brain or lung tumors, using gamma rays (Fig. 9.1). Prior to the stereotactic surgery the

R. Riener, M. Harders, *Virtual Reality in Medicine*,
DOI 10.1007/978-1-4471-4011-5_9, © Springer-Verlag London 2012

Fig. 9.1 Stereotactic
radiosurgery:
(**a**) ExacTrac®Robotics;
Brainlab AG, brainlab.com,
(**b**) Tumor treatment with
CyberKnife; Copyright
Accuray Incorporated

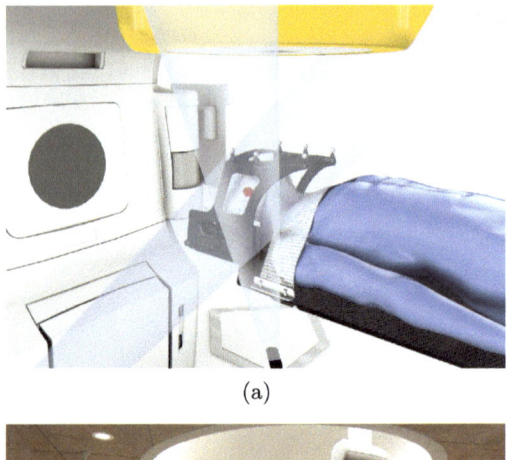

(a)

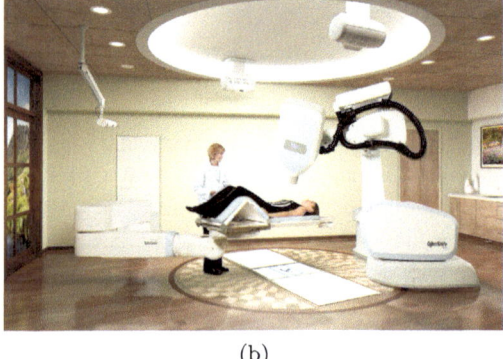

(b)

target tissue must be located in 3D and the location information must be transformed
to the coordinate frame of the radio surgery system. The treatment involves the
use of focused radiation beams. Rays are emitted via a linear accelerator to the
determined area inside the human body in order to destroy the pathological tissue.
The gamma rays are absorbed by the cells causing genetic changes in the cells,
finally leading to a degeneration of the pathologic tissue. However, also healthy
cells can suffer from the radiation. Thus, the pathological area should be hit with
the highest radiation dose, which is optimized with particular visualisation tools,
whereas healthy tissue (such as nerves, sensory organs, or blood vessels) must not
get harmed by the radiation.

With multiple cross-fired radiation beams, the gamma rays are projected from
different directions to the target tissue, causing a high radiation dose at the target
location while adjacent tissue absorb lower radiation. This technique can destroy
the target tissues without damaging other healthy tissues around the target area. For
an accurate treatment, the radiation beams have to be conformed to the (projected)
shape of the tumor tissue or lesion. In the past, a set of different fixed-shape collimators were used; each collimator is mounted to the moving linear accelerator to
hit the target area from different directions. Current radiosurgical devices use multi-
leaf collimators (Fig. 9.2), which allow a dynamic reshaping of the outline and the

Fig. 9.2 m3®
Micro-Multi-leaf Collimator;
Brainlab AG, brainlab.com

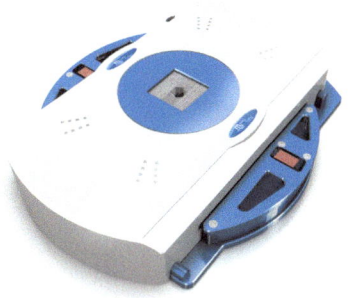

intensity of the radiation beams during the movement of the linear accelerator by changing the position of each leaf.

VR-based planning stations have been developed, which display not only the anatomical relationships but also the radiation beam and the dose distribution on the human tissue (Fig. 9.3). The technology helps neurosurgeons to view the lesion and important healthy tissue in 3D perspective. The graphical display is also used to determine the direction of the radiation beams applied during the therapy in order to avoid damaging important nerve tissue and to minimize the deterioration of surrounding healthy tissue.

9.2.2 Surgery Room Design

VR approaches can be used to simulate working environments comprised by medical equipment, machines, furniture and even patients and medical staff in order to design and optimize space and ergonomic aspects of an operating room. This can be especially helpful, if novel surgical instruments such as robotic devices have to be inserted in the operating room (Figs. 9.4 and 9.5). On the basis of an artificial

Fig. 9.3 iPlan® RT Dose;
Brainlab AG, brainlab.com

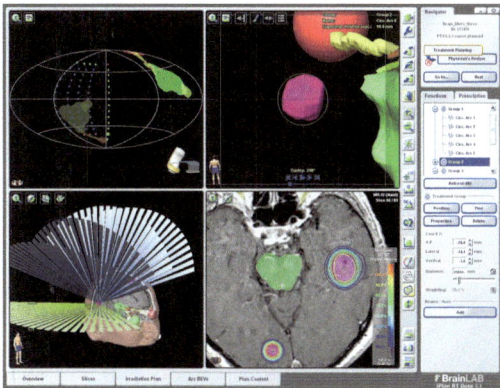

Fig. 9.4 Simulation
KISMET developed for the
design of an operation room
and planning of surgical
workflow (Origin:
Forschungszentrum
Karlsruhe, Germany)

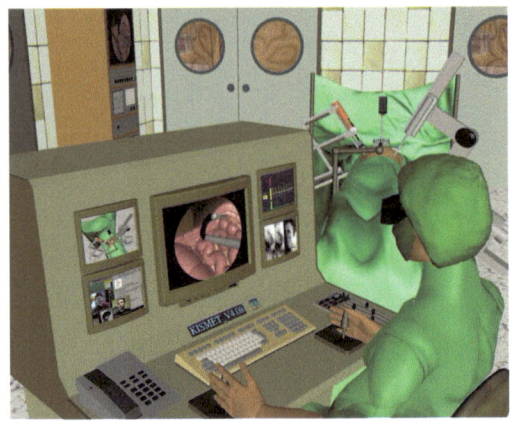

Fig. 9.5 ANYSIM
simulation environment used
to plan the spatial
arrangement of patient,
bench, operation light and
surgical robot to reduce the
risk of collisions (image
source: Dr. H. Götte, iwb, TU
München)

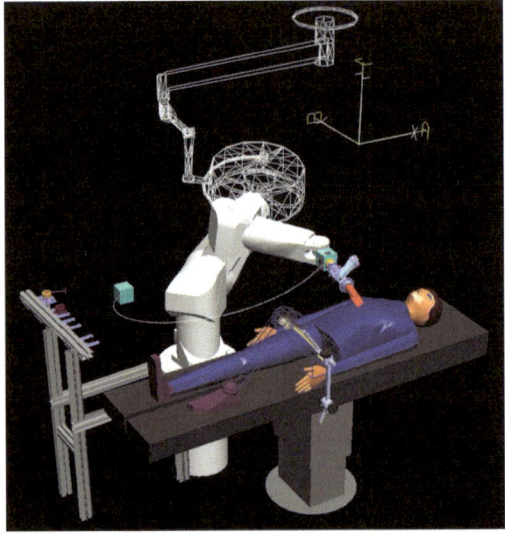

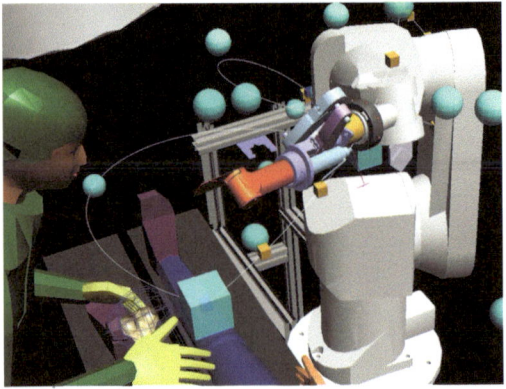

representation of the operating room, also the risk of collisions between patient, operating personnel and medical devices can be analyzed and minimized, or the lighting conditions as well as other facility design issues can be planned.

When a surgical robot is introduced in the operating room, the surgeons have to define the work steps of the surgical robot. The steps depend not only on the type of surgery and the patient specific data, but also on the structure of the robot and the surgical room environment. The range of motion and the work steps must be optimized to provide the most effective clinical workflow and avoid collisions between the robotic arm, the surgical environment and any human involved in the operation.

9.2.3 Orthopedic Surgery Planning

Particular graphical user interfaces and visual rendering methods can be applied for orthopedic surgery planning, especially when a high accuracy and quantitative planning outcome are required such as in robot-assisted endoprostheses implantations. With such a planning tool, the surgeon can decide which type and size of prosthesis should be chosen and how the robot should remove bone material through the different cutting and drilling steps in order to optimally replace the pathologic joint by the endoprosthesis. In more advanced planning tools the surgeon can even evaluate his planning result through a static anatomical hard and soft tissue viewer or a biomechanical (functional) movement animator before the surgical procedure will be executed.

9.2.4 Virtual Endoscopy

Surgical endoscopy is a non-invasive or minimally invasive therapeutic and diagnostic technique used to visualize, examine or surgically treat the interior of hollow organs. Such hollow organs can be those that can be reached from outside the body, without any incision. Examples are the colon, stomach, bladder, esophagus, tracheae or bronchial tubes. The method of virtual endoscopy is based on a 3D image reconstruction of specific organs or organ regions in such way that it allows views similar to those obtained from real endoscopy. Virtual endoscopy enables physicians to better see anatomical structures and recognize pathologic tissue in a more intuitive way. This can strengthen or confirm the diagnosis and also mean an important step when a surgical procedure has to be planned after the diagnosis. In other words, the user can interact with patient-specific data by "flying through the patient's body" in an intuitive way. Virtual endoscopy can be applied to different minimally invasive surgical fields, such as laparoscopy, colonoscopy, bronchioscopy (Fig. 9.6).

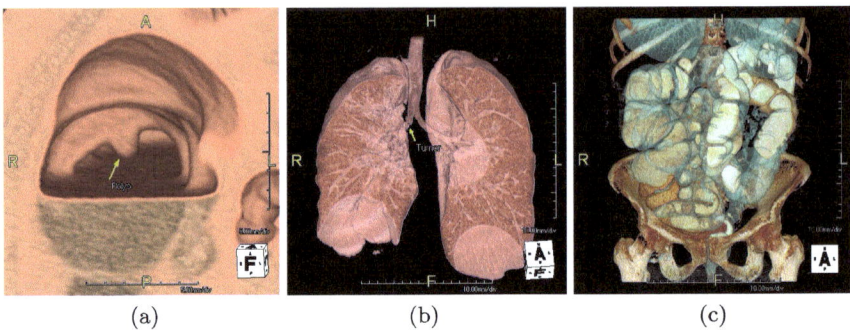

(a)   (b)   (c)

Fig. 9.6 Virtual endoscopy visualizations: (**a**) colonoscopy, (**b**) bronchoscopy, (**c**) transparent patient with colon and skeleton; by courtesy of David Vining

9.3 Augmented Reality in Surgery

9.3.1 Definition and Historical Background

While VR aims at immersing the user entirely into a computer-generated virtual world, augmented reality (AR) takes a different approach, in which virtual computer generated objects are added to the real physical space [37]. Milgram and Kishino, 1994 [22], described AR as a mixture of VR and the real world in which the real part is more dominant than the virtual one. Azuma [1, 2] described AR by its properties of aligning virtual and real objects in a real environment in real-time. Sielhorst et al., 2008 [32], claim that medical AR takes its main motivation from the need of visualizing medical data and the patient within the same physical space. It goes back to the desire of having an X-ray vision, seeing through objects, which was the goal of many medical augmented reality solutions proposed in the literature [32]. Probably the first one was Steinhaus [34], who suggested already in 1938 a method for visualizing a piece of metal inside tissue registered to its real view (see also [32]). In 1968, Sutherland [35] was the first to use a tracked head-mounted display enabling a viewpoint-dependent visualization of virtual objects. Two decades later Roberts et al., 1968 [25], developed an AR system, where segmented medical data obtained from computed tomography (CT) were integrated into the optics of an operating microscope. Movements of the microscope were recorded by an ultrasonic tracking system and used to update the image overlays in the microscopic view. In the early 1990s further AR systems were developed for several industrial applications [12, 14].

9.3.2 Classes of Medical AR Applications

Most medical AR research and development is concerned with merging a real world patient or an operating scenario with a digitally simulated environment by using

advanced graphic displays and motion tracking technologies. Medical VR operators use displays that project an artificial scene into the eyes, and allow the users
to move and manipulate the virtual objects such as a surgical instrument or human
organ. AR operators, in contrast, may use translucent or semi-transparent displays
through which they can still see the real world, while computer-generated images
are projected on top of the real view. AR users are usually interacting with real
physical objects, a real patient or physician, and a real surgical scenario, which is
augmented by medical image data or other computer-generated information. According to Sielhorst et al., 2008 [32], and Krevelen and Poelman [36] AR systems
can be grouped into different classes depending on the kind and placement of the
visual display system in relation to the patient position (Fig. 9.7). The following
classes can be distinguished:

- **HMD-based AR systems** Already the system presented by Sutherland [35] was
  based on a head-mounted display system, which combined real and virtual images
  by means of a semi-transparent mirror, also called optical see-through HMD. In
  1992 Bajura et al. [4] presented a video see-through HMD for the augmentation
  of ultrasound images. Later, this system was improved to reach better performance of the image generation [3, 33]. The first real-time (i.e. 30 fps) system,
  which allowed a synchronized display of real and virtual images, was built by
  Sauer et al. [29]. Many other groups followed that developed high-performance
  AR systems based on HMD technology (see [11, 26] for a detailed overview). The
  advantage of HMD-based AR systems is that there is no eye-to-display calibration needed as long as the position of the HMD in relation to the head/eye remains
  fixed and known. Thus, only the object (i.e. the patient, if moving) and the HMD
  must be tracked with respect to their positions in space. One of the main disadvantages, however, is that the physician has to wear a sometimes rather bulky and
  heavy, thus, uncomfortable device, which may disturb the natural view onto the
  operating scene.
- **Medical device display** Another way to augment real world scenarios with artificial images is to integrate video displays with semi-transparent mirrors into
  standard optics such as operating microscopes or operating binoculars. Like with
  the HMD-based approach, this does not require further eye-to-display calibration.
  Moreover, the operator can use his standard equipment and is not distracted by
  any artificial and uncomfortable device. Thus, augmented optics technology can
  be easily integrated into the usual surgical workflow. Kelly et al. were one of the
  first who proposed such a system and applied it in stereotactic brain surgery [18].
  The first augmented microscope was developed by Roberts et al. [25] in the mid
  eighties showing a segmented tumor slice of a computed tomography data set
  in a monocular operating microscope [32]. Later other groups presented further
  augmented optics systems that were applied to support neurosurgical interventions [13], ophthalmology [5], or maxillofacial surgery [7, 8].
- **See-through displays** A third option for in situ visualization is the use of see-
  through displays (Fig. 9.8), which are also called AR windows [32]. One of
  the first systems was developed in 1995 by Masutani et al., who used a semi-
  transparent mirror and placed it between the user and the object to be aug-

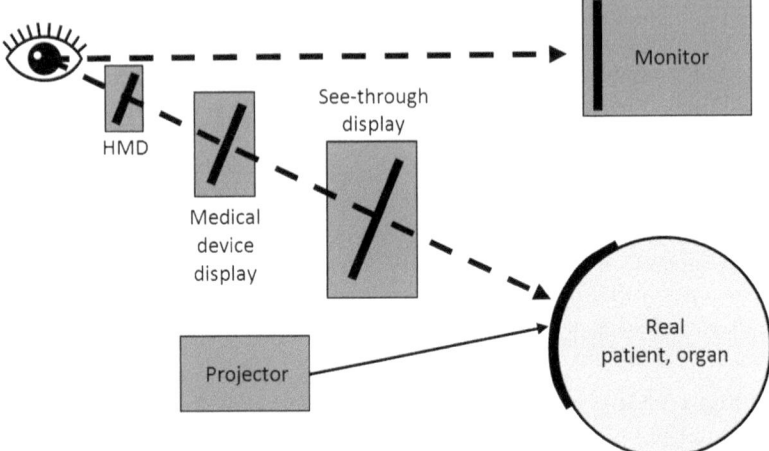

Fig. 9.7 Classes of different AR systems distinguished by the visual display technique and positioning. Visual information can be merged with real world via a head-mounted display, medical device display (e.g. microscope), see-through display, monitor, or projection onto the object (Figure adapted from [6] and [36])

mented [21]. The virtual images were created by an autostereoscopic monitor. The advantage of the autostereoscopic view is that no tracking system is required to maintain the registration after it has been established once. Disadvantages are the limited resolution and range of view. Other groups used stereo-projection systems based on ordinary monitors and semitransparent mirrors in combination with shutter glasses [9] (Fig. 9.9) or polarization glasses [16]. However, in comparison to the use of autostereoscopic monitors, they require to track the position of the user's eyes in addition to the position of the patient and the see-through display [32]. Wesarg et al., 2004, presented a see-through setup based on a monoscopic screen in combination with a transparent display [38]. The system is rather compact, since no mirror is used and no special glasses are required. However, it cannot display images in 3D quality and only one eye can see a correct image overlay [32]. Furthermore, the foci of the virtual and real image are at different distances, which makes the use of the system inconvenient and fatiguing for the eyes. A general disadvantage of all see-through displays is that distracting reflections from different light sources can occur. Furthermore, the display, which has to be placed between the patient and the user, may obstruct the surgeon's working area and view.

- **Augmented monitors** It is also possible to augment video images on ordinary monitors. The point of view is given by a tracked video camera. Lorensen et al., 1993 [20], and then Grimson et al., 1996 [17], used segmented MRI data in order to augment a live video of a surgical intervention. Sato et al., 1998 [28], published a live video augmentation of a breast cancer surgery using segmented 3D ultrasound images. The advantage of augmented monitors is that the users do not need to wear glasses or an HMD. However, the hand-eye coordination is not opti-

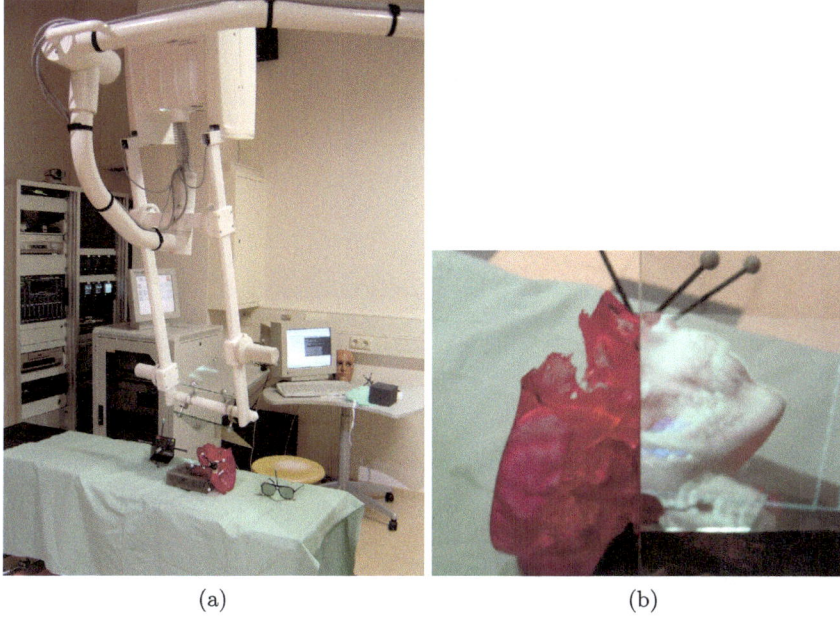

(a)   (b)

Fig. 9.8 ARSyS-Tricorder: augmented reality system for intraoperative navigation with transparent display; by courtesy of G. Goebbels

mal, as the virtual images are presented on a remote monitor and are not directly overlaid on the real objects. A special group of augmented monitors is formed by endoscopic applications, where the required camera is already part of the endoscopic system. Hence, the integration of AR technology does not necessarily introduce additional hardware into the workflow of the image-guided intervention. However, since the point of view is continuously changing, tracking of the camera (i.e. the endoscope) can be rather challenging. Endoscopic augmentation was applied to otolaryngology [15] and brain surgery [30, 31]. In these systems rigid endoscopes were tracked by infrared or magnetic tracking systems, respectively. In contrast, flexible (non-rigid) endoscopes are difficult to track. Optical tracking systems cannot be used as the inserted part of the endoscope is not visible to the tracking system and—due to the flexibility of the device—its shape is not known. A possible solution is the use of geometric knowledge and image processing [10, 23]. Other groups use magnetic tracking, which can cope with the visual obstruction of the endoscope's hidden end [19, 24]. There is a large number of different devices developed by research groups and distributed by companies that provide augmented monitor systems without life video presentation. These are so-called "image-guided" or "intra-operative navigation" systems, which do not record real images, but only track surgical instruments and the patient. They display the moving instrument positions into the static images of segmented CT, MRI or ultrasound data of the patient anatomy. More details about this group of augmented monitors is given in Sect. 9.4.

Fig. 9.9 Pelvic screw
fixation simulation using
shutter glasses (reprinted
from [9], Copyright 2000,
with permission from
Elsevier)

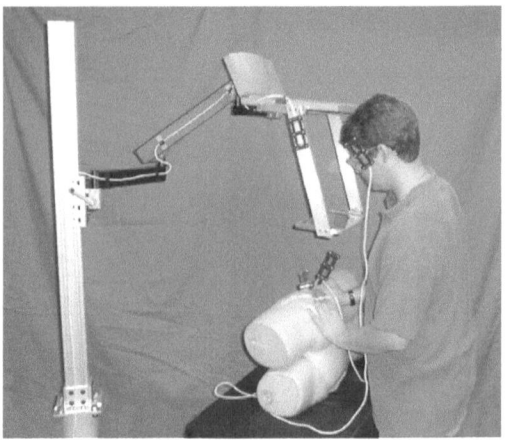

- **Projection on the patient** The last option is to augment image data directly onto the patient. The advantage is that the images are visible in situ without the need of any additional optical device such as glasses, HMD, microscope, etc. The user's head even does not need to be tracked if the displayed information is meant to be on the skin rather than beneath [32]. In such a case, the visualization can be used by multiple users. One of the first systems was introduced in 2002, by Sasama et al., [27]. They used two lasers, each of them creating a plane projected through a mirror system. The intersecting lines on the patient indicated a spot of interest, e.g. an incision point, where a trocar has to be inserted for the use of laparoscopic instruments.

9.4 Image Guided Surgery

The idea of intraoperative navigation is to assist surgeons during surgery with the presentation of image data of the human anatomy and the surgical instruments. Anatomical image data needs to be recorded by a CT or MR scanner, or any other 3D imaging device, prior to the intervention. The medical images are registered to a reference system in 3D space that can be transformed to the reference system of the surgical instruments. The instrument positions and orientations in space are recorded usually by an optical tracking system. The intraoperative navigation system then allows the surgeon to see the location of the animated surgical tool on the monitor with respect to the visually displayed anatomical images during the operation. Both tool and anatomy are displayed on a 2D or 3D screen. Passive markers have to be attached to the patient in order to allow posture determination and motion tracking of the respective body limbs.

Note that this technique cannot be used, if the human tissue deforms too much, as this can cause large deviations between the real anatomy and the virtual anatomy

Fig. 9.10 Examples of
intraoperative navigation
systems: (**a**) Frameless
Biopsy System; Brainlab AG,
brainlab.com;
(**b**) VarioGuide™, Brainlab
AG, brainlab.com

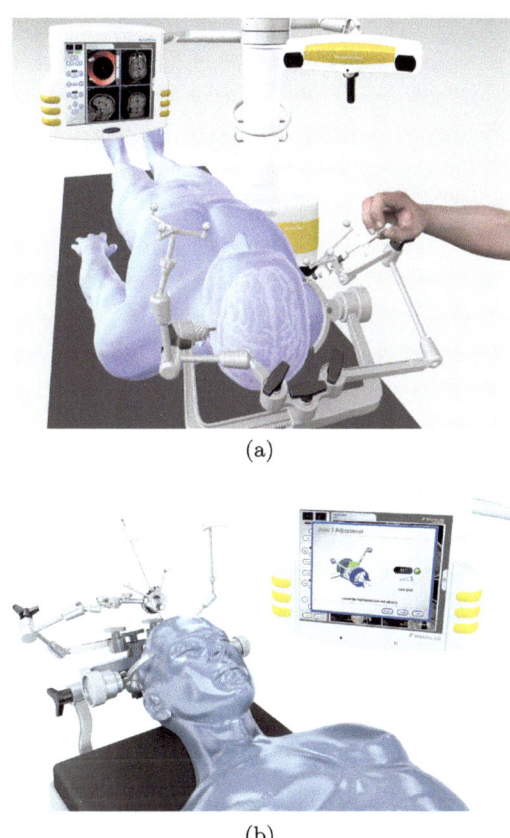

(a)

(b)

displayed on the screen. Intraoperative navigation systems are currently being applied mostly in the areas of neurosurgery, otolaryngology, and orthopedic surgery (Fig. 9.10).

According to the abovementioned definitions, image guided surgery (also called intraoperative navigation) systems can be considered as AR systems, more specifically as augmented monitors. These systems do neither require extra optical devices worn by the surgeon, nor a camera to film the patient and operation scenario. Due to their simplicity and compactness, image guided surgery systems are rather popular, with several commercial solutions available worldwide.

References

1. Azuma, R.T., et al.: A survey of augmented reality. Presence **6**(4), 355–385 (1997)
2. Azuma, R., Baillot, Y., Behringer, R., Feiner, S., Julier, S., MacIntyre, B.: Recent advances in augmented reality. IEEE Comput. Graph. Appl. **21**(6), 34–47 (2001)
3. Bajura, M., Neumann, U.: Dynamic registration correction in video-based augmented reality systems. IEEE Comput. Graph. Appl. **15**(5), 52–60 (1995). doi:10.1109/38.403828

4. Bajura, M., Fuchs, H., Ohbuchi, R.: Merging virtual objects with the real world: seeing ultra-sound imagery within the patient. In: Proceedings of the 19th Annual Conference on Computer Graphics and Interactive Techniques, vol. 26, pp. 203–210. ACM, New York (1992)

5. Berger, J.W., Shin, D.S.: Computer-vision-enabled augmented reality fundus biomicroscopy. Ophthalmology **106**(10), 1935–1941 (1999). doi:10.1016/S0161-6420(99)90404-9

6. Bimber, O., Raskar, R.: Modern approaches to augmented reality. In: Proceeding ACM SIG-GRAPH 2006 Courses. ACM, New York (2006)

7. Birkfellner, W., Huber, K., Watzinger, F., Figl, M., Wanschitz, F., Hanel, R., Rafolt, D., Ewers, R., Bergmann, H.: Development of the varioscope AR. A see-through HMD for computer-aided surgery. In: Augmented Reality, 2000 (ISAR 2000). Proceedings. IEEE and ACM International Symposium on, pp. 54–59 (2000). doi:10.1109/ISAR.2000.880923

8. Birkfellner, W., Figl, M., Huber, K., Watzinger, F., Wanschitz, F., Hummel, J., Hanel, R., Greimel, W., Homolka, P., Ewers, R., Bergmann, H.: A head-mounted operating binocular for augmented reality visualization in medicine—design and initial evaluation. IEEE Trans. Med. Imaging **21**(8), 991–997 (2002). doi:10.1109/TMI.2002.803099

9. Blackwell, M., Nikou, C., DiGioia, A.M., Kanade, T.: An image overlay system for medical data visualization. Med. Image Anal. **4**(1), 67–72 (2000)

10. Bricault, I., Ferretti, G., Cinquin, P.: Registration of real and ct-derived virtual bronchoscopic images to assist transbronchial biopsy. IEEE Trans. Med. Imaging **17**(5), 703–714 (1998). doi:10.1109/42.736022

11. Cakmakci, O., Rolland, J.: Head-worn displays: a review. J. Disp. Technol. **2**(3), 199–216 (2006). doi:10.1109/JDT.2006.879846

12. Caudell, T.P., Mizell, D.W.: Augmented reality: an application of heads-up display technology to manual manufacturing processes. In: System Sciences, 1992. Proceedings of the Twenty-Fifth Hawaii International Conference on, vol. II, pp. 659–669 (1992). doi:10.1109/HICSS.1992.183317

13. Edwards, P., Hill, D., Hawkes, D., Spink, R., Colchester, A., Strong, A., Gleeson, M.: Neurosurgical guidance using the stereo microscope. In: Computer Vision, Virtual Reality and Robotics in Medicine, pp. 555–564. Springer, Berlin (1995)

14. Feiner, S., Macintyre, B., Seligmann, D.: Knowledge-based augmented reality. Commun. ACM **36**(7), 53–62 (1993)

15. Freysinger, W., Gunkel, A.R., Thumfart, W.F.: Image-guided endoscopic ENT surgery. Eur. Arch. Oto-Rhino-Laryngol. **254**(7), 343–346 (1997)

16. Goebbels, G., Troche, K., Braun, M., Ivanovic, A., Grab, A., von Lübtow, K., Sader, R., Zeilhofer, H.F., Albrecht, K., Praxmarer, K.: Arsystricorder–development of an augmented reality system for intraoperative navigation in maxillofacial surgery. In: Proc. IEEE and ACM Int. Symp. on Mixed and Augmented Reality (ISMAR) (2003)

17. Grimson, W.E.L., Ettinger, G.J., White, S.J., Lozano-Perez, T. III, Wells, W.M., Kikinis, R.: An automatic registration method for frameless stereotaxy, image guided surgery, and enhanced reality visualization. IEEE Trans. Med. Imaging **15**(2), 129–140 (1996). doi:10.1109/42.491415

18. Kelly, P.J., Alker, G.J. Jr., Goerss, S.: Computer-assisted stereotactic microsurgery for the treatment of intracranial neoplasms. Neurosurgery **10**(3), 324 (1982)

19. Klein, T., Traub, J., Hautmann, H., Ahmadian, A., Navab, N.: Fiducial-free registration procedure for navigated bronchoscopy. In: Medical Image Computing and Computer-Assisted Intervention, pp. 475–482 (2007)

20. Lorensen, W., Cline, H., Nafis, C., Kikinis, R., Altobelli, D., Gleason, L.: Enhancing reality in the operating room. In: Visualization, 1993. Visualization '93, Proceedings. IEEE Conference on, pp. 410–415 (1993). doi:10.1109/VISUAL.1993.398902

21. Masutani, Y., Iwahara, M., Samuta, O., Nishi, Y., Suzuki, N., Suzuki, M., Dohi, T., Iseki, H., Takakura, K.: Development of integral photography-based enhanced reality visualization system for surgical support. In: Proceedings of ISCAS, vol. 95, pp. 16–17 (1995)

22. Milgram, P., Kishino, F.: A taxonomy of mixed reality visual displays. IEICE Trans. Inf. Syst. **77**(12), 1321–1329 (1994)

23. Mori, K., Deguchi, D., Hasegawa, J., Suenaga, Y., Toriwaki, J., Takabatake, H., Natori, H.: A method for tracking the camera motion of real endoscope by epipolar geometry analysis and virtual endoscopy system. In: Medical Image Computing and Computer-Assisted Intervention—MICCAI 2001, pp. 1–8. Springer, Berlin (2001)

24. Mori, K., Deguchi, D., Akiyama, K., Kitasaka, T., Maurer, C., Suenaga, Y., Takabatake, H., Mori, M., Natori, H.: Hybrid bronchoscope tracking using a magnetic tracking sensor and image registration. Med. Image Comput. Comput.-Assist. Interv. **3750**, 543–550 (2005)

25. Roberts, D.W., Strohbehn, J.W., Hatch, J.F., Murray, W., Kettenberger, H.: A frameless stereotaxic integration of computerized tomographic imaging and the operating microscope. J. Neurosurg. **65**(4), 545–549 (1986)

26. Rolland, J.P., Fuchs, H.: Optical versus video see-through head-mounted displays in medical visualization. Presence **9**(3), 287–309 (2000)

27. Sasama, T., Sugano, N., Sato, Y., Momoi, Y., Koyama, T., Nakajima, Y., Sakuma, I., Fujie, M., Yonenobu, K., Ochi, T., et al.: A novel laser guidance system for alignment of linear surgical tools: its principles and performance evaluation as a man–machine system. Med. Image Comput. Comput.-Assist. Interv. **2489**, 125–132 (2002)

28. Sato, Y., Nakamoto, M., Tamaki, Y., Sasama, T., Sakita, I., Nakajima, Y., Monden, M., Tamura, S.: Image guidance of breast cancer surgery using 3-d ultrasound images and augmented reality visualization. IEEE Trans. Med. Imaging **17**(5), 681–693 (1998). doi:10.1109/42.736019

29. Sauer, F., Wenzel, F., Vogt, S., Tao, Y., Genc, Y., Bani-Hashemi, A.: Augmented workspace: designing an AR testbed. In: Augmented Reality, 2000 Proceedings. IEEE and ACM International Symposium on, pp. 47–53 (2000). doi:10.1109/ISAR.2000.880922

30. Scholz, M., Konen, W., Tombrock, S., Fricke, B., Adams, L., Von Duering, M., Hentsch, A., Heuser, L., Harders, A.G.: Development of an endoscopic navigation system based on digital image processing. Comput. Aided Surg. **3**(3), 134–143 (1998)

31. Shahidi, R., Wang, B., Epitaux, M., Grzeszczuk, R., Adler, J.: Volumetric image guidance via a stereotactic endoscope. In: Medical Image Computing and Computer-Assisted Intervention, pp. 241–252 (1998)

32. Sielhorst, T., Feuerstein, M., Navab, N.: Advanced medical displays: a literature review of augmented reality. J. Disp. Technol. **4**(4), 451–467 (2008)

33. State, A., Livingston, M.A., Garrett, W.F., Hirota, G., Whitton, M.C., Pisano, E.D., Fuchs, H.: Technologies for augmented reality systems: realizing ultrasound-guided needle biopsies. In: Proceedings of the 23rd Annual Conference on Computer Graphics and Interactive Techniques, p. 439 (1996)

34. Steinhaus, H.: Sur la localisation au moyen des rayons x. C. R. Acad. Sci. **206**, 1473–1475 (1938)

35. Sutherland, I.E.: A head-mounted three dimensional display. In: Proceedings of the December 9–11, 1968, Fall Joint Computer Conference, Part I, AFIPS '68, pp. 757–764. ACM, New York (1968). doi:10.1145/1476589.1476686

36. van Krevelen, D.W.F., Poelman, R.: A survey of augmented reality technologies, applications and limitations. Int. J. Virtual Real. **9**(2), 1–20 (2010)

37. Wellner, P., Mackay, W., Gold, R.: Back to the real world. Commun. ACM **36**(7), 24–26 (1993)

38. Wesarg, S., Firle, E.A., Schwald, B., Seibert, H., Zogal, P., Roeddiger, S.: Accuracy of needle implantation in brachytherapy using a medical AR system—a phantom study. In: Proceedings of SPIE Medical Imaging. Citeseer, Princeton (2004)

Chapter 10
Medical Model Generation

10.1 Introduction

Model generation in VR-based applications is a necessary step in providing a simulated environment to the user. This process is in general a difficult task. The increase of computational power enabled the display of larger virtual environments, thus, reinforcing the need for improved methods for model acquisition, enhancement, optimization, and adaptation. The objects in a VR scene can usually be categorized into either man-made or natural entities. Two general strategies are followed to create these objects—artificial generation or real-world based acquisition. The former technique focuses on manual or semi-automatic design of virtual environments using computer-based modeling tools. In addition, some simple, exactly defined structures can be generated completely automatically following pre-defined procedural formalisms (see e.g. [60]). Until about a decade ago, synthetic model generation has been the preferred approach, however, recent years have witnessed a paradigm shift towards real-world based acquisition. This is mainly due to the slow, tedious, labor intensive, and costly processing of synthetic scenes. As an example, in [3] it has been reported that building a model of a house (partly at quarter-inch resolution) required three person-years of work (see Fig. 10.1). Similar times are also reported in the movie industry, where virtual scenes are generated for special effects, e.g. city models in the movie *Superman Returns* took 15 person-years to be completed. Therefore, real-world based model generation has received increasing attention recently. A typical technique in this class is the acquisition of real objects via sensors and their subsequent reconstruction (see e.g. [43, 99]). Also, obtaining volumetric representations of organs using medical imaging technology and the subsequent extraction of their surfaces based for instance on the *marching cubes* algorithm [56] falls into this category. Another possibility is the direct usage of CAD models of specific real-world counterparts. Since an increasing number of man-made entities undergo a computer-based design process, more and more highly detailed digital representations are becoming available. Finally, formal analysis of real shapes or processes in order to generate a compact mathematical description for model derivation also belongs into the second category. The resulting models

R. Riener, M. Harders, *Virtual Reality in Medicine*,
DOI 10.1007/978-1-4471-4011-5_10, © Springer-Verlag London 2012

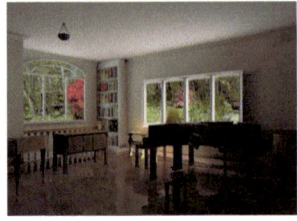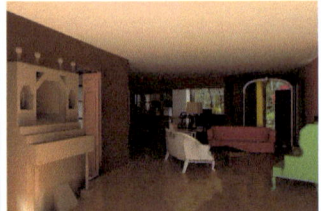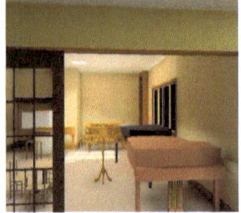

Fig. 10.1   Brooks' house model (courtesy of Frederick Brooks)

often need further processing. For instance, noise introduced during the acquisition process has to be removed, while object mesh properties are maintained, thus requiring enhanced smoothing techniques, like used in [96]. Moreover, mesh size is often quite large, making a polygon reduction step necessary. Again, during surface simplification, characteristic shape features have to be maintained (see e.g. [31]).

Several characteristics of a model generation process can play a role for deciding on an appropriate approach.

- **Modelling time** A model generation process can take from a few minutes up to several days. Often a direct trade-off between model accuracy and the modelling time is encountered. Depending on the application, a long process might not be acceptable. For instance, if a patient-specific planning of a surgical intervention should be performed, then a waiting time of several days or weeks before obtaining a model might not be appropriate.
- **Process complexity** The applied modelling technology might require specially trained personnel to be operated. This denotes the acquisition hardware as well as the processing software, e.g. sensing systems or mesh processing tools.
- **Process cost** Depending on the modelling time, the involved experts, and the applied software tools, the creation of a full 3D representation of a patient can result in considerable cost. This again is related to the application field as well as the required accuracy of the model.
- **Model quality** Different degrees of realism can be achieved in a modelling process. This is due to several factors, e.g. the quality of the data acquisition as well as any approximations made during mesh generation and simplification.
- **Model format** A final point to consider is the data format of the generated model. Depending on the application various representations can be used.

In the following, the focus will be on the steps required for building a medical model. Firstly, the input data have to be obtained based on medical imaging techniques. The latter are usually 3D cross-sectional datasets acquired via tomographic imaging. Thereafter, a segmentation is carried out to subdivide the data into meaningful entities (e.g. organs vs. background). This is necessary for any advanced data processing, visualization, or quantitative measurements. Based on the outcome of the segmentation, usually a further step is necessary: the conversion of the labeled volumes into polygon meshes. The latter then might need additional processing to reduce the number of polygons or to apply smoothing. The final step is the possible

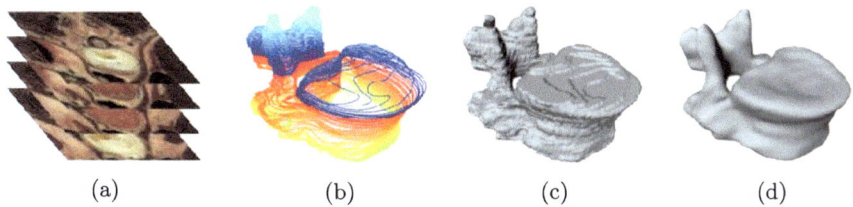

(a)   (b)   (c)   (d)

Fig. 10.2 Example process of building a medical model (from [41], courtesy of Johannes Hug).
(**a**) Initial medical input data; (**b**) Slice-based contour segmentation of anatomical structure;
(**c**) Surface reconstruction based on segmentation; (**d**) Mesh optimization via smoothing of artifacts

adaptation of the meshes for specific applications. For instance, for surgical simulation an artificial pathology might be placed into the model to create a training task
for a simulated intervention. The mentioned elements of the medical model generation will be discussed in more detail in the following. An overview of the involved
steps is shown in Fig. 10.2.

10.2 Medical Imaging

10.2.1 Overview

Medical imaging is concerned with obtaining non-invasively in-vivo information
of patient anatomy and physiology (see [5] for a broad introduction). The process
is in general based on some form of interaction of energy with matter, i.e. a patient's (or volunteer's) body. Concerning the latter process, different image formation paradigms can be identified. In *transmission*-based imaging, energy is passing
through a body; an example being X-ray imaging. In *emission*-based imaging, signals are detected from within the body; an example being positron emission tomography (PET), where radioactively marked molecules are traced. In a certain sense,
magnetic resonance imaging can also be considered in this category. Finally, in *reflection*-based techniques signals are reflected from matter; an example being ultrasound imaging. Further aspects can be considered concerning the imaging process,
such as scale (macroscopic, microscopic, molecular), dimension (from 1D length
measurements to 4D time series), image quality (signal-to-noise ratio, distortions),
or the imaging purpose (diagnostics, therapy, training, etc.). Other aspects are costs,
safety, maintenance, etc.

The focus in the following will be on imaging methods to generate anatomical
models. The first step in the geometry generation chain is the radiological acquisition of the in-vivo organ shape. Several medical imaging modalities are available
to obtain the necessary 3D anatomical data. The most suitable techniques for this
task are computed tomography (CT) and magnetic resonance imaging (MRI). 3D
ultrasound imaging (US) could also be an option, but the image quality is currently

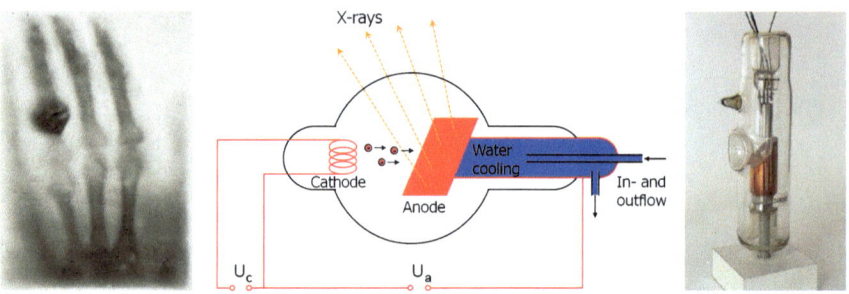

Fig. 10.3 X-ray imaging. First image taken by Roentgen of his wife's hand in 1895 (*left*). Old X-ray tube for generating X-rays (*right*) (courtesy of Udo Radtke)

still limited. In the following the different imaging techniques are explained in more detail (overviews of the methods are also provided in Tables 10.1, 10.2, 10.3).

10.2.2 X-Ray Imaging

X-rays were discovered in 1895 by Roentgen [82]. For this discovery he has been awarded the first Nobel prize in physics. Figure 10.3 shows the first image taken with this technique. X-rays are part of the electromagnetic spectrum. They have short wavelengths and are capable of penetrating matter. In order to produce X-rays for imaging, X-ray tubes are used (see Fig. 10.3). These are vacuum tubes in which electrons are emitted from a cathode filament towards an anode target. A high voltage of several keV is applied to accelerate the electrons. The latter are decelerated when hitting the anode, turning about 1% of the energy into X-ray photons, emitted perpendicular to the electron beam. This process is also known under the German term *Bremsstrahlung*.

There are some safety concerns associated with X-rays. High energy electromagnetic waves belong to the class of ionizing radiation. Photons can detach electrons from an atom, thus ionizing it. The created free radicals can result in unnatural chemical reactions inside cells. DNA chains could be damaged, which can lead to cell death or create mutated tumor cells. Since ionizing radiation is dangerous for human beings, doses and imaging times should be minimized to reduce X-ray exposure. Nevertheless, in cancer treatment very high doses of X-rays may be used to destroy pathological tissue [58] (see Sect. 9.2.1).

X-ray imaging is based on attenuation in tissue. The differences in attenuation due to varying density of body tissues (i.e. different absorption rates), are captured in a sensing system, e.g. a photographic plate. The captured intensity I_D can be expressed via the Beer-Lambert law as a line integral along the emitted ray from the source to the projection plane: $I_D(\tilde{x}, \tilde{y}) = I_O \varepsilon^{-\int \mu(x,y,z)dl}$, where I_O is the source intensity and μ the spatial attenuation coefficient of a body element. After the X-rays passed the body, they hit the detection medium, where "shadows" result at

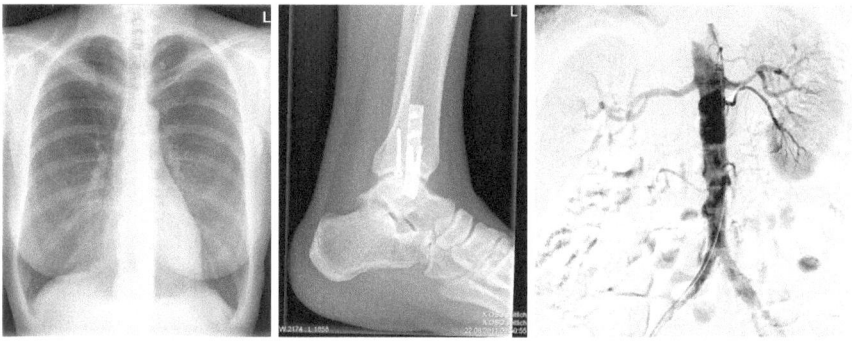

Fig. 10.4 Medical images based on X-ray imaging (courtesy of University Hospital Zurich)

Table 10.1 Overview of X-ray imaging

Discovered	1895 (Roentgen, Nobel prize 1905)
Principle	Attenuation of X-rays in tissue
Form of radiation	Electromagnetic radiation (photons)
Energy/wavelength	0.1–100 keV / 10–0.01 nm
Resolution	Very high (sub-mm, gray-levels)
Application	Mammography, lung, dentistry, gastrointestinal, orthopedics, cardiovascular
Problems	Ionizing radiation, superposition, little soft tissue contrast, not optimal for 3D

places where radiation has been attenuated. Most of the X-rays are absorbed by the Calcium of the bones, therefore the latter appear white on a photographic plate. Fat and other soft tissues absorb less X-rays, thus appearing gray. Air absorbs them the least, so lungs appear dark on X-ray film.

Different procedures can be used to examine hollow structures, such as the lungs, blood vessels, or the intestines. In these cases, contrast agents are inserted into the body, to make the organs more visible in X-ray acquisition. Figure 10.4 shows samples of typical medical imaging studies using X-rays. Unfortunately, due to the superposition effect and the 2D nature of the approach, X-ray imaging is not well suited for generating 3D models.

10.2.3 Computed Tomography

The underlying theoretical principle of this X-ray based imaging technique is the reconstruction of an object from its projections. Godfrey Hounsfield constructed the first clinically usable computed tomography (CT) scanner [38] with which he presented in 1972 cross-sectional images of the human brain. Figure 10.5 depicts

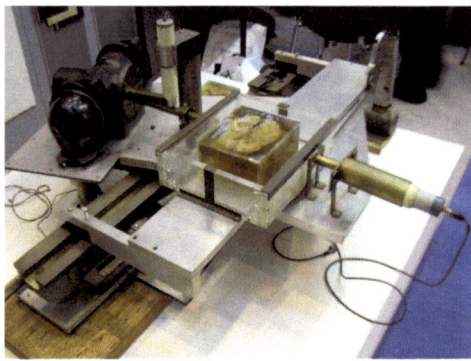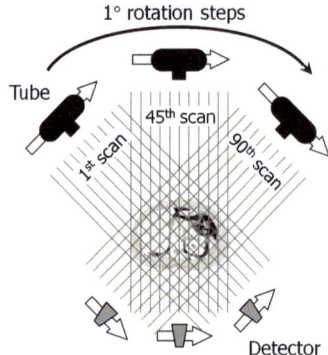

Fig. 10.5 Hounsfield laboratory prototype (picture taken at UKRC 2005 exhibition in Manchester G-MEX centre) and acquisition process in computed tomography

an early laboratory prototype and the underlying acquisition principle. A source-detector assembly is used to send parallel X-rays through a body. This is done from different positions at different rotations around the scanned object. The projections of the radiodensities in the body are acquired via the detector. Thus, one orientation gives a 1D profile of signal strengths describing the radiodensities. Several of these profiles are obtained for the different rotations around the body. The key step is then the reconstruction of the spatial radiodensities based on these profiles. Different reconstruction algorithms can be followed for this purpose.

Similar to work of Johann Radon in 1917 [79], a tomographic reconstruction algorithm has been proposed in the 1960s by Allan Cormack [13, 14]. His findings provided a solution to the problem of superposition in conventional X-ray imaging. Godfrey Hounsfield developed at the end of the 1960s an approach using the so-called inverse Radon-transformation. A simple, but effective reconstruction can be achieved by filtered back-projection. The key idea is to "smear" back the acquired projections into the image matrix. These backprojections are added up for all acquired rotations. In a final step, a high-pass filter kernel is applied to reduce blurring. The reconstruction quality can be improved by increasing the spatial resolution per scan, as well as increasing the number of obtained projections from different rotations.

The introduced principles and technologies have been continuously improved over several generations of scanners. Multi-detector-row tomographs available today are capable of acquiring isotropic imaging data during a single breath-hold in a few seconds, thus even allowing time-series of beating hearts. The number of slices is dependent on the type of study, e.g. a thorax scan might contain 500–2000 slices. Figure 10.6 shows a typical scanner used in the clinical environment (opened to show the source-detector setup). A full turn of the acquisition ring generates one slice. During the rotation the patient is moved through the scanner on a table, thus allowing to obtain several cross-sectional images. Putting together a number of such consecutive slices generates volume datasets, which allow the reconstruction of organs in 3D. The acquired image grey value data are usually expressed in

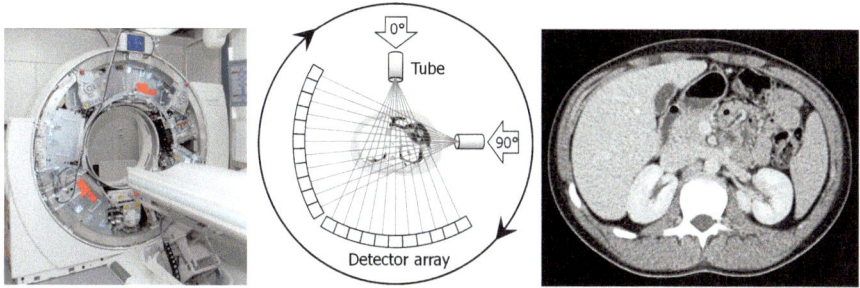

Fig. 10.6 CT imaging. Opened clinical CT scanner (*left*) (courtesy of University Hospital Zurich). Imaging principle with rotating source-detector assembly (*middle*). Horizontal abdominal CT slice (*right*) (courtesy of University Hospital Zurich)

Table 10.2 Overview of computed tomography

Discovered	1972 (Hounsfield, Nobel prize 1979)
Principle	Multiple X-ray axial slice projections & reconstruction
Form of radiation	Electromagnetic radiation
Energy/wavelength	10–100 keV / 0.1–0.01 nm
Resolution	High (mm), sub-mm slice distance
Application	Soft tissue & bone imaging (gastrointestinal, thorax, cardiovascular, joints)
Problems	Ionizing radiation, data size

the 12-bit Hounsfield scale, which typically ranges from -1024 to 3071 Hounsfield units (HU). On this scale air has a value of -1000 HU, water 0 HU, and bone >400 HU. The quality of CT scanners is continuously improving. In current systems the source-detector assembly revolves at 3 rotations per second. Newer models acquire 3×16 images per second with an in-slice resolution of 1024×1024 pixels. Slice thickness can be below 1 mm. This creates the problem of interpreting such large amounts of data. Nevertheless, in current medical practice, CT has become an indispensable imaging tool and is considered as a gold standard in the diagnosis of several pathologies.

Although high quality images can be generated with computed tomography, still a number of image artifacts can be encountered. Noise due to motion during acquisition or due to presence of metal is a typical example. Also the partial volume effect has to be taken into consideration. The latter describes the mixing of tissues in one voxel (i.e. different attenuation values) due to insufficient in-slice resolution. This leads to blurring of edges, which can cause difficulties in locating boundaries in a subsequent segmentation step. Finally, it again has to be considered that ionizing radiation is used, which poses health concerns. The exposure during a CT scan is in general higher than during X-ray imaging. Further information on computed tomography can, for instance, be found in [39].

10.2.4 *Magnetic Resonance Imaging*

Magnetic resonance imaging (MRI) is a tomographic technique that reconstructs images based on the magnetic resonance of atomic nuclei. Already in 1945 Felix Bloch [1] and Edward Purcell [77] discovered the principle of nuclear magnetic resonance (NMR). Raymond Damadian recognized the potential of NMR and suggested in 1971 its use for cancer detection [15]. In 1973 Paul Lauterbur proposed the addition of a gradient field to enable the spatial location of signals [53]. Moreover, he applied back-projection methods to create the first MRI images. Peter Mansfield provided the mathematical analysis of the gradient fields [57].

Magnetic resonance imaging is based on the magnetic properties of nuclei and their reaction to radio frequency excitation. Atomic particles exhibit a quantum property called spin. Particles with an uneven number of protons or neutrons have a non-zero spin, and thus a non-zero magnetic moment. In a simplified sense they can be considered as tiny magnets. For imaging in humans, the main target is hydrogen. Application of a strong uniform external magnetic field causes the magnetic moment vectors to align with the field. This creates a net magnetization in longitudinal direction.

The magnetic moment vectors precess around the field lines at a certain frequency. The latter is given according to the Larmor equation: $\omega_0 = \gamma B_0$, where B_0 is the magnetic field strength and γ the gyromagnetic ratio. Applying radio frequency (RF) electromagnetic pulses at this frequency in a plane orthogonal to the magnetic field causes the nuclei to temporarily assume a non-aligned high-energy state. The moment vectors are flipped into the transversal plane and rotate in phase. This creates a measurable oscillating magnetization signal in the transversal direction. When the RF excitation is removed, the nuclei start to dephase and re-align with the external field until equilibrium is again reached. Measurements can be made during this process to create the MRI images.

Several properties can be used to generate images, including proton density, spin-grid relaxation (T1), spin-spin relaxation (T2), and spin-echo techniques without refocusing (T2*). T1-weighted images are based on the time it takes until 63% of the initial longitudinal magnetization has been recovered. T2-weighted images are formed based on the decay of the transversal magnetization due to dephasing. They encode the time until 37% of the magnetization has decayed. The duration of these effects depends on the tissue properties, thus different types of tissues can be visualized in the T1- and T2-weighted images. A further point to consider is the spatial encoding of the signals. An additional gradient magnetic field can be applied to only select a desired slice through a body. In-slice encoding is finally achieved by using frequency and phase.

The most costly part of an MRI scanner is the strong magnet since it should produce a stable and homogeneous field of high Tesla. Normal field strengths are about 1–3 T, while scanners up to 9 T are used in research. Note that the Earth's magnetic field is about 50 µT, thus 1 T is 20,000 times stronger. Typically superconducting magnets are used as external magnets. It has to be considered that the main magnet is always turned on, wherefore magnetic material cannot be taken to the scanner.

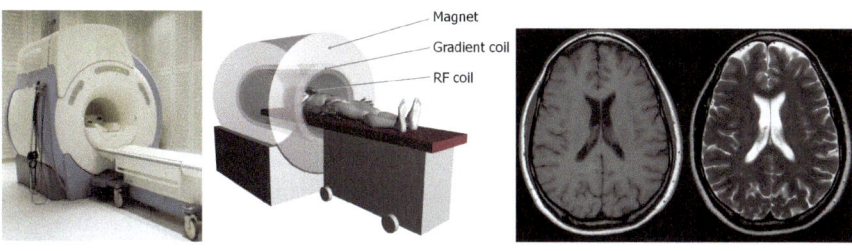

Fig. 10.7 MRI imaging. Clinical canning system (*left*) (courtesy of University Hospital Zurich). Key system components (*middle*). T1- and T2-weighted horizontal slices of human brain (*right*) (courtesy of University Hospital Zurich)

Table 10.3 Overview of magnetic resonance imaging

Discovered	1945 (Bloch, Purcell [NMR], Nobel prize 1952)/1973 (Mansfield, Lauterbur, Nobel prize 2003)
Principle	Magnetic properties of nuclei, RF excitation and relaxation
Form of "radiation"	Radio frequency (RF) pulse
Frequency/wavelength	10–100 MHz / 30–3 m
Resolution	High (mm), less than CT
Application	Anatomical and functional imaging
Problems	High magnetic field, image artifacts, acquisition time, slice thickness

A further concern is the acoustic noise during scanning due to fast changing gradient fields, which can go up to 120 dB. Also, MRI scanning takes considerable time, depending on the study 10–30 mins. Finally, MRI scanning systems have a considerably cost, with high monthly maintenance fees. Nevertheless, MRI provides excellent soft tissue resolution, with no known health risks. Using MRI, images of soft tissues as well as physiological processes can be obtained. Figure 10.7 illustrates components of MRI scanning. Complete coverage of this imaging modality is beyond the scope of this work; the reader is referred to the related literature, e.g. [2, 105].

10.2.5 Ultrasound

The physical principles of ultrasound imaging, such as the piezo-electric effect or sound propagation in materials have been discovered already in the 19th century. The first usage of ultrasound in medicine focused on therapeutic applications of high intensity pulses, for instance in neuro-surgery as an attempt to treat Parkinson's disease. In the early 1940s Karl Theo Dussik was one of the first to create ultrasound images. Since then medical sonography has evolved into the second most utilized medical imaging modality in diagnostics. Although the technique is relatively safe and inexpensive, the imaging quality is rather low due to noise and interference effects. An overview of the historical development of the technique and technical details can be found for instance in [21].

The detection of ultrasound waves reflected at borders of changing acoustic density is the key component of sonography. Sound pulses (usually 1–3 MHz) can be created by a phased array of piezoelectric transducers. The waves travel through the body, and are partially reflected at boundaries of differing acoustic impedance. Reflected waves are detected using the same piezoelectric setup. The distance from the probe to the structure is determined from the echo time assuming a constant speed of sound in tissue of about 1,540 m/s. The distances and intensities can be displayed on the screen as a two-dimensional image. An advantage of the technique is the user-controlled generation of images in real-time. Problems are encountered due to the presence of air or bones. The acoustic impedance of the former is low, thus causing mostly reflections of the signal. Therefore, air blocks the view into deeper layers. The latter has a high acoustic impedance, thus absorbing sound waves. Acquiring several two-dimensional images, by moving probes across the body surface or rotating probes, allows to combine 2D scans into 3D datasets. However, the quality of these is still limited and not sufficient for generation of high-quality medical models. Noise is mainly due to reverberation and scattering effects.

10.2.6 Visible Human Project

Apart from the standard medical imaging modalities, the acquisition of anatomical cross-sections from cadavers should also be scrutinized. While such a data source is not appropriate for acquiring several instances of anatomy, it nevertheless has been used to obtain organ models in a number of surgical simulation endeavors (see e.g. [95]). The Visible Human dataset has been created in a project by the US National Library of Medicine in 1991. In order to obtain the Visible Human data, the self-donated bodies of a 39-year old male and a 59-year old female were first imaged using CT and MRI in the unfrozen state. Thereafter, the bodies were fixated using a foaming agent as well as gelatin, and then frozen. The cryomacrotomy was performed with a specialized milling device, shaving off individual slices of the cadaver block at 1 mm or 0.33 mm intervals for male and female specimen, respectively. After each cut, color photographs of the top of the blocks were taken. This approach resulted in 1,871 (male) and 5,189 (female) axial high resolution (i.e. $0.33 \text{ mm}^2 \times 1$ mm for the male and 0.33 mm^3 for the female dataset, respectively) color images with 24 bits of color information. Further details of the acquisition process concerning the Visible Human male data are described in [91] (an overview is also provided in Table 10.4). The data are publically available and can be downloaded online from the National Library of Medicine. Research groups have used the data to create 3D models of organs. By now, the whole datasets have been completely segmented. An advantage of the cryosections is the included color information. Figure 10.8 illustrates the Visible Human datasets.

Fig. 10.8 Cryosections of the Visible Human male and female dataset (courtesy of the Visible Human Project, US National Library of Medicine)

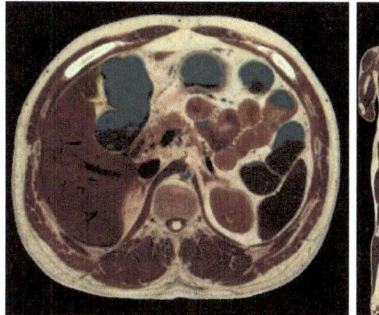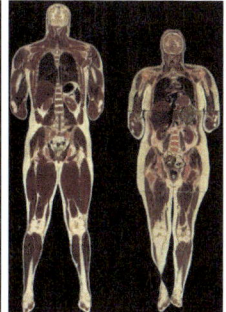

Table 10.4 Overview of visible human datasets

	Male	Female
Cryo-sections,	$0.33\ \text{mm}^2 \times 1.0\ \text{mm}$	$0.33\ \text{mm}^3$
color axial images	$1760 \times 1216 \times 1871$	$1662 \times 928 \times 5189$
Size	9.5 GB	22.4 GB
CT	512×512 axial slices	
MRI	256×256 slices in 3 modes	

10.3 Segmentation

10.3.1 Overview

Segmentation is the process of partitioning a digital image into individual components. This is typically done by assigning labels, specific to anatomical structures
or background, to all image pixels. The main target is to locate and extract objects
and/or edges, thus allowing further interpretation and analysis of the data. Current
medical tomographic imaging units provide huge amounts of high resolution three-
dimensional spatial (and in many cases also temporal) data, which require further
processing. Segmentation is in many cases the bottleneck when trying to use radiological image data in clinically important applications, such as radiological diagnosis, monitoring, radiotherapy, or surgical planning. Before any high-level reasoning
can be applied, the data have to be segmented into their major structural components. Several surveys of methods used in general or medical image analysis are
available, for instance [19, 71, 74]. The methods used in medical image segmentation can be classified with regard to their degree of automation.

- **Manual segmentation** This segmentation paradigm is based on manual identification of the object of interest on each slice by a medical expert. Typically, this is
  done by outlining the object contour. The approach is highly insensitive to noise,
  tolerant of incomplete information, and in many cases sufficiently precise. Therefore, it is often regarded as a gold standard for image segmentation. However,
  it is very time consuming, has to be done in a tedious pixel-by-pixel manner,

and lacks reproducibility. Poor reproducibility of the results also makes manual segmentation questionable for statistical studies where the correlation between morphological changes and therapeutical actions, or clinical diagnoses have to be analyzed. Moreover, it is prone to inconsistency between operators, who might have different biases. Also, the settings of the screen (e.g. contrast) used for displaying the image data can have an effect on the segmentation results.

• **Automatic segmentation** In contrast to the former, automatic segmentation refrains from using direct user interaction. It is regarded as the holy grail of medical image segmentation. Unfortunately, up to now no robust general-purpose algorithm has been found, that can segment any arbitrary dataset. A problem that was recognized in early approaches is the assumption that radiological images contain most of the information which is necessary for the identification of anatomical objects. However, a radiologist uses a broad range of related knowledge of the field of anatomy, pathology, physiology, and radiology in order to arrive at a reasonable image interpretation. Due to the difficulty of formalizing this necessary a-priori knowledge about the examined anatomical structures, automatic approaches could so far only be applied successfully within exactly defined bounds.

• **Interactive segmentation** In between the two extremes lie semi-automated or interactive algorithms, respectively, which try to merge the advantages of both worlds. Rather than attempting to duplicate the complex and not fully understood human capability to recognize objects, they provide an interactive environment in which users control the segmentation process and exploit their expert knowledge. The subtle distinction between semi-automatic and interactive segmentation approaches can be made relating to the amount of user interactivity during the segmentation. In semi-automatic methods a user might be limited to initializing or evaluating the results (possibly including manual adjustments or corrections), while interactive segmentation allows the direct intervention during the complete run-time of the algorithm.

Over the last decades, a great number of approaches were proposed for the segmentation of anatomy in 3D medical images. These methods vary widely dependent on the application and the underlying image modality. In the following section, a brief overview of the most important techniques will be given.

Present algorithms for segmentation can be coarsely divided into low-level and high-level methods. Low-level algorithms directly operate on the voxels of the given intensity images. Such algorithms are usually not sufficiently flexible to solve all problems encountered during segmentation. High-level methods include additional knowledge such as shape or appearance in a mathematical model to determine the segmentation. Frequently, low-level techniques are applied as a preprocessing step.

10.3.2 Low-Level Methods

• **Thresholding** This is one of the simplest and widely used segmentation technique, especially for extracting bones (see for instance [83] for a general

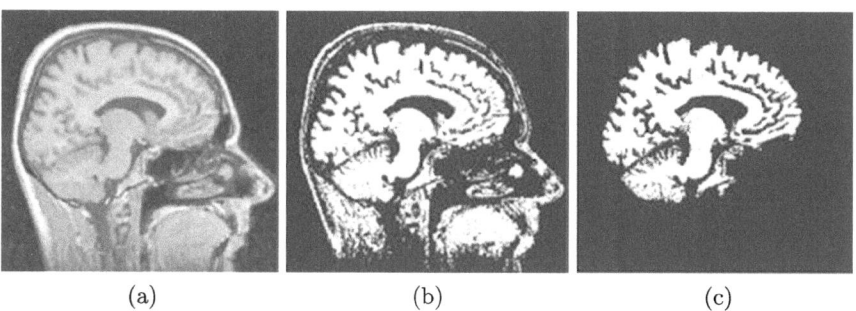

(a) (b) (c)

Fig. 10.9 Low-level segmentation methods. (**a**) Input data slice; (**b**) Thresholding of input data; (**c**) Region growing result

overview). In global thresholding, all voxels with a value below/above a globally defined threshold or within a specific interval are regarded as part of the object, whereas all other voxels are interpreted as background. Global thresholding performs poorly if the object and background intensities vary significantly throughout the image. Therefore, thresholding mostly fails in segmenting soft tissue structures. A better approach is to calculate a local threshold for each voxel based on the intensity distribution in a certain neighborhood. The appropriate threshold can be determined by statistical methods, often also incorporating prior knowledge. Nevertheless, local thresholding has the tendency to merge structures in case of weak boundaries. Figure 10.9 shows an example of thresholding on a slice image.

- **Region growing** The most common region-based segmentation algorithm is seeded region growing (see e.g. [26]). Starting from an initially defined seed, neighboring voxels are incrementally added to the region based on a user-defined similarity measure, e.g. intensity differences between neighboring voxels. The region grows until the similarity criterion is no more satisfied. Adaptive similarity measures were introduced to improve robustness in case of varying intensities or in the presence of noise. The main drawback of region-based algorithms for segmentation is their tendency to leak into neighboring tissue due to weak boundaries. Region-growing also has a bias towards merging objects which are close together. Figure 10.9 illustrates the better performance of region growing on the example data.

- **Edge-detection methods** Edges define the boundaries between homogeneous image regions. Therefore, an accurate detection of the edges of an object results in an outline of the object shape. Edge detection methods (see e.g. [62, 107] for a survery) are usually based on first- or second-order derivatives of the image intensity function. Image smoothing is often performed as a pre-processing step due to the high noise sensitivity of the discrete image derivatives. While perfect edges can be obtained on datasets with good contrast, e.g. between bones and soft tissue, the performance is poor at similar contrasts, resulting in discontinuities.

- **Watershed algorithm** The basic idea of the watershed transform (see [81] for an overview) is to interpret the image values as a height-map. The height-map is "flooded with water" from different sources, which can be local minima in the image or user-defined markers. For each source a catchment basin (i.e. labeled region) is constructed which grows during successive flooding. Watersheds, representing the segmented region boundaries, are built for adjacent basins to avoid merging. While the watershed transform is effective in separating regions, a combination with a different method such as thresholding is required to achieve a segmentation. Therefore, the watershed transform shares the problems of the applied additional segmentation method.

10.3.3 High-Level Methods

- **Deformable models** These approaches use energy minimization strategies for the segmentation. A survey is available in [59]. A 3D parametric deformable model is represented by a parameterized surface of the object being segmented. The model is deformed according to external image forces and internal forces, resulting in corresponding terms in the overall energy function. Internal energy enforces the smoothness of the surface while the surface is pulled towards the segmentation target by image forces. A deformable approach is robust against boundary discontinuities. However, in basic implementations the topology of the model cannot change.
- **Statistical models** These models are widely used for the segmentation of anatomy. A recent review can be found in [36]. In statistical approaches, prior knowledge about the shape and/or appearance of the anatomy of interest is integrated into a statistical model. In order to capture anatomical variations in shape, such a model is trained from a set of example shapes based on segmented image data. The model is set up by computing the mean shape over the training data. Additionally, observed variations are encoded in the model as a number of modes describing the most characteristic variations. In Sect. 10.7 the application of this technique to describe organ variability is outlined in more detail.

10.4 Model Conversion

10.4.1 Outline

Depending on the segmentation strategy, different representations of objects are obtained after this step. The outcome of a segmentation can be a labeled volume (in background and object voxels), 2D object contours on data slices, or even surface meshes. Typically, a further processing step is required to turn the segmentation outcome into the right format for the actual application. For surgical simulation, often labeled volume datasets have to be converted to triangular surface meshes. This is

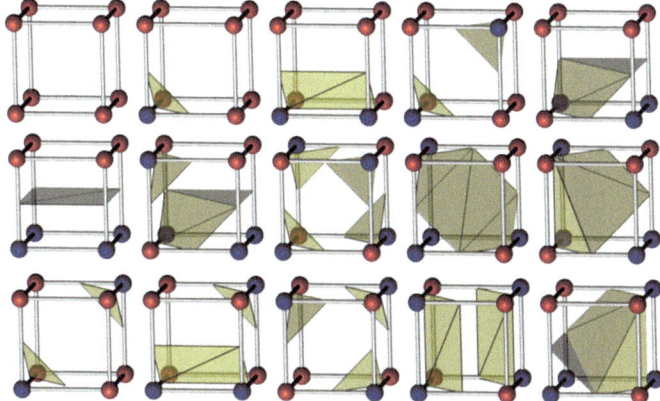

Fig. 10.10 Marching cubes lookup table with triangles for 15 unique cases of configurations of 8 voxels (*blue = inside, red = outside*)

usually done via the marching cubes algorithm (see [64] for an overview). Nevertheless, it sometimes might also be required to turn polygon meshes into voxel representations. This can be done with a voxelization algorithm (see e.g. [22, 45]). In the following the former algorithm will be introduced in more detail.

10.4.2 Marching Cubes

The marching cubes algorithm was developed by Lorensen and Cline in 1987 [56]. It is applied for creating a polygonal surface representation from volumetric (i.e. voxel) data. More specifically, it approximates an isosurface of a dataset with a polygonal mesh. To this end, each voxel in the 3D grid needs to be labeled as belonging to the object of interest or to the background. This information is usually available from the previous segmentation step. Otherwise, it is possible to carry out the labeling via an (isosurface) threshold. Any voxel with a value higher than the threshold is considered as part of the object of interest and vice versa.

In the next step, eight labeled, adjacent voxels (in a cube-shaped configuration) are processed at a time. The labeling of the voxels as *inside* or *outside* allows to determine where the isosurface should pass through within the imaginary cube. By using a lookup table, appropriate triangles and normals for the various label configurations can be retrieved. Due to rotational and reflective invariance, there are only 15 unique cases in the $2^8 = 256$ possible configurations (see Fig. 10.10).

Each case contains 0 to 4 triangles. The vertices of the triangles are all located on "edges" between voxels. In addition, the triangle normals are also given. By connecting all triangles for all consecutive groups of eight voxels, a triangulated isosurface mesh is formed. In order to further improve the mesh approximation, the positions of the vertices on the "edges" between the voxels are usually linearly

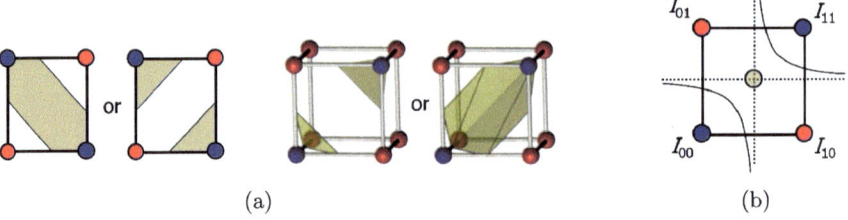

(a)   (b)

Fig. 10.11 Solving unclear connections between labeled voxels. (**a**) 2D and 3D example of ambiguity; (**b**) Solving ambiguity with asymptotic decider

interpolated taking the data values of the voxels and the isosurface threshold into account.

It has to be noted that ambiguities in the algorithm exist, in which the placement of triangles between voxels is not clear. Figure 10.11(a) depicts 2D and 3D examples of such cases. For instance, in the 2D example it can be seen that if opposite corners are labeled as belonging to the object, these could either be connected by a thin structure or be separated by a gap.

One possibility to solve this ambiguity is based on so-called asymptotic deciders [65]. This process will be outlined in detail for the 2D case. The approach is using the bilinear interpolation function of the four corner values:

$$\mathbf{I}(s, t) = (1 - s, s) \begin{bmatrix} I_{00} & I_{01} \\ I_{10} & I_{11} \end{bmatrix} \begin{pmatrix} 1 - t \\ t \end{pmatrix}. \tag{10.1}$$

The values of s and t for which the interpolation evaluates to a specific constant value α define a curve $\mathcal{C}$:

$$\mathcal{C} = \big\{(s, t)|\mathbf{I}(s, t) = \alpha\big\}. \tag{10.2}$$

The curve $\mathcal{C}$ is a rectangular hyperbola. The parameter α is given by the isosurface value of the marching cubes reconstruction. The asymptotes of the hyperbola intersect at a location $(\tilde{s}, \tilde{t})$, as shown in Fig. 10.11(b). By comparing $\mathbf{I}(\tilde{s}, \tilde{t})$ to α, a decision can be made whether a connection between the corners exists or not. If the interpolation at the intersection is larger than the isosurface value, then the corners should be connected.

Finally, it is interesting to note that the marching cubes algorithm has been patented in 1985. Therefore, it was not possible to use the approach without paying royalties. As an alternative, similar algorithms—e.g. *marching tetrahedra* (see for instance [9, 97])—have been proposed. The mentioned patent finally expired in 2005 and the technique can now be freely applied again.

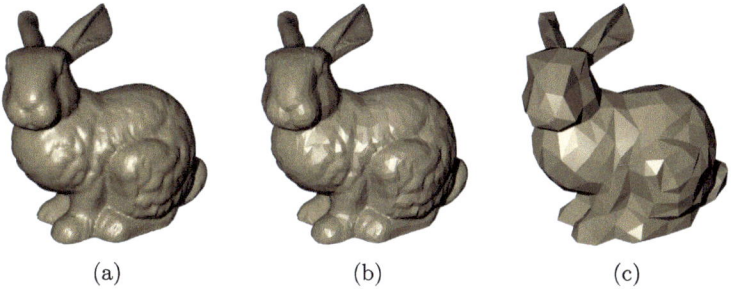

Fig. 10.12 Reduction of the polygon mesh of the Stanford bunny (courtesy of Stanford Computer Graphics Laboratory). (**a**) 69666 polygons; (**b**) 6966 polygons; (**c**) 696 polygons

10.5 Mesh Reduction and Smoothing

10.5.1 Outline

The next step in the model generation pipeline focuses on post-processing. A central target is the further optimization of triangle meshes. Different tasks have to be carried out in this context. One key element is the reduction of the model size. Meshes created with the marching cubes algorithm usually contain a large number of elements. For real-time interactive simulations this high number of triangles needs to be reduced. A further target in this context is the elimination of any redundant geometry. Polygon reduction techniques can also be used to create geometry representations at different levels of details (LOD). It is a typical technique in computer graphics to only render models with high detail when they are close, while distant objects are shown at reduced fidelity (see e.g. [11, 20]). It should be kept in mind that any mesh processing should still maintain the perceptual features of the represented object [80]. Figure 10.12 illustrates the outcomes of a reduction process. Another mesh optimization step is the smoothing of the surface. In medical model building, typical artifacts appearing during segmentation, e.g. staircase artifacts in slice-based techniques, need to be corrected. In the following, polygon reduction and mesh smoothing will be examined in more detail.

10.5.2 Polygon Reduction

Different methods exist to reduce the number of polygons in a mesh (see e.g. [10] for a survery). A simple technique is the clustering of proximate vertices. To this end, space is partitioned into a regular grid and all vertices in a cell are merged into an average vertex. Unfortunately, this method can introduce several artifacts. It can change mesh topology and violate manifold properties, as can already be seen in a simple 2D example in Fig. 10.13(a). An alternative strategy is to remove individual vertices from a mesh. Different metrics can be used to decide about vertex removal.

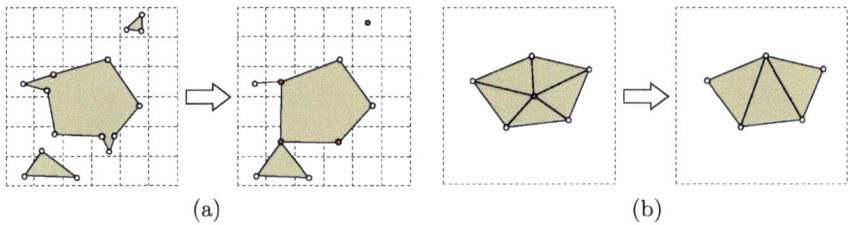

Fig. 10.13 Simple strategies for polygon reduction. (**a**) Clustering of vertices in 2D within cells in space partitioning; (**b**) Vertex/triangle removal and filling of hole with new triangles

One possibility is to examine the distance of a vertex to a plane fitted through all neighboring vertices [85]. If this distance is below a predefined threshold, then the local region is assumed to be flat. Thus, the vertex and all adjacent triangles can be removed, and the created hole be filled with new triangles, as shown in Fig. 10.13(b). Another strategy of polygon reduction is the collapse of edges (e.g. in [37, 55]). In this approach, two vertices are contracted into a new one, thus removing two triangles. Again, the decision whether to contract or not is done according to a metric. An example of this technique is the quadric-based surface simplification by Heckbert and Garland [31]. This algorithm will exemplarily be explained in more detail.

A key element of the quadric-based approach is finding vertices with minimal offset to a set of planes $\mathcal{P}$ by minimizing squared distances (i.e. errors):

$$\epsilon(\mathbf{v}) = \sum_{\mathbf{p} \in \mathcal{P}} (\mathbf{p}^T \mathbf{v})^2, \tag{10.3}$$

where vector $\mathbf{p} = (a\ b\ c\ d)^T$ with $a^2 + b^2 + c^2 = 1$ defines a plane via equation $ax + by + cz + d = 0$; and $\mathbf{v} = (x\ y\ z\ 1)^T$ is a vertex in homogeneous coordinates. The set of planes $\mathcal{P}$ associated with a vertex is given by its adjacent triangles.

The algorithm goes through all pairs of vertices connected by edges. For two considered vertices, $\mathbf{v}_1$ and $\mathbf{v}_2$, the respective two sets of planes are temporarily combined. Then a new vertex $\mathbf{v}'$ is found, which minimizes the error metric to this new set of planes and the determined minimal error is temporarily stored. Repeating this process for all possible pairs gives further minimal distances. The vertex pair ij that yields the smallest error is then finally collapsed. The vertices $\mathbf{v}_i$ and $\mathbf{v}_j$ are removed and replaced by the new vertex $\mathbf{v}'_{ij}$. The combined set of planes is assigned to the newly created node: $\mathcal{P}(\mathbf{v}'_{ij}) = \mathcal{P}(\mathbf{v}_i) \cup \mathcal{P}(\mathbf{v}_j)$. For clarification, Fig. 10.14 shows an example of this process in 2D. Note that in this case a vertex is associated with a set of lines instead of planes. Moreover, in this example only one pair is tested and then collapsed. By repeating the overall process, a mesh can be decimated further while keeping the differences to the original object small. This process is the underlying key concept of the simplification algorithm. However, a further extension has to be made.

A difficulty in the presented technique is the handling of the sets of planes. These can grow considerably, which is not optimal for the distance minimization step. The

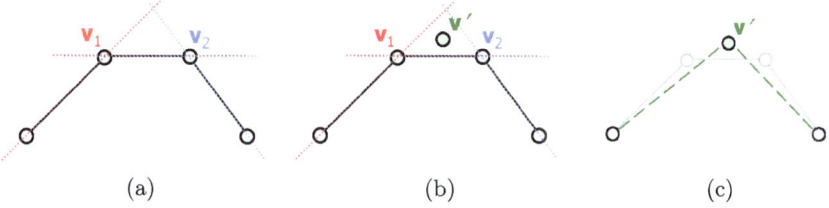

Fig. 10.14 2D example of main step in quadric-based surface simplification. (**a**) Initial vertex pair with associated lines; (**b**) New vertex minimizing distance to all lines; (**c**) Replacement of original vertices/edges by new vertex/edges

problem can be avoided by rearranging the error metric to obtain a quadric-based formulation:

$$\epsilon(\mathbf{v}) = \sum_{\mathbf{p}\in\mathcal{P}} \left(\mathbf{p}^T \mathbf{v}\right)^2 = \sum_{\mathbf{p}\in\mathcal{P}} \mathbf{v}^T \left(\mathbf{p}\mathbf{p}^T\right)\mathbf{v} = \mathbf{v}^T \left(\sum_{\mathbf{p}\in\mathcal{P}} \mathbf{K}_{\mathbf{p}}\right)\mathbf{v} = \mathbf{v}^T \mathbf{Q}\mathbf{v}, \qquad (10.4)$$

with symmetric 4×4 matrices for each plane given by:

$$\mathbf{K}_{\mathbf{p}} = \mathbf{p}\mathbf{p}^T = \begin{bmatrix} a^2 & ab & ac & ad \\ ab & b^2 & bc & bd \\ ac & bc & c^2 & cd \\ ad & bd & cd & d^2 \end{bmatrix}. \qquad (10.5)$$

By summing up all the matrices $\mathbf{K}_{\mathbf{p}}$ we obtain a single matrix $\mathbf{Q}$ describing a quadric surface. This representation allows to work conveniently with single matrices in the outlined simplification process. Minimum-distance vertices for a vertex pair are found by minimizing $\mathbf{v}^T \mathbf{Q}\mathbf{v}$. When the two vertices with the minimum overall error are combined then a new quadric surface is formed simply by addition: $\mathbf{Q}_{\mathbf{v}'} = \mathbf{Q}_{\mathbf{v}_i} + \mathbf{Q}_{\mathbf{v}_j}$. The process is again repeated as before for further polygon reduction.

10.5.3 Mesh Smoothing

Various techniques exist to smooth the geometric representations of anatomical models obtained from medical data. Perhaps the most popular method of surface smoothing is the direct application of Gaussian filtering to the underlying volume data. The basic idea is to convolve the volumetric representation of the object with a discrete Gaussian kernel. Thus, the filtering is applied to the volume, before a surface is reconstructed, e.g. using isosurface reconstruction methods. A discrete version of the 3D Gaussian

$$G(\mathbf{v}) = \frac{1}{(2\pi\sigma^2)^{\frac{3}{2}}} e^{-\frac{v^2}{2\sigma^2}} \qquad (10.6)$$

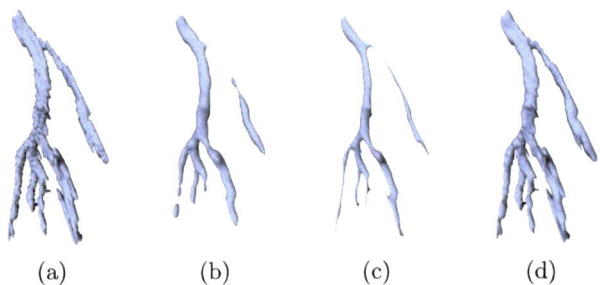

(a)   (b)   (c)   (d)

Fig. 10.15 Mesh smoothing strategies (from [41], courtesy of Johannes Hug). (**a**) Original iso-surface reconstruction; (**b**) Data convoluted with Gaussian kernel ($\sigma = 1.5$) before reconstruction; (**c**) Application of discrete Laplacian smoothing on mesh ($\lambda = 0.33, t = 90$); (**d**) Outcome after Taubin smoothing ($\kappa = 0.33, \mu = -0.34, t = 90$)

is applied in the convolution. In spite of its simplicity, this method has the disadvantage of potentially causing topological changes, which often appear as thinning effects (see [66]). As illustrated in Fig. 10.15, small objects such as vessel trees may be cut into several unconnected parts, thin surfaces such as ligaments might be perforated, or tight structures such as bowel loops might grow together.

An alternative is to perform the convolution directly on the surface itself. A discrete approximation of Gaussian filtering is carried out, also known as Laplacian smoothing [51]. The basic idea is to displace vertices in the direction of the Laplacian, thus approximating a diffusion process. To this end, an update rule is iteratively applied to all vertices.

$$\mathbf{v}^{[t+1]} = \mathbf{v}^{[t]} + \lambda \Delta \mathbf{v}^{[t]}, \quad 0 < \lambda < 1, \tag{10.7}$$

with the discrete approximation of the Laplace operator (see [102] for a broad discussion)—also called the umbrella operator—given by:

$$\Delta \mathbf{v}^{[t]} = \frac{1}{\|neigh(\mathbf{v})\|} \sum_{\mathbf{u} \in neigh(\mathbf{v})} \|\mathbf{u} - \mathbf{v}\|. \tag{10.8}$$

The parameter λ is a scaling factor. Unfortunately, the same difficulties of shrinking are encountered (see Fig. 10.15). The iterative application of the operator is equivalent to progressively reducing the surface's membrane energy and thus also leads to shrinking.

By exploiting filter design principles, Gabriel Taubin developed a fairing method that modifies Gaussian filtering such that the contraction effect is minimized [96]. The central idea is to alternate between a shrinking and an un-shrinking filter, whose scale factors are chosen at a suitable pass-band frequency. Thus, an inward and an outward diffusion is carried out which prevents shrinkage of low-frequency components. The local smoothing operator is given by:

$$\mathbf{v}^{[t+1]} = \mathbf{v}^{[t]} + s\,\Delta\mathbf{v}^{[t]}, \quad s = \begin{cases} \kappa & \text{if } t \text{ even, } 0 < \kappa < 1, \\ \mu & \text{if } t \text{ odd, } \mu < -\kappa. \end{cases} \tag{10.9}$$

10.6 Model Adaptation

The ability to present variable scenarios is a crucial component in surgical training systems. In currently existing simulators this point is often neglected. In order
to replicate the day-to-day workload of a surgeon, different patients with varying
manifestations of pathologies have to be integrated. Moreover, it should be possible to provide seldom cases. This is analogous to the scenario generation in flight
simulation, where varying weather conditions, traffic situations, airports, aircraft
types, and emergencies can be selected. Optimally, a scene would be automatically
generated according to specifications of the medical expert overseeing the training
session. This could for instance include key parameters of a patient, such as his
height, weight, or age. In the context of scene generation for surgical simulation,
in the following the main components needed to define a scenario will be examined. Different steps in the process are analyzed in detail—the generation of the
scene geometry including healthy and pathologic anatomy, the generation of vascular structures, the definition of biomechanical parameters, and the modeling of organ
surface appearance via texturing. The discussions are partly based on [33], where
additional details on surgical scene generation for VR-based training in medicine
are provided. Several of the examples are provided within the context of a specific
surgical simulator for hysteroscopic interventions (i.e. endoscopic inspection and
treatment of the uterus) [34].

10.7 Modelling Organ Variability

10.7.1 Outline

This section will focus on the derivation of a model to automatically generate varying meshes of the uterus. The shape and size of this organ varies considerably depending on different factors, such as age or number of children. The underlying
idea of the geometry generation of healthy organs is based on the derivation of a
statistical model describing the natural variability of the organ shape. The main target is to find for a given population of object instances the shape space which most
compactly describes the variations occurring in the sample dataset.

   Under the assumption that the variability of uterus shape descriptors is Gaussian and the dependencies of the shape parameters are only up to second order, the
principal component analysis (PCA) (see [42] for an introduction) can be applied to

decorrelate the parameters and reduce the dimensionality of the description. Linear transformation maps the data to a new coordinate system, thus providing a linear vector space spanned by a complete set of orthogonal basis vectors in which the main variations of object shape are separated. This technique has been applied in several research areas, for instance focusing on segmentation of medical imagery in [48, 92, 100]. A number of approaches can be followed to represent organ shape by a parametric model. Using the vertex coordinates of polygonal object representations to encode shape leads to the so-called point distribution models (PDM) [8, 12, 40].

A key requirement to obtain meaningful results from the PCA is the correspondence between the shape parameters of the individual instances of the population. In the case of PDMs, vertices located at the same anatomical feature should have the same index in all instances of the training set. Moreover, all training samples have to be expressed in the same coordinate system. Several methods have been proposed to establish the described correspondences. For instance, an automatic approach is to perform a global optimization of the determinant of the covariance matrix of the study population, as described in [52]. Also a semi-automatic paradigm can be followed, for instance focusing on initialization of subdivision surfaces by a user based on generalized landmarks [93]. Finally, directly ensuring point correspondences during the necessary segmentation process also results in a statistical shape description of reasonable quality [89]. In the following the generation of a model of organ variability is described based on the concrete example of hysteroscopy simulation.

10.7.2 Medical Data Segmentation

As a first step, medical datasets were obtained from 26 volunteers. These were selected such as to cover the range in age and number of pregnancies that is usually encountered in patients undergoing hysteroscopy. Imaging was performed with a GE 1.5 Tesla machine yielding a resolution of 0.46 mm^2 × 3 mm. Scanning time was lower than 10 mins due to the small number of slices, thus avoiding motion artifacts.

In order to maintain point correspondences, a coarse-to-fine subdivision scheme can be applied, which ensures similarity of vertex indices between different segmentations [89]. The shape extraction process starts with the rigid registration [108] of MRI datasets in order to ensure that the slices are aligned in space with sufficient accuracy. Thereafter, the segmentation process is carried out in a semi-automatic fashion. Prior knowledge about the anatomical shape of the uterus allows to provide a coarse surface mesh as an initial guess for the organ shape. This root mesh has been manually designed and contains openings for the cervix as well as the tubal ostia (Fig. 10.16). Thus, from a topological point of view, the surface is represented by two concentric spherical shapes connected by three short cylindrical tunnels. By choosing mesh dimensions according to standard anatomical measurements of the uterus, a reasonable initialization can be achieved for the subsequent steps. The initial guess is refined using a combination of interactive segmentation techniques— global free form-deformation, local mesh adaptation, and mesh optimization. The

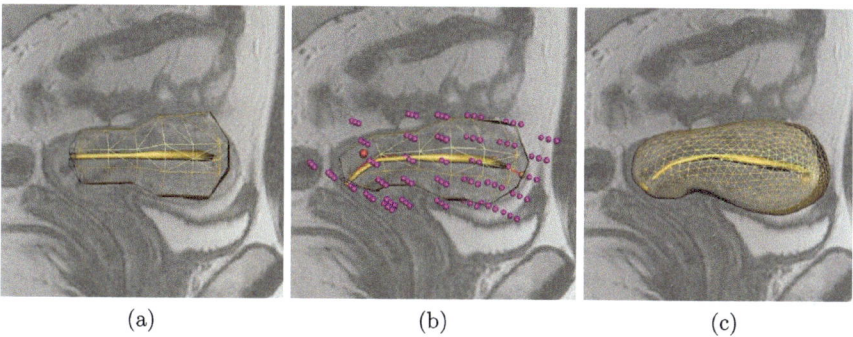

(a)   (b)   (c)

Fig. 10.16 Steps of uterus segmentation (from [33]). (**a**) Coarse mesh for initialization; (**b**) Free-form deformation; (**c**) Final segmentation after subdivision and smoothing

initial coarse mesh can be further subdivided following a quaternary scheme, during which correspondence between vertices is maintained. By combining all these steps, triangular surface meshes of the uteri have been segmented from all MRI datasets.

10.7.3 Statistical Model

Before the statistical analysis can be performed, the instances of the study population have to be transformed into a common coordinate system. The three natural orifices of the uterine cavity serve as a basis for defining a right-handed coordinate system. The origin of the system is given by the right tubal ostium. The axes are rotated such that the x-axis passes through the cervical ostium and the left tubal ostium lies on the xy-plane in negative y-direction. The z-axis is then determined by the cross-product of the other axes. Apart from defining a common coordinate frame, no spatial normalization has to be applied.

After this step, the statistical model is obtained by employing the principal component analysis (PCA) on all object instances in the database. The used population of object instances consists of the segmented surfaces of the uteri. For N instances, given as polygonal models with M vertices

$$\mathbf{p}_i = \left[x_i^{[1]}, y_i^{[1]}, z_i^{[1]}, \ldots, x_i^{[M]}, y_i^{[M]}, z_i^{[M]} \right]^T,$$

the parameter signals of the shapes are centered by calculating the average model $\bar{\mathbf{p}}$

$$\bar{\mathbf{p}} = \frac{1}{N} \sum_{i=1}^{N} \mathbf{p}_i \tag{10.10}$$

and an instance specific difference vector

$$\Delta \mathbf{p}_i = \mathbf{p}_i - \bar{\mathbf{p}}. \tag{10.11}$$

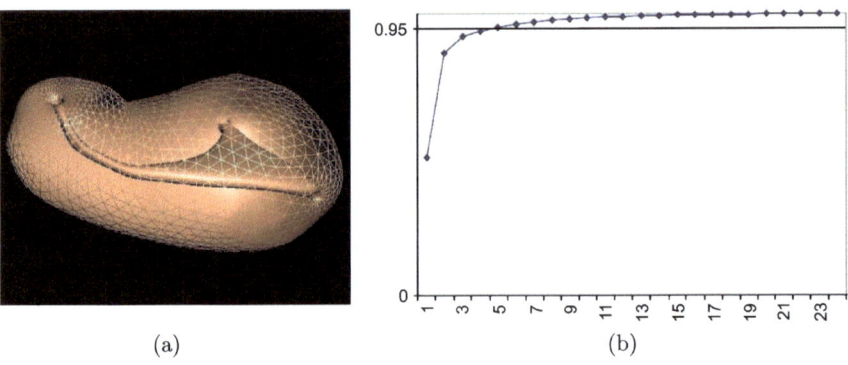

(a)   (b)

Fig. 10.17 Statistical model of natural variability (from [33]). (**a**) Mean uterus shape; (**b**) Cumulative histogram of eigenvalues

Figure 10.17 depicts the average uterus shape obtained from the input dataset. The covariance matrix Σ and the resulting PCA given by the eigensystem of that matrix can subsequently be determined according to:

$$\Sigma = \frac{1}{N-1} \sum_{i=1}^{N} \Delta \mathbf{p}_i \, \Delta \mathbf{p}_i^T \stackrel{PCA}{=} \mathbf{U} \boldsymbol{\Lambda} \mathbf{U}^T; \tag{10.12}$$

with $\boldsymbol{\Lambda} = \text{diag}(\lambda_1, \dots, \lambda_{N-1})$ containing the eigenvalues and $\mathbf{U}$ the eigenvectors (i.e. eigenshapes). This gives us a transformation of the difference vectors into shape space.

$$\mathbf{b}_i = \mathbf{U}^T \Delta \mathbf{p}_i, \quad \mathbf{b}_i = [b_{1,i}, \dots, b_{N-1,i}]. \tag{10.13}$$

The original organ instances can be reconstructed by using

$$\mathbf{p}_i = \bar{\mathbf{p}} + \mathbf{U} \mathbf{b}_i. \tag{10.14}$$

Note that this can be considered as a linear combination of the eigenvectors with parameters $b_{j,i}$ as weights. The components in PCA are ordered by variance. In general the first $k \ll N$ eigenshapes corresponding to the largest eigenvalues capture most of the shape variability. Thus, the linear combination of a small number of eigenshapes results in a compact description of the population. The shape of a new instance is fully defined by the parameter set $\mathbf{b} = \{b_1, \dots, b_k\}$. In Fig. 10.17 the influence of the eigenvalues is shown by plotting $i \rightarrow (\sum_{k=1}^{i} \lambda_k / \sum_{k=1}^{N-1} \lambda_k)$ (i.e. the ratio of the sum of the first k to the sum of all eigenvalues). As can be seen, the first five eigenshapes capture already about 95% of the overall variability.

The original organ shapes can be approximately reconstructed by only considering the first few eigenshapes.

$$\mathbf{p}_i \approx \bar{\mathbf{p}} + \sum_{j=1}^{k} b_{j,i} \mathbf{u}_j, \quad k \ll N. \tag{10.15}$$

Following this notion, it is actually possible to select different weights $\tilde{b}$ for combining the eigenvectors. This allows to derive new organ shapes that were not observed before. A new instance can be generated by a combination of weighted eigenshapes and the mean shape.

$$\tilde{\mathbf{p}} = \overline{\mathbf{p}} + \sum_{j=1}^{k} \tilde{b}_j \mathbf{u}_j. \tag{10.16}$$

The trade-off between tractability and accuracy of the model description is influenced by the number of parameters k. Unfortunately, the shape changes obtained when varying the individual parameters b_j do not necessarily map to intuitive anatomical metrics, thus making it complicated to control the object appearance based only on these parameters. Instead, it should be possible to control the shape changes by adjusting standard anatomical metrics, e.g. length, width, or depth of the uterine fundus. To achieve this, an approach of progressive elimination of variation could be followed [40].

Nevertheless, a problem is still encountered in the current formulation. The number of variables ($3M$) is much larger than the number of observations (N). Due to the linear dependency of the difference vectors $\sum_{i=0}^{N} \Delta \mathbf{p}_i = 0$, the covariance matrix is rank-deficient. In addition, due to the large number of variables, i.e. mesh vertices, the numerical methods become quite slow and unstable.

These difficulties can be avoided by following an alternative approach. The underlying idea is to determine the corresponding set of eigenvectors $\mathbf{U}$, by performing the singular value decomposition of the reduced $N \times N$ covariance matrix

$$\tilde{\Sigma} = \frac{1}{N-1} \Delta \mathbf{P}^T \Delta \mathbf{P} \stackrel{\text{PCA}}{=} \tilde{\mathbf{U}} \tilde{\mathbf{\Lambda}} \tilde{\mathbf{U}}^T. \tag{10.17}$$

From this alternative formulation, the sought-after eigenvalues are given directly by $\mathbf{\Lambda} = \tilde{\mathbf{\Lambda}}$. The corresponding eigenvectors can also be determined according to $\mathbf{U} = \frac{1}{(N-1)\lambda^{\frac{1}{2}}} \Delta \mathbf{P} \tilde{\mathbf{U}}$. Note that the scaling factor is necessary to normalize the vectors.

10.8   Integration of Pathologies

10.8.1   Outline

After the generation of new instances of the healthy organ, the pathological variation needs to be added. For this, there are a number of requirements which have to be met. The main target is to generate a realistic geometric representation—optimally in an automatic process according to medical terms. Moreover, to accommodate for repeated training, some degree of randomness during the generation process has to be included. In addition to this, during the model development, it should be possible to track and/or include further information, such as surface textures, blood perfusion, and biomechanical properties. Finally, the seamless integration into the healthy organ model also has to be ensured. In the following an example will be given how to model the growth of a myoma, i.e. a benign tumor in the uterus, using cellular automata.

10.8.2 Cellular Automata Growth Model

Cellular automata were initially introduced in the late 1940s by John von Neumann [101]. However, the first practical application of the theory is probably the renowned *Game of Life* by John Horton Conway (see e.g. [30]). In general, cellular automata are used for modeling discrete dynamical processes without explicitly relying on differential equations. An advantage of cellular automata is their simplicity and extendibility. The growth process can be described based on a small number of rules acting on a regular lattice. In addition, all intermediate stages of the evolution can be observed if desired. Moreover, simulation with cellular automata is intrinsically stable.

The modeling of tumor growth with cellular automata has been an active topic of research for more than a decade [44, 78, 103]. In the following a possible approach to using cellular automata for modelling tumor growth [88] will be described. It should be noted, that the number of actual cells in a myoma is too large to be handled at interactive rates. Therefore, individual cells are not simulated, but instead conglomerations of cells. Thus, in the following the term *cell* will denote a node of the cellular automaton, and not a single biological cell.

Individual nodes (i.e. cells) of the cellular automaton are located at positions $\mathbf{p} = (x, y, z)$ on a regular, three-dimensional cubic lattice $\mathcal{L}$. At a specific time step t during the simulation each cell at position $\mathbf{p}$ has two characteristic states associated with it—a *tumor* and a *tissue* state. The former is described by the discrete value $S_{tumor}^{t}(\mathbf{p}) \in \{0, \frac{1}{n}, \frac{2}{n}, \ldots, 1\}$, while the latter is represented by a continuous value $S_{tissue}^{t}(\mathbf{p}) \in [0, 1]$. These states are altered during the simulation by a set of predefined rules. Based on the states, three different cell classes can exist. Positions with $S_{tumor}^{t}(\mathbf{p}) = 1$ are considered to be part of the tumor. The remaining cells having $S_{tissue}^{t}\mathbf{p} > 0$ are part of the healthy tissue, while the rest is background, i.e. free space inside the uterine cavity.

The dynamic evolution of the system is controlled by local space- and time-independent transition rules R. The latter can be either deterministic or probabilistic. In order to model tumor growth, the conventional cellular automaton is extended by introducing a global rule R_{global}, which controls the application of the rules. The former is time-dependent, thus allowing to change the sequence of application of the rules R during tumor evolution. The individual rules are applied simultaneously on all cells at every time step. The interaction neighborhood $\mathcal{N}(\mathbf{p})$ defines the set of neighboring nodes which will be considered when one of the rules is applied to position $\mathbf{p}$. Typical neighborhoods used in 3D are the von Neumann neighborhood $\mathcal{N}_6$ or the Moore neighborhood $\mathcal{N}_{26}$.

Four specific rules are sufficient to model the growth process of a myoma. The first rule of the tumor growth automaton describes the growth of the cancerous tissue. The tumor state of a cell at location $\mathbf{p}$ is increased if one of the nodes $\mathbf{q}$ in its neighborhood has a non-zero tumor state.

$$R_{grow}: \quad S_{tumor}^{t+1}(\mathbf{p}) = \min\left[1, S_{tumor}^{t}(\mathbf{p}) + \frac{1}{n}\right],$$

(10.18)

$$\text{if } S_{tumor}^{t}(\mathbf{q}) > 0, \quad \mathbf{q} \in \mathcal{N}_{26}(\mathbf{p}).$$

In order to introduce some randomness in this process, the rule is only applied with a certain probability depending on the neighbor location. If $\mathbf{q}$ is in $\mathcal{N}_6$, then the probability is high, otherwise low.

The next rule models the migration of the tumor inside the healthy tissue. The tumor states of all cells are moved in one of the six major directions based on a global cost function determined by the tissue states.

$$R_{move}: \quad S_{tumor}^{t+1}(\mathbf{p}) = S_{tumor}^{t}(\mathbf{p} - \mathbf{d})$$

$$\underset{\mathbf{d}}{\arg\min}\, C(\mathbf{d}), \quad \mathbf{d} = (\mathbf{q} - \mathbf{p}), \quad \mathbf{q} \in \mathcal{N}_6(\mathbf{p}).$$

The global cost function C sums up the tissue states of the neighbors of all cells with $S_{tumor} > 0$ in one of the six major directions. Thus, there are accordingly six different associated costs.

The displacement of healthy tissue by the growing tumor is produced by the third rule. The neighbor of a current cell position with the largest tumor value moves its tissue to the latter.

$$R_{displace}: \quad \tilde{\mathbf{q}} = \underset{\mathbf{q} \in \mathcal{N}_{26}(\mathbf{p})}{\arg\max}\, S_{tumor}^{t}(\mathbf{q})$$

$$S_{tissue}^{t+1}(\mathbf{p}) = \min\left[1, S_{tissue}^{t}(\tilde{\mathbf{q}}) + S_{tissue}^{t}(\mathbf{p})\right]$$

(10.19)

$$S_{tissue}^{t+1}(\tilde{\mathbf{q}}) = 0.$$

After the displacement the tissue states are smoothed with a Gaussian filter. Thereafter, a final rule R_{close} ensures that all tumor cells are covered by a cell layer of healthy tissue.

For the growth simulation, the automaton is initialized by defining background and tissue cells. The states of the tissue cells are set proportional to the normalized distance from their position to the tissue/background interface (i.e. $0 < S_{tissue}^{0} < 1$). One of the tissue cells is then initialized with a non-zero tumor state. By placing this single tumor cell into the layer of healthy cells representing the myometrium the growth is started.

According to R_{global} different growth intervals are specified. At the start of the simulation a faster movement of the tumor is allowed. As its size increases the application of R_{move} can be reduced. The tumor volume can be approximately determined by multiplying R_{grow} with the respective probability of $\mathcal{N}_6$. This measure

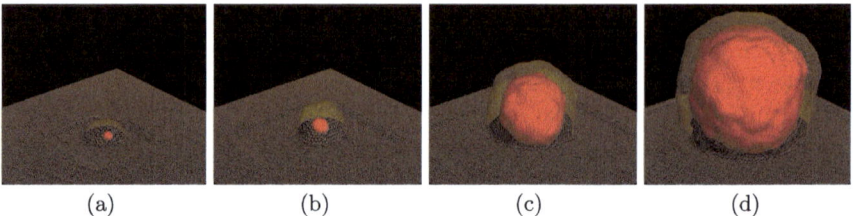

| (a) | (b) | (c) | (d) |

Fig. 10.18 Steps of cellular automata based myoma growth (outer tissue surface shown in *beige wireframe*, inner tumor surface in *solid red*) (from [33]). (**a**) Iteration $t = 20$; (**b**) Iteration $t = 30$; (**c**) Iteration $t = 40$; (**d**) Iteration $t = 50$

can also be used as a stopping criterion for the algorithm. An example of a growth process for a myoma based on the described cellular automaton on a 100^3 lattice is shown in Fig. 10.18. Note that the depicted surfaces have been extracted from the volumetric lattice using the marching cubes algorithm.

The described approach is able to simulate the growth of different kinds of myoma. A medical expert has to define the starting location of the tumor growth as well as the desired size. Thereafter, the generation process runs automatically. Nevertheless, a number of limitations exist. As mentioned, the outcome of the algorithm is a volume of labeled voxels describing the pathology. For visualization purposes first a surface has to be extracted. Moreover, the generated geometry has to be merged with that of the healthy anatomy. One viable approach to this task would be to voxelize the part of the cavity, where the tumor is going to be located. After the growth process, a surface mesh could be obtained and merged with the remaining parts. However, due to the involved voxelization step some surface detail might be lost depending on the underlying lattice resolution. Figure 10.19 shows examples of generated (and textured) myomas, as well as real myomas encountered during actual interventions.

10.9 Generation of Vascular Structures

10.9.1 Outline

A further component of a surgical scene definition scheme is the generation and integration of vascular structures. Blood vessels affect surgical simulation on several levels. Firstly, they are the carrier of blood circulation and thus an integral part of a patient physiology model. Moreover, they affect the visual appearance of organ surfaces and thus have to be included into the texturing process, since vascular patterns contain vital information for a surgeon. Moreover, vessel trees also have to be treated as geometric entities. This is necessary during cutting procedures, to determine the source of bleeding as well as to obtain further information affecting the rendering of the blood flow. Also, processes such as the intravasation occurring in

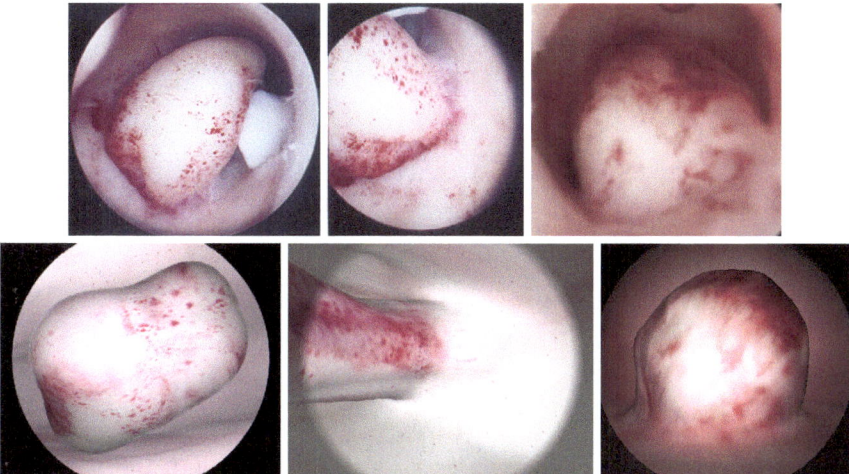

Fig. 10.19 Pathologies in the uterus—real (*top*) vs. generated (*bottom*)

hysteroscopy [98] require a vascular model. Finally, larger vessels even have to be treated as deformable objects during tool-tissue interaction.

Since vessel structures are usually too complex to be synthesized with texture generation approaches and, moreover, have to be included in the simulation as geometric objects, a specialized generation process is required. In the past a number of methods for modeling of vascular systems have been suggested [84, 94]. As a possible approach for vessel tree generation, L-systems (Lindenmayer systems) will be introduced.

10.9.2 Lindenmayer Systems

L-systems were proposed in 1968 by Aristid Lindenmayer as a mathematical model for describing cellular interaction during growth [54]. An L-system is essentially a context free grammar within the Chomsky hierarchy (in the theory of formal languages). It is a parallel rewriting system consisting of an initial state and a set of rewriting rules or productions.

An L-system is given by a tuple $L = (V, \omega, P)$, where V are the variables, ω the axiom, i.e. the initial state, and P the production rules. Starting with the first axiom, symbols are converted into new symbols or strings of symbols according to the production rules. This parallel substitution is repeated recursively several times. By assigning geometrical semantics to the different symbols, for instance following the paradigm of turtle graphics, one can interpret the final string as a spatial object. Throughout the past years, L-system have become a very useful and popular tool for generating artificial plants [75] in computer graphics. By following similar strategies, also vessel systems can be generated.

Fig. 10.20 Drawings obtained by L-system after 1, 2, and 3 recursive applications of the rule $F \rightarrow F + F - - F + F$

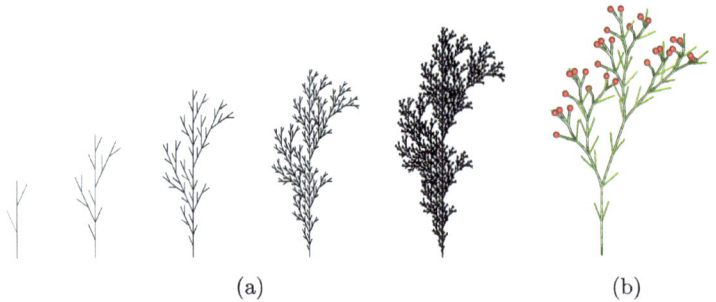

(a)   (b)

Fig. 10.21 Generation of plant-like structures via L-systems with memory. (**a**) Results of the first five applications of the production rule $F \rightarrow F[-F]F[+F][F]$; (**b**) Plant generated with L-system

As an example, an L-system will be presented which produces a variant of a Koch curve. Consider the L-system consisting of the variable F and the constants $+$ and $-$. With the production rule $F \rightarrow F + F - - F + F$ and the axiom F the mentioned Koch curve can be created. The latter is done following the turtle graphics paradigm. In the latter an oriented cursor is placed on the Cartesian plane, which can be moved and rotated, while it is also used for drawing lines. Interpreting F as [*draw a line forward*], $+$ as [*turn left by 60 degrees*], and $-$ as [*turn right by 60 degrees*], we obtain the curves shown in Fig. 10.20 in the first three iterations. Note that the drawings are normalized in size. Starting instead with the axiom $F - - F - - F$ would create the actual closed Koch curve (known as Koch snowflake).

By extending the formalism more complex structures can be created. For instance, by introducing a positional memory, branching structures can be generated. Interpreting the symbol [as [*store current position and orientation*] and] as [*restore previous position and orientation*], allows to generate plant-like objects by recursively applying the production rule $F \rightarrow F[-F]F[+F][F]$. Figure 10.21(a) shows the (scaled) outcome of the first five applications of this production rule. Extending this to 3D, adding leaves at branchings as well as flowers at the terminals, and coloring the components, already convincing models of plants can be created, as shown in Fig. 10.21(b). Further examples can be found in [76].

10.10 Biomechanical Parameters

An important element of any deformation simulation module is the determination of appropriate material parameters. Living tissue is a non-linear, inhomogeneous, anisotropic material with viscoelastic, and in some cases also viscoplastic, properties. Moreover, soft organs are usually layered, with each layer exhibiting different mechanical properties. In addition, considerable variation between healthy and pathological tissue can be encountered. In the past, several experimental methodologies have been proposed for the mechanical testing of soft tissues to acquire appropriate tissue parameters. These can be categorized into ex- and in-vivo approaches.

10.10.1 Ex-vivo Measurements

First steps aiming at the measurement of mechanical properties of living tissue have been undertaken in [106] and [27]. Geometrically well-defined samples were excised from a body and examined using standard material testing methods, usually tension or compression tests with known boundary conditions [23]. Inflation and indentation experiments have also been carried out [16]. Due to well-defined experimental conditions, stress and strain values can easily be obtained. However, several short-comings limit the ex-vivo approach. As shown in [47] and [69] the mechanical behavior of tissue after excision is much different from the in-vivo case. This is for instance due to loss of perfusion or muscle tone, dehydration or temperature changes. To alleviate this problem an approach has been suggested, where porcine liver is kept in quasi-in-vivo physiologic conditions during ex-vivo testing [49]. First results showed better approximations of the in-vivo state, however, further research in this direction is needed.

10.10.2 In-vivo Measurements

Due to the mentioned limitations of ex-vivo testing, several approaches focus instead on in-vivo acquisition of soft tissue parameters. These follow either an indirect strategy via non-invasive imaging techniques or a direct one via invasive in-vivo testing. The latter can be further classified with regard to the selected access method to the organs—either during open surgery or minimally-invasive procedures.

Non-invasive acquisition A holy grail of in-vivo tissue property measurement is the non-invasive acquisition via imaging technology. Methods have been developed using MRI [25, 61] or US imaging [67]. Strain images are acquired which allow to map and quantify small displacements, caused by propagating harmonic mechanical waves. Unfortunately, only elastic moduli can be obtained this way due to the constriction to small deformations. Thus, the initial slope of the stress-strain curve can be determined, however, non-linear behavior at large strains cannot be obtained. Nevertheless, recent studies indicate that an extension to the non-linear case could be possible [90]. A problem that remains with these approaches is, however, the undetermined boundary conditions during the measurements.

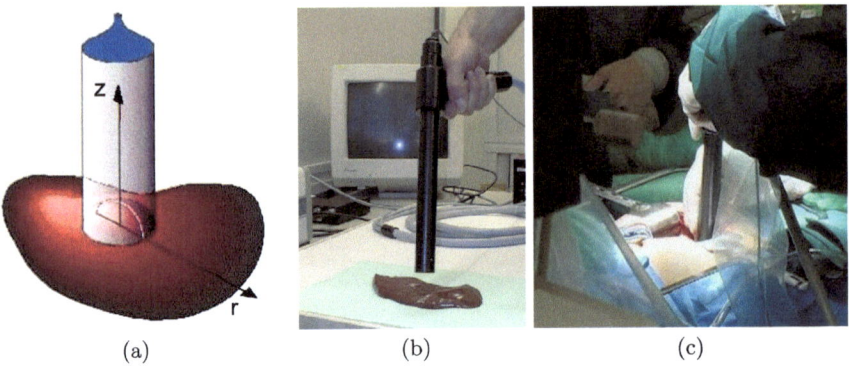

Fig. 10.22 Overview of tissue aspiration device (from [46]). (**a**) Measurement principle based on aspiration; (**b**) Aspiration device; (**c**) Application of device during open surgery

Invasive acquisition In invasive methods, measurements are acquired via direct contact with organs. The easiest access to the latter is during open surgery, since less restrictions exist regarding the size of the testing devices [6, 50]. A less invasive approach is the acquisition during minimally invasive procedures [4, 68].

As an example of an in-vivo acquisition technique a device developed at ETH Zurich will be discussed in more detail [47]. Using the setup, tissue parameters can be derived by carrying out in-vivo aspiration experiments on human tissue during open surgeries. Figure 10.22 visualizes components of the aspiration hardware.

The approach involves placing a tube against the target tissue and producing a weak vacuum in the tube. The vacuum fixes the organ to the latter, thus setting well-defined boundary conditions, and causes small deformation of the tissue, which is sucked into the tube. During this procedure, the applied pressure as well as the resulting deformation is tracked. Assuming axisymmetry and homogeneous tissue in the portion covered by the aspiration tube, a complete description of the deformation is given by the profile of the aspirated tissue. An explicit axisymmetric finite element simulation of the aspiration experiment is used together with a Levenberg-Marquardt optimization to estimate the material model parameters in an inverse parameter determination process. Tissue properties of the uterus, kidney, and liver in healthy as well as pathological condition could for instance be obtained with this technique [63].

10.11 Organ Texture Generation

Modelling of organ appearance in the virtual scene is the next element of the scenario generation process. Realism of rendered scenes demands complexity, or at least appearance of complexity [35]. Therefore, it is desirable to enhance the visual richness of the surface triangle models generated in the previous steps by adding further detail. The application of surface textures to geometric models—also referred

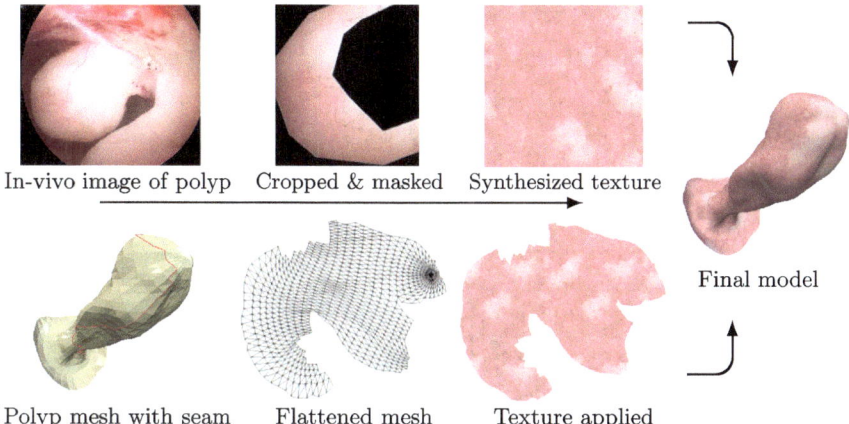

In-vivo image of polyp **Cropped & masked** **Synthesized texture**

Final model

Polyp mesh with seam **Flattened mesh** **Texture applied**

Fig. 10.23 Texturing process for hysteroscopy simulation (from [70])

to as *texturing*—is currently one of the key technique in interactive computer graphics to add complexity and thus realism to visual rendering [7]. With this approach, representation of minute object detail with geometric information can be avoided. Moreover, texture mapping only requires little additional computational effort in the rendering process.

Especially in the limited views of minimally-invasive settings, where the surgical site is accessed through natural orifices or small incisions in the skin, texture contains several cues facilitating spatial navigation. Changes in texture characteristics according to perspective distortion provide knowledge about depth and orientation. Since endoscopic interventions are usually performed with monoscopic cameras, these monocular depth cues contain significant additional semantic information. Apart from this, different kinds of texture of various organs provide further cues for orientation. This is especially true for laparoscopic procedures in the human abdomen, where a large variety of structures is present. Typical organ surface textures allow a surgeon to infer his position from the limited endoscopic view.

There are two key steps to texture a surface mesh—the generation of a texture as well as the mapping of it to the mesh (see Fig. 10.23 for an overview). Concerning the former, generally, two different strategies could be followed: empirical procedural texture generation based on closed mathematical formulations (see e.g. [29, 72, 73]) or analytical approaches applying example-based synthesis (see e.g. [18, 28, 104]). Mainly the latter are used in the scenario definition process, since procedural methods suffer from several limitations, such as the non-intuitive control of the algorithms.

The underlying idea of approaches falling into the synthesis category is texture creation from example. A sample is supplied to an algorithm, analyzed, and then a new texture is automatically created resembling the original one. Different strategies can be used to ensure the similarity between the in- and output texture. Texture synthesis methods originate from diverse underlying ideas and follow different strategies. A distinction of the approaches is not straight-forward, since often a

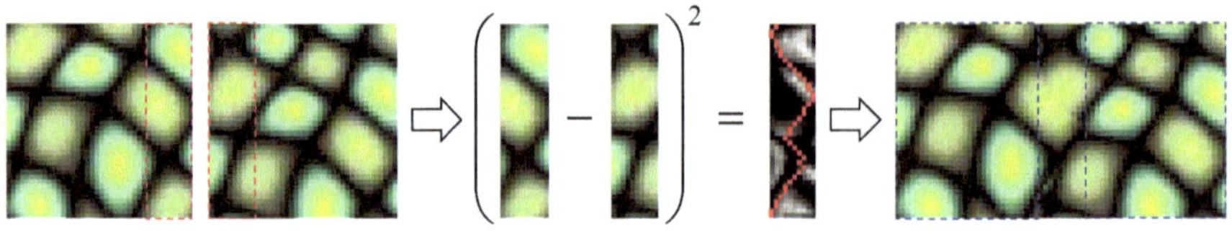

Fig. 10.24 Overview of texturing via image quilting

combination of methods is used. One possible categorization discriminates between pixel- and patch-oriented synthesis. The former synthesizes a pixel at a time, while the latter pastes complete patches into the new texture. In the following, an example for the latter technique shall be given.

A patch-based synthesis process termed *image quilting* has been proposed by Efros et al. in [17]. New textures are synthesized one patch at a time in scanline order by placing overlapping square samples from a source image into the new texture. Candidate patches are selected randomly from the source such as to minimize the L2 norm for pixels in the overlapping area. Once a square patch has been found, an optimal cutting path between adjacent patches is determined. Dynamic programming can be applied to perform this minimum error boundary cut. Figure 10.24 briefly outlines the main steps in image quilting.

After the synthesis step, the textures have to be mapped to object geometries. If the texture is built as a bivariate field, then a bijective mapping function has to be determined, relating 3D points on a mesh surface to the parametric 2D texture space.

A mapping M between two surfaces S_1 and S_2 is called isometric, if the geodesic distances d_{geo} between arbitrary points is maintained.

$$\forall \mathbf{p}_i, \mathbf{p}_j \in S_1 : d_{geo}(\mathbf{p}_i, \mathbf{p}_j) = d_{geo}(M(\mathbf{p}_i), M(\mathbf{p}_j)). \qquad (10.20)$$

In this case, the surface S_1 is also called developable. Gaussian curvature at a point $\mathbf{p}$ on surface S is defined as

$$K = \frac{1}{R_1 R_2}, \qquad (10.21)$$

where R_1 and R_2 are the largest and the smallest principle radii of curvature of the respective osculating circles. A sphere has, for instance, a constant positive Gaussian curvature, while that of a cylinder is everywhere zero. Already Carl Friedrich Gauss stated that an isometric mapping of surfaces with unequal Gaussian curvatures K is not possible [32]. Thus, distortions are inevitable when mapping from 2D texture patches with zero curvature to 3D surfaces with non-zero curvature. Thus, a method has to be found to minimize these distortions.

The key step for texture mapping is the parametrization of the objects meshes (an extensive overview of current techniques can be found in [24]). The meshes are represented as piecewise linear triangular surfaces $S_{\mathcal{T}}$, defined by a set of triangles $\mathcal{T} = \{T_1, \ldots, T_N\}$. For the parameterization, a piecewise linear mapping

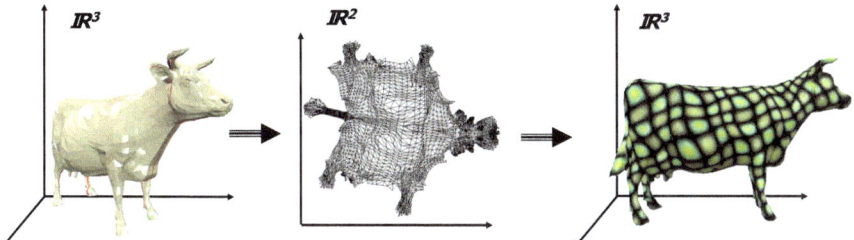

Fig. 10.25 Overview of texture mapping via 3D-2D parameterization

$f : S_{\mathcal{T}} \rightarrow S^*$ of the surface $S_{\mathcal{T}} \in \mathbb{R}^3$ into the planar domain $S^* \in \mathbb{R}^2$ has to be found. As discussed above, distortions are usually introduced in this step. A mapping can either be conformal, i.e. angle-preserving, or equiareal, i.e. area-preserving. An isometric mapping is conformal and equiareal; however, since for our meshes such a mapping cannot be found, angle and area distortion should be minimized.

A surface can only be mapped to a plane, if it is homomorphic to a disk. Thus, a number of cases can be encountered, where a surface has to be cut before the mapping step. The genus G of a closed surface is defined by the Euler-Poincare formula

$$G = \frac{1}{2}E - V - F - B + 2, \qquad (10.22)$$

where V, E, and F are the number of mesh vertices, edges, and faces, respectively, and B the number of boundary loops. The genus of a surface can be regarded as the number of holes or handles in a 2-manifold mesh. Surfaces with non-zero genus are not homomorphic to a disk, and thus have to be cut to reduce the genus. The same is true for a manifold mesh with a boundary. If interior holes are present, then these surfaces also have to be separated. Apart from this, the introduction of additional seams by subdivision of an already disk-like mesh can be applied to further reduce distortion (see e.g. [86]).

For the mesh cutting, surfaces are separated along existing edges according to quality metrics. Firstly, a visibility measure for mesh edges is calculated by rendering the scene from different viewpoints and marking of visible elements. Secondly, distortion of mesh nodes is determined by estimating the Gaussian curvature. The 3D surface is then separated along nodes and seams with high distortion, but minimal visibility. Thereafter, the actual parameterization step can be carried out, i.e. the mesh is flattened into the 2D plane. This can be done by using *angle based flattening* [87]. In this process, a functional is minimized according to differences between 2D and 3D mesh angles. This robust and efficient method generates provable conformal mappings with low stretch and no flipped triangles. In 2D the texture is applied and finally mapped back to the 3D mesh. Figure 10.25 illustrates the steps in this process.

References

1. Bloch, F.: Nuclear induction. Phys. Rev. **70**(7–8), 460–474 (1946)
2. Boesiger, P.: Kernspin-Tomographie Für die Medizinische Diagnostik. Teubner, Leipzig (1985)
3. Brooks, F.P.: What's real about virtual reality? IEEE Comput. Graph. Appl. **19**(6), 16–27 (1999)
4. Brown, J.D., Rosen, J., Kim, Y.S., Chang, L., Sinanan, M., Hannaford, B.: In-vivo and in-situ compressive properties of porcine abdominal soft tissues. In: Westwood, J.D., et al. (eds.) Medicine Meets Virtual Reality, vol. 11, pp. 26–32 (2003)
5. Bryan, N.R. (ed.): Introduction to the Science of Medical Imaging. Cambridge University Press, Cambridge (2009)
6. Carter, F.J., Frank, T.G., Davies, P.J., McLean, D., Cuschieri, A.: Measurement and modelling of the compliance of human and porcine organs. Med. Image Anal. **5**(4), 231–236 (2001)
7. Catmull, E.E.: A subdivision algorithm for computer display of curved surfaces. PhD thesis, Department of Computer Science, Univ. of Utah (1974)
8. Caunce, A., Taylor, C.J.: 3D point distribution models of the cortical sulci. In: Proceeding of Sixth International Conference on Computer Vision, pp. 402–407 (1998)
9. Chan, S.L., Purisima, E.O.: A new tetrahedral tesselation scheme for isosurface generation. Comput. Graph. **22**(1), 83–90 (1998)
10. Cignoni, P., Montani, C., Scopigno, R.: A comparison of mesh simplification algorithms. Comput. Graph. **22**, 37–54 (1997)
11. Clark, J.H.: Hierarchical geometric models for visible surface algorithms. Commun. ACM **19**(10), 547–554 (1976)
12. Cootes, T.F., Taylor, C.J.: Active shape models—smart snakes. In: Proc. British Machine Vision Conf., pp. 266–275 (1992)
13. Cormack, A.M.: Representation of a function by its line integrals, with some radiological applications. I. J. Appl. Phys. **34**(9), 2722–2727 (1963)
14. Cormack, A.M.: Representation of a function by its line integrals, with some radiological applications. II. J. Appl. Phys. **35**(10), 2908–2913 (1964)
15. Damadian, R.: Tumor detection by nuclear magnetic resonance. Science **171**(3976), 1151–1153 (1971)
16. Davies, P.J., Carter, F.J., Cuschieri, A.: Mathematical modelling for keyhole surgery simulations: a biomechanical model for spleen tissue. J. Appl. Math. **67**(1), 41–67 (2002)
17. Efros, A.A., Freeman, W.T.: Image quilting for texture synthesis and transfer. In: Proceedings of the 28th Annual Conference on Computer Graphics and Interactive Techniques, pp. 341–346 (2001)
18. Efros, A.A., Leung, T.: Texture synthesis by non-parametric sampling. In: Computer Vision, 1999. The Proceedings of the Seventh IEEE International Conference on, vol. 2, pp. 1033–1038 (1999)
19. El-Baz, A.S., Acharya, U.R., Laine, A.F., Suri, J.S. (eds.): Multi Modality State-of-the-Art Medical Image Segmentation and Registration Methodologies, vol. 2. Springer, Berlin (2011)
20. Erikson, C., Manocha, D., Baxter III, W.V.: HLODs for faster display of large static and dynamic environments. In: 2001 ACM Symposium on Interactive 3D Graphics, pp. 111–120 (2001)
21. Erikson, K.R., Fry, F.J., Jones, J.P.: Ultrasound in medicine-a review. IEEE Trans. Sonics Ultrason. **21**(3), 144–170 (1974)
22. Fang, S., Chen, H.: Hardware accelerated voxelization. Comput. Graph. **24**(3), 433–442 (2000)
23. Farshad, M., Barbezat, M., Flüeler, P., Schmidlin, F., Graber, P., Niederer, P.: Material characterization of the pig kidney in relation with the biomechanical analysis of renal trauma. J. Biomech. **32**(4), 417–425 (1999)

24. Floater, M.S., Hormann, K.: Surface parameterization: a tutorial and survey. In: Floater, M.S., Sabin, M.A. (eds.) In Advances in Multiresolution for Geometric Modelling, pp. 259–284. Springer, Berlin (2004)

25. Fowlkes, J.B., Emelianov, S.Y., Pipe, J.G., Skovoroda, A.R., Adler, R.S., Carson, P.L., Sarvazyan, A.P.: Magnetic resonance imaging techniques for detection of elasticity variation. Med. Phys. **22**(11), 1771–1778 (1995)

26. Freixenet, J., Munoz, X., Raba, D., Marti, J., Cufi, X.: Yet another survey on image segmentation: region and boundary information integration. In: ECCV, pp. 408–422 (2002)

27. Fung, Y.C.: Biomechanics: Mechanical Properties of Living Tissues. Springer, Berlin (1993)

28. Gagalowicz, A., Ma, S.D.: Sequential synthesis of natural textures. Comput. Vis. Graph. Image Process. **30**(3), 289–315 (1985)

29. Gardner, G.Y.: Simulation of natural scenes using textured quadric surfaces. In: Proceedings of the 11th Annual Conference on Computer Graphics and Interactive Techniques, pp. 11–20 (1984)

30. Gardner, M.: The fantastic combinations of John Conways's new solitaire game of life. Sci. Am. **223**(4), 120–123 (1970)

31. Garland, M., Heckbert, P.: Surface simplification using quadric error metrics. In: Proceedings of the 24th Annual Conference on Computer Graphics and Interactive Techniques, pp. 206–216 (1997)

32. Gauss, C.F.: Disquisitiones generales circa superficies curva (1828)

33. Harders, M.: Surgical Scene Generation for Virtual Reality-based Training in Medicine. Springer, Berlin (2008)

34. Harders, M., Bachofen, D., Bajka, M., Grassi, M., Heidelberger, B., Sierra, R., Spaelter, U., Steinemann, D., Teschner, M., Tuchschmid, S., Zatonyi, J., Székely, G.: Virtual reality based simulation of hysteroscopic interventions. Presence **17**(5), 441–462 (2008)

35. Heckbert, P.S.: Survey of texture mapping. IEEE Comput. Graph. Appl. **6**(11), 56–67 (1986)

36. Heimann, T., Meinzer, H.-P.: Statistical shape models for 3D medical image segmentation: a review. Med. Image Anal. **13**(4), 543–563 (2009)

37. Hoppe, H., DeRose, T., Duchamp, T., McDonald, J., Stuetzle, W.: Mesh optimization. In: Proceedings of the 20th Annual Conference on Computer Graphics and Interactive Techniques, SIGGRAPH '93, pp. 19–26 (1993)

38. Hounsfield, G.N.: Computerised transverse axial scanning (tomography): Part 1. Description of system. Br. J. Radiol. **46**, 1016–1022 (1973)

39. Hsieh, J.: Computed Tomography: Principles, Design, Artifacts, and Recent Advances, vol. PM114. SPIE Press, Bellingham (2003)

40. Hug, C., Brechbühler, J., Székely, G.: Model-based initialisation for segmentation. In: Proceedings 6'th European Conference on Computer Vision—ECCV 2000, Part II, pp. 290–306 (2000)

41. Hug, J.: Semi-automatic segmentation of medical imagery. PhD thesis, ETH Zurich (2001)

42. Jolliffe, I.T.: Principal Component Analysis. Springer, Berlin (2002)

43. Kalberer, G.A., Van Gool, L.: Realistic face animation for speech. J. Vis. Comput. Animat. **13**(2), 97–106 (2002)

44. Kansal, A.R., Torquato, S., Harsh, G.R., Chiocca, E.A., Deisboeck, T.S.: Simulated brain tumor growth dynamics using a three-dimensional cellular automaton. J. Theor. Biol. **203**(4), 367–382 (2000)

45. Karabassi, E.-A., Papaioannou, G., Theoharis, T.: A fast depth-buffer-based voxelization algorithm. J. Graph. Tools **4**, 5–10 (1999)

46. Kauer, M.: Inverse finite element characterization of soft tissues with aspiration experiments. PhD thesis, ETH Zurich (2001)

47. Kauer, M., Vuskovic, V., Dual, J., Szekely, G., Bajka, M.: Inverse finite element characterization of soft tissues. Med. Image Anal. **6**(3), 275–287 (2002)

48. Kelemen, A., Szekely, G., Gerig, G.: Elastic model-based segmentation of 3-D neuroradiological data sets. IEEE Trans. Med. Imaging **18**(10), 828–839 (1999)

49. Kerdok, A.E., Ottensmeyer, M.P., Howe, R.D.: Effects of perfusion on the viscoelastic characteristics of liver. J. Biomech. **39**(12), 2221–2231 (2006)
50. Kim, J., Tay, B.K., Stylopoulos, N., Rattner, D.W., Srinivasan, M.A.: Characterization of intra-abdominal tissues from in vivo animal experiments for surgical simulation. In: Medical Image Computing and Computer-assisted Intervention, pp. 206–213 (2003)
51. Kobbelt, L., Campagna, S., Vorsatz, J., Seidel, H.-P.: Interactive multi-resolution modeling on arbitrary meshes. In: Proceedings of the 25th Annual Conference on Computer Graphics and Interactive Techniques, pp. 105–114 (1998)
52. Kotcheff, A.C.W., Taylor, C.J.: Automatic construction of eigenshape models by direct optimization. Med. Image Anal. **2**(4), 303–314 (1998)
53. Lauterbur, P.C.: Image formation by induced local interactions: examples employing nuclear magnetic resonance. Nature **242**, 190–191 (1973)
54. Lindenmayer, A.: Mathematical models for cellular interaction in development: Parts I and II. J. Theor. Biol. **18**(3), 300–315 (1968)
55. Lindstrom, P., Turk, G.: Fast and memory efficient polygonal simplification. In: Proceedings of the Conference on Visualization '98, VIS '98, pp. 279–286 (1998)
56. Lorensen, W.E., Cline, H.E.: Marching cubes: a high resolution 3D surface construction algorithm. In: Proceedings of the 14th Annual Conference on Computer Graphics and Interactive Techniques, vol. 21, pp. 163–169 (1987)
57. Mansfield, P.: Multi-planar image formation using NMR spin echoes. J. Phys. C, Solid State Phys. **10**(3), 55–58 (1977)
58. Mayles, P., Nahum, A., Rosenwald, J.C.: Handbook of Radiotherapy Physics: Theory and Practice. Taylor and Francis, London (2007)
59. McInerney, T., Terzopoulos, D.: Deformable models in medical image analysis: a survey. Med. Image Anal. **1**(2), 91–108 (1996)
60. Mueller, P., Wonka, P., Haegler, S., Ulmer, A., Van Gool, L.: Procedural modeling of buildings. ACM SIGGRAPH 2006 Pap. **25**(3), 614–623 (2006)
61. Muthupillai, R., Lomas, D.J., Rossman, P.J., Greenleaf, J.F., Manduca, A., Ehman, R.L.: Magnetic resonance elastography by direct visualization of propagating acoustic strain waves. Science **269**(5232), 1854–1857 (1995)
62. Nadernejad, E., Sharifzadeh, S., Hassanpour, H.: Edge detection techniques: evaluations and comparisons. Appl. Math. Sci. **2**(31), 1507–1520 (2008)
63. Nava, A., Mazza, E., Kleinermann, F., Avis, N.J., McClure, J.: Evaluation of the mechanical properties of human liver and kidney through aspiration experiments. Technol. Health Care **12**(3), 269–280 (2004)
64. Newman, T.S., Yia, H.: A survey of the marching cubes algorithm. Comput. Graph. **30**(5), 854–879 (2006)
65. Nielson, G.M., Hamann, B.: The asymptotic decider: resolving the ambiguity in marching cubes. In: Proceedings of the 2nd Conference on Visualization '91, pp. 83–91 (1991)
66. Oliensis, J.: Local reproducible smoothing without shrinkage. IEEE Trans. Pattern Anal. Mach. Intell. **15**(3), 307–312 (1993)
67. Ophir, J., Cespedes, I., Ponnekanti, H., Yazdi, Y., Li, X.: Elastography: a method for imaging the elasticity of biological tissues. Ultrason. Imaging **13**(2), 111–134 (1991)
68. Ottensmeyer, M.P.: In vivo measurement of solid organ visco-elastic properties. In: Medicine Meets Virtual Reality, vol. 85, pp. 328–333 (2002)
69. Ottensmeyer, M.P., Kerdok, A.E., Howe, R.D., Dawson, S.: The effects of testing environment on the viscoelastic properties of soft tissues. In: Medical Simulation, vol. 3078, pp. 9–18 (2004)
70. Paget, R., Harders, M., Szekely, G.: A framework for coherent texturing in surgical simulators. In: Proceedings of the 13th Pacific Conference on Computer Graphics and Applications, pp. 112–114 (2005)
71. Pal, N.R., Pal, S.K.: A review on image segmentation techniques. Pattern Recognit. **26**(9), 1277–1294 (1993)

72. Peachey, D.R.: Solid texturing of complex surfaces. In: Proceedings of the 12th Annual Conference on Computer Graphics and Interactive Techniques, pp. 279–286 (1985)
73. Perlin, K.: An image synthesizer. In: Proceedings of the 12th Annual Conference on Computer Graphics and Interactive Techniques, pp. 287–296 (1985)
74. Pham, D.L., Xu, C., Price, J.: A survey of current methods in medical image segmentation. Annu. Rev. Biomed. Eng. **2**, 315–338 (2000)
75. Prusinkiewicz, P., Hanan, J., Mech, R.: An l-system-based plant modeling language. In: Proceedings of the International Workshop on Applications of Graph Transformations with Industrial Relevance, AGTIVE '99, pp. 395–410 (2000)
76. Prusinkiewicz, P., Lindenmayer, A.: The Algorithmic Beauty of Plants. Springer, Berlin (1990)
77. Purcell, E.M., Torrey, H.C., Pound, R.V.: Resonance absorption by nuclear magnetic moments in a solid. Phys. Rev. **69**(1–2), 37–38 (1946)
78. Qi, A.S., Zheng, X., Du, C.Y., An, B.S.: A cellular automaton model of cancerous growth. J. Theor. Biol. **161**(1), 1–12 (1993)
79. Radon, J.: Über die Bestimmung von Funktionen durch ihre Integralwerte längs gewisser Mannigfaltigkeiten. Rep. Proc. Sax. Acad. Sci. **69**, 262–277 (1917)
80. Reddy, M.: SCROOGE: Perceptually-driven polygon reduction. Comput. Graph. **15**(4), 191–203 (1996)
81. Roerdink, J.B.T.M., Meijster, A.: The watershed transform: definitions, algorithms and parallelization strategies. Fundam. Inform. **41**, 187–228 (2000)
82. Röntgen, W.C.: Über Eine Neue Art Von Strahlen. Sitzungsberichte der Würzburger Physik.-medic. Gesellschaft (1895)
83. Sahoo, P.K., Soltani, S., Wong, A.K.C., Chen, Y.C.: A survey of thresholding techniques. Comput. Vis. Graph. Image Process. **41**(2), 233–260 (1988)
84. Schreiner, W., Buxbaum, P.F.: Computer optimization of vascular trees. IEEE Trans. Biomed. Eng. **40**(5), 482–491 (1993)
85. Schroeder, W.J., Zarge, J.A., Lorensen, W.E.: Decimation of triangle meshes. Comput. Graph. **26**, 65–70 (1992)
86. Sheffer, A., Hart, J.C.: Seamster: inconspicuous low-distortion texture seam layout. In: Proceedings of the Conference on Visualization '02, pp. 291–298 (2002)
87. Sheffer, A., Levy, B., Mogilnitsky, M., Bogomyakov, A.: ABF++: fast and robust angle based flattening. ACM Trans. Graph. **24**(2), 311–333 (2005)
88. Sierra, R., Szekely, G., Bajka, M.: Generation of pathologies for surgical training simulators. In: Proceedings of Medical Image Computing and Computer-assisted Intervention, vol. 2, pp. 202–210 (2002)
89. Sierra, R., Zsemlye, G., Szekely, G., Bajka, M.: Generation of variable anatomical models for surgical training simulators. Med. Image Anal. **10**(2), 275–285 (2006)
90. Sinkus, R., Weiss, S., Wigger, E., Lorenzen, J., Dargatz, M., Kuhl, C.: Non-linear elastic tissue properties of the breast measured by mr-elastography—initial in-vitro and in-vivo results. In: ISMRM 10th Annual Meeting, p. 33 (2002)
91. Spitzer, V., Ackerman, M.J., Scherzinger, A.L., Whitlock, D.: The visible human male: a technical report. J. Am. Med. Inform. Assoc. **3**(2), 118–130 (1996)
92. Staib, L.H., Duncan, J.S.: Boundary finding with parametrically deformable models. IEEE Trans. Pattern Anal. Mach. Intell. **14**(11), 1061–1075 (1992)
93. Styner, M.A., Rajamani, K.T., Nolte, L.P., Zsemlye, G., Szekely, G., Taylor, C.J., Davies, R.H.: Evaluation of 3D correspondence methods for model building. In: Information Processing in Medical Imaging, vol. 18, pp. 63–75 (2003)
94. Szczerba, D., Szekely, G.: Macroscopic modelling of vascular systems. In: Medical Image Computing and Computer-Assisted Intervention, pp. 284–292 (2002)
95. Szekely, G., Bajka, M., Brechbuehler, C., Dual, J., Enzler, R., Haller, U., Hug, J., Hutter, R., Ironmonger, N., Kauer, M., Meier, V., Niederer, P., Rhomberg, A., Schmid, P., Schweitzer, G., Thaler, M., Vuskovic, V., Troester, G.: Virtual reality-based simulation of endoscopic surgery. Presence **9**(3), 310–333 (2000)

96. Taubin, G.: Curve and surface smoothing without shrinkage. In: Fifth International Conference on Computer Vision, pp. 852–857 (1995)

97. Treece, G.M., Prager, R.W., Gee, A.H.: Regularised marching tetrahedra: Improved isosurface extraction. Comput. Graph. **23**(4), 583–598 (1998)

98. Tuchschmid, S., Bajka, M., Szczerba, D., Lloyd, B., Szekely, G., Harders, M.: Modelling intravasation of liquid distension media in surgical simulators. In: Medical Image Computing and Computer-Assisted Intervention, vol. 4791, pp. 717–724 (2007)

99. Van Gool, L., Defoort, F., Hug, J., Kalberer, G.A., Koch, R., Martens, D., Pollefeys, M., Proesmans, M., Vergauen, M., Zalesny, A.: Image-based 3D modeling: modeling from reality. In: Leonardis, A., Solina, F., Bajcsy, R. (eds.) Confluence of Computer Vision and Computer Graphics, vol. 84, pp. 161–178. Kluwer, Dordrecht (2000)

100. Vemuri, B.C., Radisavljevic, A.: Multiresolution stochastic hybrid shape models with fractal priors. ACM Trans. Graph. **13**(2), 177–207 (1994)

101. von Neumann, J.: Theory of Self-reproducing Automata. University of Illinois Press, Champaign (1966)

102. Wardetzky, M., Mathur, S., Kälberer, F., Grinspun, E.: Discrete Laplace operators: no free lunch. In: Proceedings of the Fifth Eurographics Symposium on Geometry Processing, vol. 19, pp. 33–37 (2007)

103. Wasserman, R., Acharya, R.: A patient-specific in vivo tumor model. Math. Biosci. **136**(2), 111–140 (1996)

104. Wei, L.-Y., Levoy, M.: Fast texture synthesis using tree-structured vector quantization. In: Proceedings of the 27th Annual Conference on Computer Graphics and Interactive Techniques, pp. 479–488 (2000)

105. Weishaupt, D., Koechli, V.D., Marincek, B.: How Does MRI Work? An Introduction to the Physics and Function of Magnetic Resonance Imaging, 2nd edn. Springer, Berlin (2003)

106. Yamada, H.: Strength of Biological Materials. Williams and Wilkins Company, Baltimore (1970)

107. Ziou, D., Tabbone, S.: Edge detection techniques—an overview. Int. J. Pattern Recognit. Image Anal. **8**, 537–559 (1998)

108. Zitova, B.: Image registration methods: a survey. Image Vis. Comput. **21**(11), 977–1000 (2003)

Chapter 11
Soft Tissue Deformation

11.1 Introduction

The computation of soft tissue behavior is a central topic of biomedical simulation. Numerous methods to model soft tissue have been proposed in the past. The key tradeoff to be considered is usually the real-time capability vs. the deformation accuracy. As discussed in [16], this tradeoff relates to the targeted application. Scientific analysis of biomedical material and instruments, for instance for the design of new products, requires a high level of accuracy. Thus, in this context offline calculations of high computational cost are usually required. In contrast to this, in surgical planning the requirements can be relaxed. This allows to increase the interactivity of planning systems, while the overall precision is reduced. This is usually accepted, since input data—such as the organ mechanical properties of a specific patient—are often not, or only approximately known. Finally, VR-based surgical simulation requires real-time updates of the computed scene. Therefore, the accuracy of deformations can often only be roughly approximated. This is referred to in the field as the computation of *physically-plausible* behavior. A point to consider in this context is the goal of a surgical simulation: in general the target is to achieve a training effect. This might not require a highly accurate reproduction of minute details of material behavior. Nevertheless, it is still an unsolved research question how realistic a deformation model has to be in a surgical simulator to achieve a certain training effect. Still, large inaccuracies in tissue behavior can potentially lead to negative training effects. Therefore, the selection of an appropriate deformation model is a key step in building a simulation system.

As already discussed in Sect. 10.10, mechanical tissue behavior is highly complex, and often only partly understood. Due to the complexity of soft tissue, the formulation of an appropriate mathematical model is a difficult task. The requirements of interactive real-time simulation have to be met, sometimes making additional simplifications and optimizations of the underlying models necessary. A further point to consider is the capability of a tissue model to allow stable, interactive cutting. After selecting an adequate mathematical model to simulate the soft

R. Riener, M. Harders, *Virtual Reality in Medicine*,
DOI 10.1007/978-1-4471-4011-5_11, © Springer-Verlag London 2012

tissue biomechanics, real tissue should be measured and analyzed in order to extract the main parameters characterizing the tissue deformations. Finally, after the full deformation model has been formulated, a validation process should be carried out in order to test and validate the behavior and to determine the limits of the model.

In the following, first an overview of common soft tissue deformation models used in surgical simulation will be provided. This will be followed by the presentation of two common approaches used in the field—namely mass-spring systems and finite element models. The former is a phenomenological approach that targets physically-plausible simulation, while the latter is more common in continuum mechanical analysis.

11.2 Overview

Realistic behavior and real-time capability are two main features required for surgical training simulators. These contradictory requirements pose a major problem to soft tissue modeling. While high accuracy is needed to achieve realism, highly complex models usually lead to increased computation times. In addition to this, simulation stability as well as the complexity of interactive topology modifications need to be taken into account. Several approaches have been proposed to model soft tissue in the past, which will be briefly reviewed in the following. Comprehensive reviews of the field are also available in [21, 31].

- **Finite Element Method** The first approach is the finite element method (FEM), which provides a rigorous representation of soft tissue physics with well-defined boundary conditions based on continuum mechanics [3]. In this approach, a body is subdivided into a number of finite elements (e.g. hexahedra or tetrahedra in 3D, quadrilaterals or triangles in 2D). Displacements and positions in an element are interpolated from discrete nodal values. For every element, the partial differential equations governing the motion of material points of a continuum are formulated, resulting in a discrete system of differential equations:

$$\mathbf{M\ddot{u} + C\dot{u} + K\delta u = f - r},\qquad(11.1)$$

  where $\mathbf{u}$ is the vector of nodal displacements, $\mathbf{M}$ the mass matrix, $\mathbf{C}$ the damping matrix, $\mathbf{K}$ the stiffness matrix, and $\mathbf{f}$ the vector of external and $\mathbf{r}$ the vector of internal node forces, respectively. All these matrices may be time dependent. In order to simplify the calculation, a quasi-static solution is often attempted, where the dynamic part of the equations is neglected ($\mathbf{\ddot{u} = \dot{u} = 0}$). Different levels of accuracy for deformation simulation have been realized with this method, ranging from linear elastic [22] to non-linear anisotropic systems [36]. An advantage of FEM is that only a few material parameters are required to describe the response of a physical system. These material parameters can be obtained from soft tissue measurements and be directly integrated into the calculation. Nevertheless, high computation times still remain an obstacle for real-time applicability of the method. Moreover, if cutting procedures are to be allowed, which require a modification of mesh topology, element mass and stiffness matrices may have to be fully recalculated during the simulation, which is computationally intensive. Pre-computation and condensation have been suggested as a remedy to some of these problems [10].

- **Boundary Element Method** Similar to FEM, this method is also based on continuum mechanics, however, the underlying partial differential equations are formulated as integral equations in boundary integral form. Boundary element methods (BEM) [9] have received increased attention since the 1980s. BEM reduces the computational complexity of the solution, since only a discretization of the object boundary is required. The degrees of freedom of the surface elements represent displacements and tractions, which are piecewise interpolated between the element vertices. The application of this method to the real-time simulation of linear elastic deformable objects has been discussed in [24, 29]. Using Green's functions as fundamental solution to the elastic problem, a system of equations results:

$$\mathbf{H}\mathbf{u} = \mathbf{G}\mathbf{t}, \tag{11.2}$$

where $\mathbf{H}$ and $\mathbf{G}$ are non-sparse $3N \times 3N$ matrices, $\mathbf{u}$ the vector of nodal displacements, and $\mathbf{t}$ the vector of nodal tractions at N nodes. A drawback of the method is the modeling based on linear elasticity, thus not accommodating for large displacements. Moreover, the objects are considered as homogeneous and isotropic. Nevertheless, the computation time is reduced. By using pre-computation and superposition techniques, haptic update rates can be achieved [23].

- **Long Element Method** A three-dimensional object is modeled as a collection of two-dimensional elements filled with an incompressible fluid in the long element method (LEM). A static solution for elastic global deformations is obtained based on Hooke's law, Pascal's principle, and the principle of volume conservation [12]. An advantage of the approach is reduced computational complexity, since the meshes are one order of magnitude smaller than tetrahedral or cubic geometries. Also, inhomogeneities in the direction of the elements can be easily represented. Nevertheless, the LEM only yields accurate results for small deformations. Large strains lead for instance to difficulties in volume conservation. A solution would be to update the object discretization at each time step, which is a bottleneck for real-time performance.

- **Tensor-Mass Model** A simplification of FEM techniques can be found in the tensor-mass model (TMM), which pairs continuum mechanics' linear elasticity with mass lumping [13]. First, the object is discretized into a tetrahedral mesh. Linear elastic forces are then determined following an energy-based continuum mechanical formulation. The movement of mesh vertices is computed according to Newton's law of motion. The force computation is independent of mesh topology, thus allowing an easy integration of interactive modifications such as cutting or tearing. Moreover, computational complexity is linear in the number of edges, making TMM faster than FEM approaches. The original model is based on linear elasticity and hence only capable of simulating small deformations. However, a modification of the model has been proposed in [35], which accommodates large displacements by using non-linear strain tensors and anisotropic material laws.

- **Mass-Spring Model** In this method, deformable objects are represented by a network of point masses connected via springs. The force applied on a mass-point is given by rest length l^0, current length l, and spring constant k, according to Hooke's law $f = k(l^0 - l)$. The spring force acting on a point i due to j connected springs is:

$$\mathbf{f}_i = \sum_j k_{ij} \big(\|\mathbf{x}_j - \mathbf{x}_i\| - l_{ij}^0 \big) \frac{\mathbf{x}_i - \mathbf{x}_j}{\|\mathbf{x}_j - \mathbf{x}_i\|}. \tag{11.3}$$

Mass-spring models (MSM) have been widely used in surgical simulation since the pioneering work by Terzopoulos [39]. The system solution is relatively easy to obtain because the equations of motion do not have to be constructed explicitly. However, a MSM is a discrete approach that only roughly approximates the true physics governing the deformation of an elastic object. Moreover, the integration of realistic tissue properties into these models is not straightforward, often necessitating manual parameter tuning. In addition, the resulting physical behavior depends on the connectivity of the point-masses. Nevertheless, topology modifications pose less problems to MSM. Besides the springs directly connecting two nodes, other relations among a number of mesh entities can also be considered to derive forces. This way forces which compensate for orientation change (e.g. torsional springs as described in [25]), area change, volume change, or other arbitrary constraints can be modelled (see [40]).

- **Meshless Methods** Recent advances in the surgical simulation field focus on mesh-free deformation paradigms [6]. One example is the point-associated finite field (PAFF) approach, which is also know as the method of finite spheres, introduced in [14]. An object is approximated by a set of points without explicit connectivity. As in classical FEM, a Galerkin formulation is applied to discretize the partial differential equations governing the deformation behavior. The displacement field is approximated using shape functions with local spherical support. A major advantage of the method is the object representation via points, thus rendering an explicit meshing step unnecessary. The technique supports the simulation of large deformations as well as topology modifications like cutting. Unfortunately, the straightforward implementation of the approach is computationally intensive, thus requiring localized solutions [15]. However, such a step compromises computational accuracy.

- **Geometrical Methods** Early applications which modelled the behavior of soft bodies were based on geometrical modifications of the surface mesh, i.e. by repositioning the vertices of the elastic object in a visually plausible manner. For instance, in [4] the surface nodes of a flexible body were displaced using 3D profile functions tuned by experts. Similarly, [2] used second order polynomial functions, fitted to empirical data, to translate the vertices of organs in the vicinity of a contact point along the direction of the virtual tool.

Fig. 11.1 2D example of
mass spring system
approximating an object.
Mass points and springs are
arranged in triangular
configuration (however, note
that the method does not
reply on actual elements)

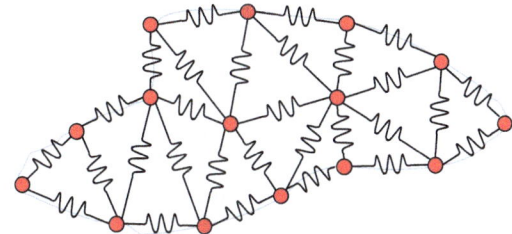

- **ChainMail Algorithms** Deformations of volumetric objects, modelled by the
  motion of linked elements similar to chains, was introduced in [20]. The movement of a single element within a certain limit does not affect the neighboring
  links in the structure. Links, which are stretched or compressed to their limits,
  drag or push their neighbors in the desired direction, propagating the deformation
  through the volume. One of the disadvantages of this approach is the dependence
  of the resulting deformation shape on the sequence of the applied forces. To avoid
  this, [34] proposed to always compute the deformations from the rest shape of the
  object. This allows to retain the rest shape of the modelled geometry, if the applied displacement is reversed.

11.3 Mass Spring Models

Mass spring systems are frequently used to simulate deformable objects because
of their conceptual simplicity and computational speed. Since the early work by
Terzopoulos et al. [38, 39] mass spring models have been a standard tool to model
deformable objects in surgical simulations (see e.g. [8, 30, 37]).

Mass spring systems require the discretization of an object into mass points connected by elastic links (see Fig. 11.1). The discretization can be defined on the surface or in the volume of the object. A typical choice of the elastic links is linear
springs based on Hooke's law to compute the forces. The global deformation behavior is determined by solving differential equations derived from Newton's second law of motion.

11.3.1 Model Formulation

In the following we introduce the formulation of a mass spring model following
[1] and [40]. The approach derives forces based on potential energy functions. Note
that this is only one possible approach for deriving the underlying mathematical
relations.

For the following, we assume that our deformable object is discretized into
masses and springs in a tetrahedral configuration (thus in a sense it is composed
of tetrahedral elements; however, in mass spring systems the focus is in general on

the mass points and springs, not on actual elements). For the links connecting the point masses a so-called Kelvin-Voigt material approach is used, which comprises linear elastic springs in parallel with purely viscous dampers.

As a first step, the inner forces of the model will be derived. This is done using potential energy functions. To this end, we consider constraints $\mathcal{C}(\mathbf{x})$, which are scalar functions depending on the mass positions $\mathbf{x} = \{\mathbf{x}_1, \ldots, \mathbf{x}_N\}$. These functions evaluate to zero in the undeformed state. In order to compute forces based on these constraints we consider potential energies of the form

$$E(\mathbf{x}) = \frac{1}{2}k\,\mathcal{C}(\mathbf{x})^2, \tag{11.4}$$

where k is a material stiffness constant that has to be defined for each type of energy function. The force is given as the negative gradient, with respect to the positions of the nodes:

$$\mathbf{f}_i = -\frac{\partial E}{\partial \mathbf{x}_i} = -k\,\mathcal{C}(\mathbf{x})\frac{\partial \mathcal{C}(\mathbf{x})}{\partial \mathbf{x}_i}. \tag{11.5}$$

The direction of the force $\mathbf{f}$ corresponds to the negative gradient of E. Therefore, a dynamic simulation resulting from these forces will reduce the deformation energy of the object.

We will now define two concrete constraint type energy functions for the elastic forces—linear spring forces acting between nodes and volume preserving forces defined for sets of nodes in tetrahedral configuration. Adding the latter helps in preserving mesh volume, and thus enhances the realism during large deformations.

The spring force function penalizes the deviation of the distance between two mass points $l_{ij} = \|\mathbf{x}_i - \mathbf{x}_j\|$ from the initial rest length l_0. Formulating this as a constraint function gives:

$$\mathcal{C}_s = \|\mathbf{x}_i - \mathbf{x}_j\| - l_0. \tag{11.6}$$

By derivation, we obtain the elastic spring force $\mathbf{f}_{i,s}$ acting on vertex i due to the spring connection ij to a neighboring vertex:

$$\mathbf{f}_{i,s} = -k_s\big(\|\mathbf{x}_i - \mathbf{x}_j\| - l_0\big)\frac{(\mathbf{x}_i - \mathbf{x}_j)}{\|\mathbf{x}_i - \mathbf{x}_j\|}. \tag{11.7}$$

Note that this corresponds to a linear elastic springs following Hooke's law ($\mathbf{f} = k\mathbf{x}$). Similar to the derivation above, the damping force defined for the spring ij and acting at vertex i can be obtained as:

$$\mathbf{f}_{i,d} = -k_d\frac{(\mathbf{v}_i - \mathbf{v}_j)\cdot(\mathbf{x}_i - \mathbf{x}_j)}{\|\mathbf{x}_i - \mathbf{x}_j\|}\frac{(\mathbf{x}_i - \mathbf{x}_j)}{\|\mathbf{x}_i - \mathbf{x}_j\|}, \tag{11.8}$$

where $\mathbf{v}_i, \mathbf{v}_j$ denote the velocities of the respective nodes. Note that in the formulas k_s, k_d define spring stiffness and spring damping, respectively.

Next, we derive volume preserving forces. The constraint function is based on the absolute difference of the current volume tet_{ijkl} of a tetrahedra formed by four mass points and its initial volume v_0:

$$C_v = \frac{1}{6}(\mathbf{x}_i - \mathbf{x}_j) \cdot \left((\mathbf{x}_l - \mathbf{x}_j) \times (\mathbf{x}_k - \mathbf{x}_j)\right) - v_0. \tag{11.9}$$

Note that the current volume of the tetrahedra is expressed by the mixed product rule. The force $\mathbf{f}_{i,v}$, applied at node i of the tetrahedron tet_{ijkl}, which penalizes the change in volume is therefore:

$$\mathbf{f}_{i,v} = -\frac{k_v}{6}\left(\frac{1}{6}(\mathbf{x}_i - \mathbf{x}_j) \cdot \left((\mathbf{x}_l - \mathbf{x}_j) \times (\mathbf{x}_k - \mathbf{x}_j)\right) - v_0\right)$$
$$\cdot \left((\mathbf{x}_l - \mathbf{x}_j) \times (\mathbf{x}_k - \mathbf{x}_j)\right). \tag{11.10}$$

Note that since we use absolute (and not relative) differences in distance or volume calculation, the stiffness coefficients are not scale invariant.

One of the problems when using mass spring systems is that the springs sometimes do not maintain their orientation with respect to the neighboring nodes. Under high load it can occur that springs flip or tetrahedra invert, in order to relieve the strain at the springs. The application of volume preserving forces mitigates this effect, as these are dependent on the positions of more than two points. Especially, the signed volume of the constraint function, as calculated in Eq. (11.9), plays a key role in this respect. Forces preserve the initial orientation of the vectors in the mixed product. If a tetrahedron is inverted and the orientation of these vectors changes, the sign of the volume represented with the mixed product changes accordingly. Thus, inverting a tetrahedron results in forces that restore its original orientation.

A further point to consider is the setting of the model parameters. Generally, only little attention is paid to specifying parameters that provide realistic behavior. Typically, stiffness, damping, and viscosity parameters are manually tuned for all springs and nodes. Quite often spring parameters are set to equal values in an attempt to ease this cumbersome process; however, that results in less realistic material behavior.

Alternative approaches have been suggested to derive more accurate parameters. These include optimization techniques (e.g. [7, 18]) as well as analytical derivations (e.g. [26, 41]). A typical approach is to minimize the difference between the stiffness matrices of a reference FEM system and corresponding matrices of the mass spring system. According to [26], in a regular tetrahedral configuration the following formalisms for setting stiffness parameters of the springs and the volume preserving forces can be used:

$$k_s = \frac{2\sqrt{2}}{21}\sum_{ij} El_{ij}\frac{4}{5}, \qquad k_v = \frac{2}{35}v_{tet}^3 E, \tag{11.11}$$

where l_{ij} denotes the length between two mass points in a configuration of a regular tetrahedron and E the Young's Modulus of the material.

Setting the masses of the nodes can be done by redistributing the overall mass of the simulated object, according to [18]. To this end, mass moments of the discretised body up to the second order are matched to exact mass moments of the simulated object, corresponding to the given geometry and mass distribution. This results in a good approximation of the true mass distribution. Thus, point masses can be set according to

$$m_i = \rho \frac{1}{4} \sum_{tet \ni i} v_{tet}. \tag{11.12}$$

11.3.2 Dynamic Simulation

The deformation of the soft tissue model is simulated dynamically according to Newton's second law of motion.

$$M \frac{\partial^2 \mathbf{x}}{\partial t^2} + D \frac{\partial \mathbf{x}}{\partial t} + \mathbf{f}_{int} = \mathbf{f}_{ext}, \tag{11.13}$$

where M is the mass matrix of the model, D the nodal damping matrix, and $\mathbf{f}$ represents internal or external forces, respectively. The internal forces are expressed in terms of the defined spring and volume preserving forces according to Eqs. (11.7), (11.8) and (11.10): $\mathbf{f}_{int} = -(\mathbf{f}_s + \mathbf{f}_d + \mathbf{f}_v)$. Damping matrix D represents viscous damping applied at each node of the mesh. For mass spring systems the matrices M and D are usually diagonal with entries m_i and d_i, respectively. In order to update the node positions and velocities, different numerical integration schemes can be applied.

11.3.3 Numerical Integration

Given the positions $\mathbf{x}_i(t)$ and velocities $\mathbf{v}_i(t)$ of a point at time t, new positions $\mathbf{x}_i(t + h)$ and velocities $\mathbf{v}_i(t + h)$ need to be determined for the next timestep of the simulation $t + h$, according to the equations of motion.

For this, we first transform Eq. (11.13) into a first order differential equation:

$$\frac{\partial}{\partial t} \begin{pmatrix} \mathbf{x} \\ \mathbf{v} \end{pmatrix} = \begin{pmatrix} \mathbf{v} \\ \mathbf{f}_{ext} - D\mathbf{v} - \mathbf{f}_{int}(\mathbf{x}, \mathbf{v}) \end{pmatrix}. \tag{11.14}$$

In the following we will present typical numerical algorithms for solving Eq. (11.14). The solvers are usually initialized with starting positions $\mathbf{x}_i^0$ and velocities $\mathbf{v}_i^0$. Given the applied external forces at each time step, a piecewise linear trajectory for each mass point is computed. Note that for simplicity in the following the label *int* will be omitted for the internal forces as well as the index for a node i. Time will be denoted in subscript.

11.3.3.1 Explicit Integration

The simplest method of numerical integration is the explicit (forward) Euler scheme, which uses the positions, velocities, and external forces at the current time step to compute the corresponding values of the following step. The explicit Euler scheme is given by the update rules:

$$\mathbf{a}_t = \frac{\mathbf{f}_{ext,t} - d\mathbf{v}_t + \mathbf{f}_t}{m}$$

$$\mathbf{x}_{t+h} = \mathbf{x}_t + h\mathbf{v}_t \tag{11.15}$$

$$\mathbf{v}_{t+h} = \mathbf{v}_t + h\mathbf{a}_t,$$

where $\mathbf{a}$ expresses the accelerations of the nodes due to the applied internal and external forces. This scheme guarantees first order precision of the computed positions and velocities.

A solution using the explicit Euler scheme is quite unstable and exhibits inferior accuracy. The time step h controls stability and speed of the computation. The smaller the time step, the higher the stability, the longer the computation, and vice versa. Higher order explicit integration methods such as the Runge-Kutta schemes improve the numerical integration. Larger time steps can be possible and an error prediction of the selected time step can also be made. One of the difficulties of deformation simulation using explicit integration is to find a trade-off between speed and stability. It should also be noted, that the parameters and the topology of the mass spring system have also an important influence on the simulation.

Better results than with the previous method can be obtained using the Velocity Verlet scheme, which ensures second order precision of the positions as well as velocities:

$$\mathbf{a}_t = \frac{\mathbf{f}_{ext,t} - d\mathbf{v}_t + \mathbf{f}_t}{m}$$

$$\mathbf{x}_{t+h} = \mathbf{x}_t + h\mathbf{v}_t + h^2\frac{\mathbf{a}_t}{2} \tag{11.16}$$

$$\mathbf{v}_{t+h} = \mathbf{v}_t + h\frac{\mathbf{a}_t + \mathbf{a}_{t+h}}{2}.$$

Note that for the actual computation the equations are split further. First a half-step velocity is determined using force and velocity at time step t. This allows to update the positions and then forces. Based on these the half-step velocity is thereafter updated to the full-step velocity for $t + h$. The Velocity Verlet scheme is often applied in dynamic simulations, since it provides acceptable results and a good ratio between the maximum possible time step and the computation time, if compared to other explicit integration methods. Other alternatives for explicit integration applied in interactive simulation are the Beeman [5] or the Newmark scheme [32]. However, the general problem of using explicit integration methods is that a stable behavior can only be reached for very small time steps. An alternative is using implicit integration schemes which enable unconditionally stable integration.

11.3.3.2 Implicit Integration

Implicit schemes assume for the solution of the next simulation state that future variables are known, e.g. positions $\mathbf{p}_{t+h}$ or velocities $\mathbf{v}_{t+h}$ of the next time step.

One of the simplest implicit integration schemes is the implicit (backward) Euler scheme:

$$\mathbf{v}_{t+h} = \mathbf{v}_t + h \frac{\mathbf{f}_{ext} - d\mathbf{v}_{t+h} + \mathbf{f}_{t+h}}{m} \tag{11.17}$$

$$\mathbf{x}_{t+h} = \mathbf{x}_t + h\mathbf{v}_{t+h}. \tag{11.18}$$

In order to compute the unknown force $\mathbf{f}_{t+h}$ at time step t a first order approximation of the Taylor series is applied:

$$\mathbf{f}_{t+h} = \mathbf{f}_t + \frac{\partial \mathbf{f}_t}{\partial \mathbf{x}}(\mathbf{x}_{t+h} - \mathbf{x}_t) + \frac{\partial \mathbf{f}_t}{\partial \mathbf{v}}(\mathbf{v}_{t+h} - \mathbf{v}_t). \tag{11.19}$$

Using Eq. (11.18) the implicit integration step for the velocities is given as:

$$\hat{M}\mathbf{v}_{t+h} = h\hat{\mathbf{f}},$$

$$\hat{M} = M + hD - h\frac{\partial \mathbf{f}_t}{\partial \mathbf{v}} - h^2 \frac{\partial \mathbf{f}_t}{\partial \mathbf{x}}, \tag{11.20}$$

$$\hat{\mathbf{f}} = \mathbf{f}_{ext} + \mathbf{f}_t + \left(\frac{M}{h} - \frac{\partial \mathbf{f}_t}{\partial \mathbf{v}} \right)\mathbf{v}_t.$$

Note that the external forces $\mathbf{f}_{ext}$ are assumed to be constant during each time step, therefore the partial derivatives of the external forces with respect to positions or velocities vanish. The terms $\frac{\partial \mathbf{f}_t}{\partial \mathbf{x}}$ and $\frac{\partial \mathbf{f}_t}{\partial \mathbf{v}}$ represent the Jacobians of the internal elastic and damping forces, respectively. We will denote these as $J_{\mathbf{x},ij}$ and $J_{\mathbf{v},ij}$, respectively. For elastic forces, the Jacobians are also referred to as negated Hessians of the mass spring system [17], since they are defined as a negated gradient of a corresponding energy function.

In Eq. (11.20), the integration scheme is expressed in matrix notation. Because the equations of motion for the mass nodes are coupled, the involved matrices are not diagonal. In order to determine the unknown velocities, a linear system of equations has to be solved at each iteration step. Using implicit integration, therefore, involves a linearisation of the applied forces (i.e. construction of the Jacobian matrices) at each time step. This poses a considerable computational burden on interactive applications.

As already introduced above, a commonly used alternative approach to compute deformations is the finite element method. This technique will be explained in more detail below. However, first the underlying theory of continuum mechanics will be introduced.

Fig. 11.2 Transformation of
body from reference (K_0) to
deformed configuration (K_t)

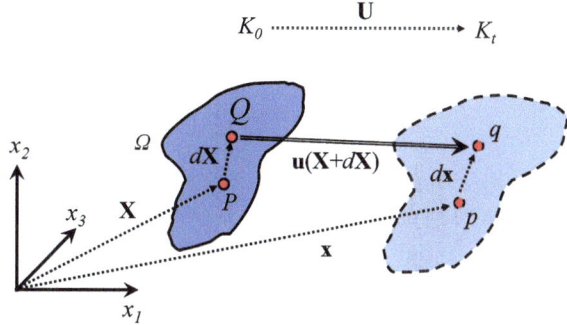

11.4   Continuum Mechanics

In continuum mechanics the behavior of a body is modelled assuming continuous
matter instead of a discrete particle view. In order to derive the FEM formalism, we
first will introduce key notions of elasticity theory, such as displacements, strains,
and stresses. Note that in the scope of this book only a general introduction is possible. For more detailed information, see for instance [27, 28, 33].

11.4.1 Concept of Strain

Assume that a body Ω is deformed from a reference configuration K_0 at time $t = 0$
to a deformed configuration K_t at a time $t > 0$. A point P in the body in the undeformed state is defined by a position vector $\mathbf{X}$ in the reference coordinate system.
Due to the deformation, the point P moves to a new position $\mathbf{x}$. Thus, a displacement has taken place, which is denoted by the vector $\mathbf{u} = \mathbf{x} - \mathbf{X}$ (see Fig. 11.2). The
displacements of all points in a body due to a deformation are denoted as displace-
ment field $\mathbf{U}$. A key target of the deformation computation via FEM is to determine
(an approximation) of this displacement field.

At this point also note that two primary ways of defining reference frames exist—
the material (Lagrangian) frame of reference and the spatial (Eulerian) frame of
reference. Simply speaking, in the first the point of view moves, while in the second
the point of view remains fixed.

Next, we will derive a formula for strain. The latter is a normalized measure
characterizing the relative change in shape or size due to external loads. Note that
strain is dimensionless. For the derivation, we consider two closely located points P
and Q in the undeformed body which are given by position vectors $\mathbf{X}$ and $(\mathbf{X} + d\mathbf{X})$.
In the deformed state these map into new points p and q at locations $\mathbf{x}$ and $(\mathbf{x} + d\mathbf{x})$,
respectively. The displacement due to the deformation is given for Q by

$$\mathbf{u}(\mathbf{X} + d\mathbf{X}) = (\mathbf{x} + d\mathbf{x}) - (\mathbf{X} + d\mathbf{X}). \tag{11.21}$$

Rearranging this gives a relation between the point distances $d\mathbf{x}$ and $d\mathbf{X}$ in the deformed and undeformed state:

$$d\mathbf{x} = \left(\mathbf{I} + \frac{\mathbf{u}(\mathbf{X} + d\mathbf{X}) - \mathbf{u}(\mathbf{X})}{d\mathbf{X}} \right) d\mathbf{X}. \tag{11.22}$$

Using differential calculus we thus can employ the displacement gradient tensor to map differential vectors from K_0 to K_t:

$$d\mathbf{x} = (\mathbf{I} + \nabla_{\mathbf{X}}\mathbf{u}) d\mathbf{X}. \tag{11.23}$$

This relationship can also be expressed using the (material) deformation gradient tensor $\mathbf{F}$:

$$d\mathbf{x} = \mathbf{F} d\mathbf{X} = \left[\frac{\partial x_i}{\partial X_i} \right] d\mathbf{X}. \tag{11.24}$$

Next, we examine the squared length of a segment $d\mathbf{x}$ in the deformed state.

$$d\mathbf{x}^2 = d\mathbf{x}^T d\mathbf{x} = d\mathbf{X}^T \mathbf{F}^T \mathbf{F} d\mathbf{X} = d\mathbf{X}^T \mathbf{C} d\mathbf{X}, \tag{11.25}$$

where $\mathbf{C} = \mathbf{F}^T \mathbf{F}$ is the right Cauchy-Green deformation tensor. It allows us to define the finite Green-Lagrange strain tensor:

$$\mathbf{E} = \frac{1}{2} \left(\mathbf{F}^T \mathbf{F} - \mathbf{I} \right) = \frac{1}{2} (\mathbf{C} - \mathbf{I}). \tag{11.26}$$

This strain measure characterizes how much a deformation differs locally from a rigid body movement. Note that if no deformation is present then $\mathbf{F}^T \mathbf{F} = \mathbf{I}$ and therefore the strain becomes zero.

The second-order deformation gradient tensor is nonsingular and thus can be expressed (according to the polar decomposition theorem) by a pure rotation tensor $\mathbf{R}$ and a (right or left) pure stretch tensor:

$$\mathbf{F} = \mathbf{R} \mathbf{U} = \mathbf{V} \mathbf{R}. \tag{11.27}$$

Note that $\mathbf{R}^T \mathbf{R} = 1$ and $\mathbf{U}^T = \mathbf{U}$ as well as $\mathbf{V}^T = \mathbf{V}$. This allows us to show that the Green-Lagrange strain tensor only depends on stretch and not on rotation, since:

$$\mathbf{C} = \mathbf{F}^T \mathbf{F} = (\mathbf{R} \mathbf{U})^T (\mathbf{R} \mathbf{U}) = \mathbf{U}^2. \tag{11.28}$$

The invariants of $\mathbf{C}$ are often employed to define strain energy density functions. The latter are scalar functions that denote the internal mechanical energy stored in a body due to a deformation. This is done by setting up a relation between the strain energy density and the deformation gradient. This will be discussed in more detail below.

Next, we consider the finite Green-Lagrange strain tensor in terms of the displacement gradients:

$$\mathbf{E} = \frac{1}{2} \left(\mathbf{F}^T \mathbf{F} - \mathbf{I} \right) \tag{11.29}$$

$$= \frac{1}{2}\left((\mathbf{I} + \nabla_{\mathbf{X}}\mathbf{u})^T(\mathbf{I} + \nabla_{\mathbf{X}}\mathbf{u}) - \mathbf{I}\right) \tag{11.30}$$

$$= \frac{1}{2}\left(\nabla_{\mathbf{X}}\mathbf{u} + \nabla_{\mathbf{X}}\mathbf{u}^T + \nabla_{\mathbf{X}}\mathbf{u}^T\nabla_{\mathbf{X}}\mathbf{u}\right). \tag{11.31}$$

Note that the strain tensor contains a quadratic product of the displacement gradient thus making it non-linear. No assumptions about the magnitude of the rotations and strains is made in this case; these can be arbitrarily large. In continuum mechanics this approach is denoted as the finite strain theory.

In contrast to this in the infinitesimal strain theory it is assumed that only very small deformations are applied. Due to this the deformation gradients are very small, i.e. $\nabla\mathbf{u} \ll 1$, which enables us to formulate a linearized small strain tensor:

$$\epsilon = \frac{1}{2}\left(\nabla\mathbf{u} + \nabla\mathbf{u}^T\right). \tag{11.32}$$

The components of the linear strain tensor can be written as:

$$\epsilon_{ij} = \frac{1}{2}\left(\frac{\partial u_j}{\partial x_i} + \frac{\partial u_i}{\partial x_j}\right). \tag{11.33}$$

Or expressed in tensor matrix notation:

$$\epsilon = \begin{bmatrix} \epsilon_{11} & \epsilon_{12} & \epsilon_{13} \\ \epsilon_{21} & \epsilon_{22} & \epsilon_{23} \\ \epsilon_{31} & \epsilon_{32} & \epsilon_{33} \end{bmatrix} = \begin{bmatrix} \frac{\partial u_1}{\partial x_1} & \frac{1}{2}\left(\frac{\partial u_1}{\partial x_2} + \frac{\partial u_2}{\partial x_1}\right) & \frac{1}{2}\left(\frac{\partial u_1}{\partial x_3} + \frac{\partial u_3}{\partial x_1}\right) \\ \frac{1}{2}\left(\frac{\partial u_2}{\partial x_1} + \frac{\partial u_1}{\partial x_2}\right) & \frac{\partial u_2}{\partial x_2} & \frac{1}{2}\left(\frac{\partial u_2}{\partial x_3} + \frac{\partial u_3}{\partial x_2}\right) \\ \frac{1}{2}\left(\frac{\partial u_1}{\partial x_3} + \frac{\partial u_3}{\partial x_1}\right) & \frac{1}{2}\left(\frac{\partial u_2}{\partial x_3} + \frac{\partial u_3}{\partial x_2}\right) & \frac{\partial u_3}{\partial x_3} \end{bmatrix}. \tag{11.34}$$

Note that the diagonal terms of the tensor denote the normal strain, while the non-diagonal ones denote the shear strain.

In the infinitesimal strain theory the difference in the material and spatial coordinates of a given material point are small, i.e. $\mathbf{X} \approx \mathbf{x}$ and thus the displacement gradients are approximately equal. The assumption of small strains and deformations results in geometric linearity. Thus, the linear strain assumption reduces the complexity of the deformation computation. However, it is only accurate for small deformations. Note also that the strain tensor is also not rotationally invariant anymore. Next, the concept of stress will be introduced.

11.4.2 Concept of Stress

Stress denotes a measure of internal force intensity due to external loads. It has the unit of force per area. For the derivation, consider an arbitrary cut through a body at a material point P. At this point a force $\mathbf{f}$ is acting on a small surface ΔA with

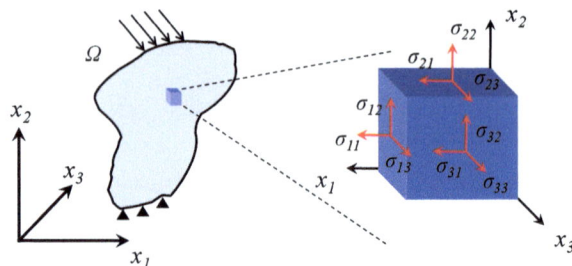

normal unit vector **n**. This results in a stress vector:

$$\mathbf{t_{(n)}} = \lim_{\Delta A \to \infty} \frac{\Delta \mathbf{f}}{\Delta A} = \frac{d\mathbf{f}}{dA}. \tag{11.35}$$

Note that the stress vector does not have to be perpendicular to the surface area.
It usually consists of a normal and a shear component. According to Cauchy's stress
theorem the stress vector can be defined via a second-order symmetric tensor $\boldsymbol{\sigma}$ and
the normal vector:

$$\mathbf{t_{(n)}} = \boldsymbol{\sigma}\mathbf{n}. \tag{11.36}$$

This tensor is called the Cauchy stress tensor. The relation implies that a stress
vector associated with an arbitrary plane given by a normal vector can be expressed
based on stress vectors on planes perpendicular to the coordinate axes. In matrix
notation the tensor is given as:

$$\boldsymbol{\sigma} = \begin{bmatrix} \sigma_{11} & \sigma_{12} & \sigma_{13} \\ \sigma_{21} & \sigma_{22} & \sigma_{23} \\ \sigma_{31} & \sigma_{32} & \sigma_{33} \end{bmatrix}, \tag{11.37}$$

where the diagonal terms are the normals stresses and the non-diagonal ones the
shear stresses (see also Fig. 11.3). Further useful stress tensors are the Piola-
Kirchhoff stress tensors. These express the stress relative to the reference configuration, whereas the Cauchy stress tensor expresses stress in relation to the deformed
state.

The first Piola-Kirchhoff stress tensor **P** relates forces in the present configuration
to areas in the reference configuration:

$$\mathbf{P} = J\boldsymbol{\sigma}\mathbf{F}^{-T}, \tag{11.38}$$

where $J = \det(\mathbf{F})$ is the Jacobian determinant of the deformation gradient **F**. Based
on this we can define the second Piola-Kirchhoff stress tensor **S**, which relates forces
in the reference configuration to areas in the reference configuration:

$$\mathbf{S} = J\mathbf{F}^{-1}\boldsymbol{\sigma}\mathbf{F}^{-T} = \mathbf{F}^{-1}\mathbf{P}. \tag{11.39}$$

The Cauchy stress tensor can be expressed based on the Piola-Kirchhoff stress tensors:

$$\sigma = J^{-1}\mathbf{P}\mathbf{F}^T = J^{-1}\mathbf{F}\mathbf{S}\mathbf{F}^T. \tag{11.40}$$

Up to this point we have introduced the concept of strains and stresses in separate. The final step is to formulate their interdependencies via constitutive relations.

11.4.3 Constitutive Material Laws

The relation between stress and strain in a general elastic material is formulated in a constitutive equation. Thus, the behavior of a specific material can be included into the model by selecting an appropriate relation. A purely elastic material stores strain energy under load. In case of a hyperelastic (homogeneous, continuous) material this behavior is captured by formulating a scalar strain energy function W.

If the strain energy function W is defined based on the deformation gradient $\mathbf{F}$, then the first Piola-Kirchhoff stress tensor is obtained by differentiation:

$$\mathbf{P} = \frac{\partial W(\mathbf{F})}{\partial \mathbf{F}}. \tag{11.41}$$

Similarly, if the strain energy function is defined based on the finite strain tensor $\mathbf{E}$, then we obtain the second Piola-Kirchhoff stress tensor by differentiation with respect to the finite strain tensor:

$$\mathbf{S} = \frac{\partial W(\mathbf{E})}{\partial \mathbf{E}}. \tag{11.42}$$

Note that a strain energy function cannot become negative, and should evaluate to zero if no deformation is present. It also only depends on the stretch component, but not on the rotation component of a deformation. Therefore, the strain energy function can also be written in terms of the right Cauchy-Green deformation tensor.

For an isotropic hyperelastic material, the strain energy function can be expressed based on the three independent invariants of the right Cauchy-Green deformation tensor:

$$W = W(\mathbf{C}) = W(I_1, I_2, I_3), \tag{11.43}$$

with the invariants of the tensor given as

$$I_1 = \text{tr}(\mathbf{C}), \qquad I_2 = \frac{1}{2}\left(\text{tr}(\mathbf{C}^2) - \text{tr}(\mathbf{C})^2\right), \qquad I_3 = \det(\mathbf{C}). \tag{11.44}$$

Note that for incompressible material there is no volume change between the reference and the deformed configuration, and thus $I_3 = \det(\mathbf{C}) = 1$. Differentiation of the strain energy function with respect to the right Cauchy-Green deformation tensor gives a general form of elasticity:

$$\frac{\partial W(\mathbf{C})}{\partial \mathbf{C}} = \alpha_1 \mathbf{I} + \alpha_2 \mathbf{C} + \alpha_3 \mathbf{C}^2, \tag{11.45}$$

where the scalar coefficients α_i are functions of the invariants I_1, I_2, I_3.

The simplest hyperelastic constitutive material law is given by the Saint Venant-Kirchhoff model. The strain energy density function is defined as

$$W(\mathbf{E}) = \frac{\lambda}{2} \left(\text{tr}(\mathbf{E})\right)^2 + \mu\,\text{tr}\!\left(\mathbf{E}^2\right), \tag{11.46}$$

where λ and μ are the Lamé constants describing the material. As we will see below the Saint Venant-Kirchhoff model is an extension of the basic linear material model to the non-linear domain.

Another typical example of a strain energy function is given by a Mooney-Rivlin material, defined as

$$W(\mathbf{C}) = \frac{\mu_1}{2}(I_1 - 3) - \frac{\mu_2}{2}(I_2 - 3), \tag{11.47}$$

with the μ_i being material constants that have to be determined experimentally. The Mooney-Rivlin material description was originally developed to represent rubber. Nevertheless, it also has been applied to model incompressible soft tissue.

Note that in the so far presented general models there exist material non-linearities due to the coefficients and quadratic terms in the material equations, as well as geometric non-linearities in the strain tensors. A simplification of this is the theory of linear elasticity, on which we will focus in the following.

11.4.4 Linear Elasticity

In linear elasticity two simplifications are made to avoid the non-linearities. A linear relationship between stresses and strains is assumed, and only infinitesimal strains and small deformations are allowed. Also note that material failure or plastic changes are not considered. In this case the energy density function is given as

$$W = \frac{\lambda}{2} \left(\text{tr}(\boldsymbol{\epsilon})\right)^2 + \mu\,\text{tr}\!\left(\boldsymbol{\epsilon}^2\right). \tag{11.48}$$

Note the similarity to the non-linear Saint Venant-Kirchhoff model. Also in the linear case the material behavior is characterized by two Lamé coefficients λ and μ. Derivation with respect to the infinitesimal strain tensor gives the relation to the

Cauchy stress tensor:

$$\sigma = \frac{\partial W}{\partial \epsilon} = \lambda\big(\mathrm{tr}(\epsilon)\big)\mathbf{I} + 2\mu\,\epsilon. \tag{11.49}$$

Note that this is Hooke's law for isotropic materials, expressed in direct tensor notation. It can also be written using vector notation. To this end, first consider that in Voigt notation the strain tensor can be transformed into a vector, by exploiting symmetries:

$$\begin{bmatrix} \epsilon_{11} \\ \epsilon_{22} \\ \epsilon_{33} \\ 2\epsilon_{12} \\ 2\epsilon_{23} \\ 2\epsilon_{13} \end{bmatrix} = \begin{bmatrix} \frac{\partial}{\partial x_1} & 0 & 0 \\ 0 & \frac{\partial}{\partial x_2} & 0 \\ 0 & 0 & \frac{\partial}{\partial x_3} \\ \frac{\partial}{\partial x_2} & \frac{\partial}{\partial x_1} & 0 \\ 0 & \frac{\partial}{\partial x_3} & \frac{\partial}{\partial x_2} \\ \frac{\partial}{\partial x_3} & 0 & \frac{\partial}{\partial x_1} \end{bmatrix} \begin{bmatrix} u_1 \\ u_2 \\ u_3 \end{bmatrix} = \mathbf{Du}. \tag{11.50}$$

Similarly, the stress tensor can be given as a vector. This allows us to specify the linear elastic constitutive relationship as:

$$\begin{bmatrix} \sigma_{11} \\ \sigma_{22} \\ \sigma_{33} \\ \sigma_{12} \\ \sigma_{23} \\ \sigma_{13} \end{bmatrix} = \begin{bmatrix} \lambda+2\mu & \lambda & \lambda & 0 & 0 & 0 \\ \lambda & \lambda+2\mu & \lambda & 0 & 0 & 0 \\ \lambda & \lambda & \lambda+2\mu & 0 & 0 & 0 \\ 0 & 0 & 0 & \mu & 0 & 0 \\ 0 & 0 & 0 & 0 & \mu & 0 \\ 0 & 0 & 0 & 0 & 0 & \mu \end{bmatrix} \begin{bmatrix} \epsilon_{11} \\ \epsilon_{22} \\ \epsilon_{33} \\ 2\epsilon_{12} \\ 2\epsilon_{23} \\ 2\epsilon_{13} \end{bmatrix}. \tag{11.51}$$

Instead of using the Lamé coefficients, a linear elastic material can also be characterized by the Young's Modulus E and the Poisson ratio v. The former is defined by the ratio of uniaxial tensile stress vs. uniaxial tensile strain, whereas the latter is defined by transversal contraction strain vs. axial elongation strain. The theoretical limits of the Poisson ratio are given as $-1 < v \le 0.5$. For a nearly-incompressible material such as biological tissues, often a Poisson ratio of $v = 0.49$ is applied. Young's Modulus and Poisson ratio are directly related to the Lamé coefficients via:

$$\mu = \frac{E}{2(1+v)}, \qquad \lambda = \frac{Ev}{(1+v)(1-2v)}. \tag{11.52}$$

The linear elastic constitutive relationship can also be given in terms of Young's Modulus and Poisson ratio:

$$
\begin{bmatrix} \sigma_{11} \\ \sigma_{22} \\ \sigma_{33} \\ \sigma_{12} \\ \sigma_{23} \\ \sigma_{13} \end{bmatrix}
= \frac{E}{(1+v)(1-2v)}
\begin{bmatrix}
1-v & v & v & 0 & 0 & 0 \\
v & 1-\mu & v & 0 & 0 & 0 \\
v & v & 1-v & 0 & 0 & 0 \\
0 & 0 & 0 & \frac{1-2v}{2} & 0 & 0 \\
0 & 0 & 0 & 0 & \frac{1-2v}{2} & 0 \\
0 & 0 & 0 & 0 & 0 & \frac{1-2v}{2}
\end{bmatrix}
$$

$$
\times
\begin{bmatrix} \epsilon_{11} \\ \epsilon_{22} \\ \epsilon_{33} \\ 2\epsilon_{12} \\ 2\epsilon_{23} \\ 2\epsilon_{13} \end{bmatrix}. \tag{11.53}
$$

Using Voigt vector notation this can be written in short form as

$$
\sigma = \mathbf{E}\epsilon, \tag{11.54}
$$

with $\mathbf{E}$ being the elasticity matrix.

As already indicated, linear elasticity uses several simplifying assumptions. Whether this is appropriate for a specific soft tissue simulation or not depends on the application. If only very small deformations take place (e.g. less than 5%) then this approach might be sufficient. Nevertheless, in general soft tissue behaves strongly non-linear, wherefore more complex formulations need to be used to avoid errors.

11.5 Finite Element Method

Apart from very simple cases, the partial differential equations resulting from the continuum mechanical formulations can only be solved using numerical techniques. Finite element methods have become a standard tool for solving continuum mechanical problems with complex geometries and material laws. FEM is widely applied in computer-based simulation in engineering. The key notion of the method is the approximation of the analyzed body Ω by a set (i.e. a mesh) of smaller elements with regular shape (see Fig. 11.4). Values within the elements are approximated based on nodal values via interpolation (using so-called shape functions). Due to

Fig. 11.4 2D example of finite element mesh approximating an object. 3-node linear triangular elements are used for the discretization

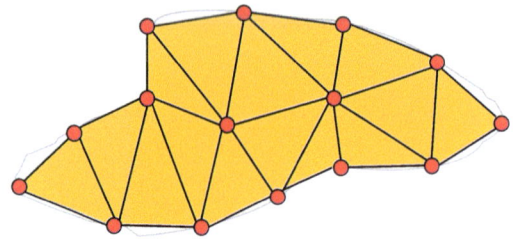

this the continuous problem is reduced to a finite problem. Note that the precision can be improved by increasing either the number of elements or the degree of interpolation. In the following we will derive the FEM model for the small-strain, linear, static case. Further, more general information can for instance be found in [11, 42].

In structural mechanics the total potential energy Π of a body is given by the internal and external energies. The former denotes the elastic strain energy stored in the deformed body and the latter the potential energy due to forces. The potential energy functional is given by:

$$\Pi = \int_\Omega \frac{1}{2} \epsilon^T \sigma \, d\Omega - \int_\Omega \mathbf{u}^T \mathbf{b} \, d\Omega - \int_\Gamma \mathbf{u}^T \mathbf{q} \, d\Gamma, \tag{11.55}$$

where σ and ϵ are vectors of the stress and strain components in Voigt notation, $\mathbf{u}$ are the displacements, $\mathbf{b}$ the vector of body forces, and $\mathbf{q}$ the vector of surface tractions. The first term represents the internal energies, the second and third the external energies. The principle of minimum potential energy states that the potential energy functional is minimized by the actual displacement field.

As indicated above, in FEM a continuous body is subdivided into a set of elements. This allows to represent the continuous displacement field using interpolation of nodal displacements. Thus, displacements are approximated via:

$$\mathbf{u} = \mathbf{N}\tilde{\mathbf{u}}, \tag{11.56}$$

where $\mathbf{N}$ is a matrix containing the interpolating shape functions and $\tilde{\mathbf{u}}$ is the vector of (unknown) nodal displacements. Note that the shape functions differ depending on the type of element selected for the mesh (e.g. tetrahedra vs. hexahedra in 3D).

Using Eq. (11.50), we can express the strain vector now in terms of the nodal displacements:

$$\epsilon = \mathbf{D}\mathbf{u} = \mathbf{D}\mathbf{N}\tilde{\mathbf{u}} = \begin{bmatrix} \frac{\partial}{\partial x_1} & 0 & 0 \\ 0 & \frac{\partial}{\partial x_2} & 0 \\ 0 & 0 & \frac{\partial}{\partial x_3} \\ \frac{\partial}{\partial x_2} & \frac{\partial}{\partial x_1} & 0 \\ 0 & \frac{\partial}{\partial x_3} & \frac{\partial}{\partial x_2} \\ \frac{\partial}{\partial x_3} & 0 & \frac{\partial}{\partial x_1} \end{bmatrix} \mathbf{N}\tilde{\mathbf{u}} = \mathbf{B}\tilde{\mathbf{u}}, \tag{11.57}$$

where $\mathbf{B}$ is a strain-displacement matrix that transforms nodal displacements to strains at any point.

In order to illustrate this process in more detail let us consider a specific case. We will derive the strain-displacement matrix for linear (4-node) tetrahedral elements (see Fig. 11.5). Displacements are interpolated from the nodal values of the four

Fig. 11.5 Linear 4-node
tetrahedral element

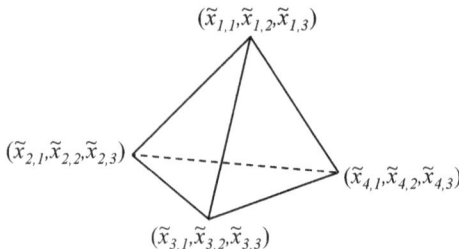

element vertices via four shape functions:

$$
\begin{bmatrix} u_1 \\ u_2 \\ u_3 \end{bmatrix} =
\begin{bmatrix}
N_1 & 0 & 0 & N_2 & 0 & 0 & N_3 & 0 & 0 & N_4 & 0 & 0 \\
0 & N_1 & 0 & 0 & N_2 & 0 & 0 & N_3 & 0 & 0 & N_4 & 0 \\
0 & 0 & N_1 & 0 & 0 & N_2 & 0 & 0 & N_3 & 0 & 0 & N_4
\end{bmatrix}
$$

$$
\times
\begin{bmatrix}
\tilde{u}_{1,1} \\
\tilde{u}_{1,2} \\
\tilde{u}_{1,3} \\
\tilde{u}_{2,1} \\
\tilde{u}_{2,2} \\
\tilde{u}_{2,3} \\
\tilde{u}_{3,1} \\
\tilde{u}_{3,2} \\
\tilde{u}_{3,3} \\
\tilde{u}_{4,1} \\
\tilde{u}_{4,2} \\
\tilde{u}_{4,3}
\end{bmatrix}.
\tag{11.58}
$$

In order to find the interpolation functions, we consider the representation of a
vertex $[x_1, x_2, x_3]$ via nodal coordinates. We will use the same shape functions to
interpolate coordinates and displacements. Using this so-called isoparametric formulation (see [19]) we can define the relation:

$$
\begin{bmatrix} 1 \\ x_1 \\ x_2 \\ x_3 \end{bmatrix} =
\begin{bmatrix}
1 & 1 & 1 & 1 \\
\tilde{x}_{1,1} & \tilde{x}_{2,1} & \tilde{x}_{3,1} & \tilde{x}_{4,1} \\
\tilde{x}_{1,2} & \tilde{x}_{2,2} & \tilde{x}_{3,2} & \tilde{x}_{4,2} \\
\tilde{x}_{1,3} & \tilde{x}_{2,3} & \tilde{x}_{3,3} & \tilde{x}_{4,3}
\end{bmatrix}
\begin{bmatrix} N_1 \\ N_2 \\ N_3 \\ N_4 \end{bmatrix},
\tag{11.59}
$$

where a vertex j of the tetrahedral element is given by coordinates $[\tilde{x}_{j,1}, \tilde{x}_{j,2}, \tilde{x}_{j,3}]$.
Note that $N_j = 1$ at node j and $N_j = 0$ at the three others. The above 4×4 matrix
is called the Jacobian matrix of the linear tetrahedron. Inversion gives:

$$
\begin{bmatrix} N_1 \\ N_2 \\ N_3 \\ N_4 \end{bmatrix} =
\frac{1}{6V}
\begin{bmatrix}
a_1 & b_1 & c_1 & d_1 \\
a_2 & b_2 & c_2 & d_2 \\
a_3 & b_3 & c_3 & d_3 \\
a_4 & b_4 & c_4 & d_4
\end{bmatrix}
\begin{bmatrix} 1 \\ x_1 \\ x_2 \\ x_3 \end{bmatrix},
\tag{11.60}
$$

where V is the volume of the element. The values a_i, b_i, c_i, d_i are derived from the node coordinates, for instance

$$b_1 = -\det \begin{bmatrix} 1 & \tilde{x}_{2,2} & \tilde{x}_{2,3} \\ 1 & \tilde{x}_{3,2} & \tilde{x}_{3,3} \\ 1 & \tilde{x}_{4,2} & \tilde{x}_{4,3} \end{bmatrix}. \tag{11.61}$$

A shape function for a linear tetrahedron is thus given as:

$$N_j = \frac{1}{6V}(a_j + b_j x_1 + c_j x_2 + d_j x_3). \tag{11.62}$$

Finally applying the matrix of differential operators we obtain the specific strain-displacement matrix for our selected element type:

$$\mathbf{B} = \frac{1}{6V} \begin{bmatrix} b_1 & 0 & 0 & b_2 & 0 & 0 & b_3 & 0 & 0 & b_4 & 0 & 0 \\ 0 & c_1 & 0 & 0 & c_2 & 0 & 0 & c_3 & 0 & 0 & c_4 & 0 \\ 0 & 0 & d_1 & 0 & 0 & d_2 & 0 & 0 & d_3 & 0 & 0 & d_4 \\ c_1 & b_1 & 0 & c_2 & b_2 & 0 & c_3 & b_3 & 0 & c_4 & b_4 & 0 \\ 0 & d_1 & c_1 & 0 & d_2 & c_2 & 0 & d_3 & c_3 & 0 & d_4 & c_4 \\ d_1 & 0 & b_1 & d_2 & 0 & b_2 & d_3 & 0 & b_3 & d_4 & 0 & b_4 \end{bmatrix}. \tag{11.63}$$

Next, we will consider the potential energy in a single element. Due to the discretization of the body via a set of elements, the total potential energy is approximated by the contributions of all individual elements.

$$\Pi = \sum_e \Pi_e. \tag{11.64}$$

We can now write the potential energy of an element, using the stress-strain relationship of Eq. (11.54) and the strain-displacement relationship of Eq. (11.57), as

$$\Pi_e = \frac{1}{2}\int_{\Omega_e} (\mathbf{B}\tilde{\mathbf{u}})^T \mathbf{E}(\mathbf{B}\tilde{\mathbf{u}})\, d\Omega_e - \int_{\Omega_e} (\mathbf{N}\tilde{\mathbf{u}})^T \mathbf{b}\, d\Omega_e - \int_{\Gamma} (\mathbf{N}\tilde{\mathbf{u}})^T \mathbf{q}\, d\Gamma. \tag{11.65}$$

Note that the right term relating to surface tractions is only present if the element is actually on Γ. By rearranging the equation we obtain:

$$\Pi_e = \frac{1}{2}\tilde{\mathbf{u}}^T \underbrace{\left(\int_{\Omega_e} \mathbf{B}^T \mathbf{E}\mathbf{B}\, d\Omega_e\right)}_{\mathbf{K}_e} \tilde{\mathbf{u}} - \tilde{\mathbf{u}}^T \underbrace{\left(\int_{\Omega_e} \mathbf{N}^T \mathbf{b}\, d\Omega_e + \int_{\Gamma} \mathbf{N}^T \mathbf{q}\, d\Gamma\right)}_{\mathbf{f}}, \tag{11.66}$$

where $\mathbf{K}_e$ is the element stiffness matrix and $\mathbf{f}$ the external forces. From the principle of minimum potential energy we finally have:

$$\frac{\partial \Pi_e}{\partial \tilde{\mathbf{u}}} = \mathbf{K}_e \tilde{\mathbf{u}} - \mathbf{f} = \mathbf{0}. \tag{11.67}$$

Since matrix $\mathbf{B}$ is constant with respect to the coordinates for the 4-node tetrahedron and the elastic moduli do not vary over the element, the 12×12 element stiffness matrix is constant and can be precomputed following:

$$\mathbf{K}_e = \mathbf{B}^T \mathbf{E} \mathbf{B} V, \tag{11.68}$$

where $V = \int_{\Omega_e} d\Omega_e$ is the volume of the element. Note that in general evaluating the integral requires numerical quadrature. Further, note that the element stiffness matrix is symmetric, square, and singular.

Finally, the stiffness matrix of the complete mesh is obtained by summing up all the element stiffness matrices:

$$\mathbf{K} = \sum_e \mathbf{K}_e. \tag{11.69}$$

Note that the global system stiffness matrix is also singular, unless sufficient boundary conditions (e.g. fixed nodes) are applied. By gathering all external forces and nodal displacements in global vectors, we arrive at the final static FEM equation:

$$\mathbf{K}\tilde{\mathbf{u}} = \mathbf{f}. \tag{11.70}$$

Given appropriate external forces the system of linear equations can be solved for the resulting node displacements. After determining these, other quantities such as stresses or strains can be computed. Note again that the presented derivation used the small-strain assumption.

11.6 Advantages and Disadvantages of MSM and FEM

A typical advantage of a mass spring system is that it is usually fast enough for real-time computation. Additionally, it is not difficult to include geometrical modifications in the model during simulation. A disadvantage is that in the standard formulation there is no volume preservation which is unrealistic, since soft tissue is nearly incompressible. Additionally, the deformation is topology dependent and the parameters of the model are unknown and difficult to select.

The advantages of the finite element method are that it is virtually independent of the geometry of the mesh and the loading. It can handle different complex analysis types, and has a solid theoretical background. On the other hand, potential disadvantages are longer computation times, unless linearizations are used. The method can also be somewhat more difficult to implement and requires experience for defining the problem (e.g. mesh generation). In addition, geometry modifications (such as cutting operations) are more complicated to represent and often require a remeshing step.

Although the FEM is usually considered to be of higher accuracy than a MSM, it still should be noted that several simplifications are made and that various sources of possible error exist. This includes uncertainty of the physical model, possible discretization errors, parameter uncertainty, as well as numerical errors in the computation. In general, it can be stated that FEM techniques require more experience to be used correctly.

References

1. Baraff, D., Witkin, A.: Large steps in cloth simulation. In: Proceedings of the 25th Annual Conference on Computer Graphics and Interactive Techniques vol. 32, pp. 43–54 (1998)
2. Basdogan, C., Ho, C.-H., Srinivasan, M.A., Small, S.D., Dawson, S.L.: Force interactions in laparoscopic simulations: haptic rendering of soft tissues. In: Proceedings of the Medicine Meets Virtual Reality Conference, pp. 385–391 (1998)
3. Bathe, K.J.: Finite Element Procedures. Prentice Hall, New York (1996)
4. Baur, C., Guzzoni, D., Georg, O.: VIRGY: a virtual reality and force feedback based endoscopic surgery simulator. In: Westwood, J.D., Hoffman, H.M., Stredney, D., Weghorst, S.J. (eds.) Medicine Meets Virtual Reality Art, Science, Technology: Healthcare (R)evolution, pp. 110–116 (1998)
5. Beeman, D.: Some multistep methods for use in molecular dynamics calculations. J. Comput. Phys. **20**(2), 130–139 (1976)
6. Belytschko, T., Krongauz, V., Organ, D., Fleming, M., Krysl, P.: Meshless methods: an overview and recent developments. Comput. Methods Appl. Mech. Eng. **139**(1–4), 3–47 (1996)
7. Bianchi, G., Solenthaler, B., Szekely, G., Harders, M.: Simultaneous topology and stiffness identification for mass-spring models based on fem reference deformations. In: Medical Image Computing and Computer-Assisted Intervention MICCAI 2004, vol. 2, pp. 293–301 (2004)
8. Bielser, D.: A framework for open surgery simulation. PhD thesis, Department of Computer Science, ETH Zürich (2003)
9. Brebbia, C.A.: The Boundary Element Method for Engineers. Pentech Press, London (1978)
10. Bro-Nielsen, M., Cotin, S.: Real-time volumetric deformable models for surgery simulation using finite elements and condensation. Comput. Graph. Forum **15**(3), 57–66 (1996)
11. Cook, R.D., Malkus, D.S., Plesha, M.E., Witt, R.J.: Concepts and Applications of Finite Element Analysis. Wiley, New York (2002)
12. Costa, I.F., Balaniuk, R.: LEM-an approach for real time physically based soft tissue simulation. In: International Conference on Robotics and Automation, vol. 3, pp. 2337–2343 (2001)
13. Cotin, S., Delingette, H., Ayache, N.: A hybrid elastic model allowing real-time cutting, deformations and force-feedback for surgery training and simulation. Vis. Comput. **16**(8), 437–452 (2000)
14. De, S., Bathe, K.J.: The method of finite spheres. Comput. Mech. **25**(4), 329–345 (2000)
15. De, S., Lim, Y.-J., Manivannan, M., Srinivasan, M.A.: Physically realistic virtual surgery using the point-associated finite field (paff) approach. Presence **15**(3), 294–308 (2006)
16. Delingette, H.: Towards realistic soft tissue modeling in medical simulation. In: Proceedings of the IEEE, pp. 512–523 (1998)
17. Desbrun, M., Schröder, P., Barr, A.: Interactive animation of structured deformable objects. In: Proceedings of the 1999 Conference on Graphics Interface '99, pp. 1–8 (1999)
18. Deussen, O., Kobbelt, L., Tücke, P.: Using simulated annealing to obtain good nodal approximations of deformable bodies. In: Sixth Eurographics Workshop on Simulation and Animation (1995)
19. Felippa, C.A., Clough, R.W.: The finite element method in solid mechanics. In: Numerical Solution of Field Problems in Continuum Physics, pp. 210–252. SIAM-AMS, Providence (1969)
20. Gibson, S.F.: 3D ChainMail: a fast algorithm for deforming volumetric objects. In: Proceedings of the 1997 Symposium on Interactive 3D Graphics, pp. 149–154 (1997)

21. Gibson, S.F., Mirtich, B.: A survey of deformable modeling in computer graphics. Technical Report TR97-19, MERL—Mitsubishi Electric Research Laboratories, Cambridge, USA (1997)
22. Gladilin, E., Zachow, S., Deuflhard, P., Hege, H.C.: A biomechanical model for soft tissue simulation in craniofacial surgery. In: Medical Imaging and Augmented Reality (MIAR), pp. 137–141 (2001)
23. James, D., Pai, D.K.: A united treatment of elastostatic and rigid contact simulation for real time haptics. Haptics-e **2**(1) (2001)
24. James, D.L., Pai, D.K.: ArtDefo—accurate real time deformable objects. In: Proceedings of the 26th Annual Conference on Computer Graphics and Interactive Techniques, pp. 65–72 (1999)
25. Jeong, I.K., Lee, I.H.: An oriented particles and generalized spring model for fast prototyping deformable objects. In: Eurographics 2004 (2004)
26. Lloyd, B., Szekely, G., Harders, M.: Identification of spring parameters for deformable object simulation. IEEE Trans. Vis. Comput. Graph. **13**(5), 1081–1094 (2007)
27. Mal, A.K., Singh, S.J.: Deformation of Elastic Solids, p. 341. Prentice-Hall, New York (1990)
28. Malvern, L.E.: Introduction to the Mechanics of a Continuous Medium, p. 713. Prentice-Hall, New York (1969)
29. Monserrat, C., Meier, U., Alcañiz, M., Chinesta, F., Juan, M.C.: A new approach for the real-time simulation of tissue deformations in surgery simulation. Comput. Methods Programs Biomed. **64**(2), 77–85 (2001)
30. Montgomery, K., Bruyns, C., Brown, J., Thonier, G., Tellier, A., Latombe, J.-C.: Spring: a general framework for collaborative, real-time surgical simulation. In: Medicine Meets Virtual Reality (2001)
31. Nealen, A., Müller, M., Keiser, R., Boxerman, E., Carlson, M.: Physically based deformable models in computer graphics (state of the art report). In: Proc. Eurographics 2005, pp. 71–94 (2005)
32. Newmark, N.M.: A method of computation for structural dynamics. ASCE J. Eng. Mech. **85**(EM3), 67–94 (1959)
33. Ogden, R.W.: Non-linear Elastic Deformations. Dover Publications, New York (1997)
34. Park, J., Kim, S.-Y., Son, S.-W., Kwon, D.-S.: Shape retaining chain linked model for real-time volume haptic rendering. In: Proceedings of the 2002 IEEE Symposium on Volume Visualization and Graphics, pp. 65–72 (2002)
35. Picinbono, G., Delingette, H., Ayache, N.: Real-time large displacement elasticity for surgery simulation: non-linear tensor-mass model. In: Medical Image Computing and Computer-Assisted Intervention, pp. 643–652 (2000)
36. Picinbono, G., Delingette, H., Ayache, N.: Non-linear and anisotropic elastic soft tissue models for medical simulation. In: IEEE International Conference Robotics and Automation, vol. 2, pp. 1370–1375 (2001)
37. Tendick, F., Downes, M., Goktekin, T., Cavusoglu, M.C., Feygin, D., Wu, X., Eyal, R., Hegarty, M., Way, L.W.: A virtual environment testbed for training laparoscopic surgical skills. Presence **9**, 236–255 (2000)
38. Terzopoulos, D., Fleischer, K.: Modeling inelastic deformation: viscolelasticity, plasticity, fracture. Comput. Graph. **22**, 269–278 (1988)
39. Terzopoulos, D., Platt, J., Barr, A., Fleischer, K.: Elastically deformable models. In: Proceedings of the 14th Annual Conference on Computer Graphics and Interactive Techniques, vol. 21, pp. 205–214 (1987)
40. Teschner, M., Heidelberger, B., Mueller, M., Gross, M.: A versatile and robust model for geometrically complex deformable solids. In: Computer Graphics International 2004, pp. 312–319 (2004)
41. Van Gelder, A.: Approximate simulation of elastic membranes by triangulated spring meshes. J. Graph. Tools **3**(2), 21–42 (1998)
42. Zienkiewicz, O.C., Taylor, R.L.: The Finite Element Method. McGraw-Hill, New York (1989)

Index

R. Riener, M. Harders, *Virtual Reality in Medicine*,
DOI 10.1007/978-1-4471-4011-5, © Springer-Verlag London 2012